Georg Rajka

Essential Aspects
of Atopic Dermatitis

With 47 Figures, some in color
and 63 Tables

Springer-Verlag Berlin Heidelberg New York
London Paris Tokyo Hong Kong

Professor Dr. GEORG RAJKA
Department of Dermatology, Rikshospitalet
Pilestredet 32, N-0027 Oslo 1
Norway

ISBN 3-540-51165-2 Springer-Verlag Berlin Heidelberg New York
ISBN 0-387-51165-2 Springer-Verlag New York Berlin Heidelberg

Library of Congress Cataloging in Publication Data
Rajka, Georg.
Essential aspects of atopic dermatitis / Georg Rajka. p. cm.
Includes bibliographical references.
ISBN 0-387-51165-2 (U. S. : alk. paper)
1. Atopic dermatitis. I. Title.
RC593.A8R35 1989
616.5′21--dc20 89-21702

© Springer-Verlag Berlin Heidelberg 1989
Printed in Germany

Typesetting, printing and binding: Appl, Wemding
2127/3145-543210 Printed on acid-free paper

Acknowledgments

I am greatly indebted to
Mrs. Grete Frövig
and G. Ryen Eriksen
for generous assistance in the
secretarial work.
I would also like to express
my indebtedness to Dr. J. Wieczorek
and to the Publishers, who did me the
honor of asking me to write this
monograph.

Dedications

This book is dedicated to
many people: to my wife Susanne,
whose help made it possible for me
to work;
to my former teachers:
to the memory of my father,
the late Professor E. Rajka
(Budapest);
to Professor Å. Nilzén,
former Head of the Clinic of Allergy,
Karolinska sjukhuset (Stockholm);
and to Dr. A. Rook, who asked me to
write my first monograph on AD.
Last but not least, this work is
dedicated to the new generation
of Norwegian medical students,
including my son, Thomas.

Preface

> *"Le secret d'ennuyer est*
> *celui de tout dire."*
>
> Voltaire (Discours sur l'homme)

Atopic dermatitis (AD) is frequently seen by dermatologists and pediatricians, by allergologists, and by many practitioners. The amount of data on AD is vast as it has been recognized for a very long time, has a worldwide distribution, and has a chapter or section devoted to it in every textbook or review of skin diseases. Difficulty arises in evaluating certain aspects of this complex disease, for many studies have been concerned with only some of its facets and with small numbers of patients. In addition a monograph on AD should also try to encompass the important theoretical aspects of this fascinating disease. Therefore, the problem in presenting a monograph on AD lies more in the critical selection than in the gathering of information, much of which is conflicting. This applies both to basic data and to details. Furthermore, the many divergent opinions in almost every field make it extremely difficult to draw unanimous conclusions. Consequently, the author has no option but to quote antagonistic views, try to make a compromise between these, and express his own opinion based on clinical experience and fundamental literary work.

Much of the information available is derived from AD cases irrespective of coexistent respiratory atopy, but as those cases with respiratory manifestations differ, especially immunologically, from those without, it is necessary in this book to consider only those without associated respiratory atopy; these are referred to as "pure" AD cases. If, however, a trait of the skin disease under consideration is unaffected by the presence of respiratory atopy, it is permissible to take such combined cases into account.

There is detailed discussion of the complex etiology of AD, and of several experimental findings which cannot at present be clearly interpreted; among these are the immunological aspects which are of great interest because of the far-reaching consequences of the progress in immunological research in recent years. Also, in reviewing the often neglected nonimmunological aspects of the disease, the concept of AD as merely an "allergic disease" is refuted.

A separate chapter is devoted to pruritus, as the author believes this symptom to be of primary importance in AD.

It would be pointless to discuss therapeutic measures in detail, for each reader is conversant with the pharmacopeias of his own country and has his own experience with different treatments; therefore only widely accepted principles are considered.

Perhaps the most difficult problem has been the selection of references. Data from various studies are mentioned but reference could be made only to selected basic or thought-provoking reports. It is inevitable that many contributions to journals of dermatology and of pediatrics, to reviews for practitioners, and not least to national periodicals in different languages, have to be omitted from a work of this size. These omissions, however, have been made for practical reasons only and do not represent a judgment on their scientific value. As "Hell hath no fury like that of a scientist uncited" (Butcher and Hittelman, 1971), the author wishes to pay tribute to all those authors who, in spite of valuable contributions to research on AD, are not mentioned in this work.

Reference

Butcher RW, Hittelman KJ (1971). In: Austen KE, Becker EL (eds) Biochemistry of the Acute Allergic Reactions. Blackwell, Oxford London, p 141

Table of Contents

Abbreviations

ACTH	adrenocorticotropic hormone
AD	atopic dermatitis
ADCC	antibody-dependent cellular cytotoxicity
ASO	antistreptolysin O
Asta	antistaphylotoxin
ATP	adenosine triphosphate
cAMP	cyclic adenosine 3′,5′-monophosphate
CMI	cell-mediated immunity
ConA	concanavalin A
DNA	deoxyribonucleic acid
ECP	eosinophilic cationic protein
HSF	histamine-suppressor factor
Ig	immunoglobulin
IRC	interdigitating reticulum cell
LT	leukotriene
MBP	major basic protein
NK	natural killer
PAF	platelet activating factor
PDE	phosphodiesterase
PG	prostaglandin
PHA	phytohemagglutinin
PRIST	radioimmunosorbent test (Phadebas)
PUVA	psoralen UV-A combined therapy
PWM	pokeweed mitogen
RAST	radioallergosorbent test
RIST	radioimmunosorbence technique
TWL	transepidermal water loss
UV	ultraviolet
VIP	vasoactive intestinal polypeptide

1 History and Nomenclature

1.1 History

Controversy over and discussion of minutiae between different schools of dermatology are the predominant ingredients of the history of AD. As these do not lend themselves well to precise chronological arrangement, a short historical survey is a more suitable approach.

The first description of a possible case of AD was given by the historian Suetonius. The Roman emperor Augustus showed traits which may be interpreted as corresponding to respiratory and skin atopy (Ring 1985). Willan (1808) gave the first decriptions of prurigo and of prurigo-like conditions, remarking on their characteristic itchiness. Von Hebra (1884) gave a simpler account in which he distinguished between prurigo simplex and itchy pruriginous conditions, and he postulated that the papule preceded the itch. Other dermatologists, particularly the French, took the contrary view that itch is the initial event and, by emphasizing the nervous component of prurigo, they were the originators of the term neurodermatitis (Brocq and Jacquet 1891). Jacquet, even at this time, believed that "Ce n'est pas l'élément éruptif qui est prurigineux, c'est le prurit qui est éruptif." This opinion was published in 1904 (Jacquet 1904) and became the most frequently quoted definition of the role of itching in this disease. Besnier (1892) distinguished the prurigo group of diseases and described their clinical features; in addition to skin involvement, he listed emphysema, bronchial asthma, hay fever, and, more rarely, gastrointestinal disturbances as members of the group. Furthermore, he suggested that the disease tended to be familial and to occur in the constitutionally predisposed. He agreed with Jacquet when he stressed that "le symptome premier et le premier symptome est le prurit." His term for the disease - prurigo diathèsique - was soon changed to Besnier's prurigo (Rasch 1903). The basic discovery of the concept of allergy by von Pirquet (1906) and its consequent results formed the next milestone; advances in the concept of allergy were to follow.

"Atopy," a word of Greek derivation, was introduced by Coca and Cooke (1923) to connote a strange disease. It was applied to some clinical manifestations of eczema and certain varieties of drug and food idiosyncrasy. Two years later, Coca (1925) included in his definition of atopy those specific reaginic antibodies which are transferable by the Prausnitz-Küstner method, and the redefinition was clearly expressed in a later work (Coca et al. 1931). The constitutional stigmata which distinguish atopic skin disease from other eczemas were summarized by Rost and Marchionini (1932), while "atopic dermatitis" was introduced by Wise and Sulzberger (1933) and Hill and Sulzberger (1935) as the term befitting this concept.

In 1953 Coca again modified his definition: "Atopy comprises a group of allergic diseases that are subject to a common hereditary influence and in which the atopic reagins are often demonstrable." However, even after the discovery of IgE as the earlier postulated reagin, the definition is still being discussed. Since nonatopic subjects also develop IgE antibody, it is important to point out Pepys' (1975) view, that such subjects produce it solely in response to peculiarly potent allergenic exposures, whereas atopics readily produce it in response to ordinary exposure to the common allergens of the subject's environment (see also Sect. 5.5.5.2).

1.2 Nomenclature

Many terms are of historical interest. Besnier's prurigo and "diffuse neurodermatitis" have already been mentioned in a historical context, and these and synonyms of similar background have been, and remain, in frequent use. *"Früh- und spätexsudatives Eczematoid"* was introduced by Rost (1928), while "asthma-eczema" owes its origin to the frequent association with asthma. *"Endogenes Ekzem,"* a term previously used in a broader sense, was chosen by Korting (1954) to characterize the disease, and "neurodermatitis constitutionalis sive atopica" was favored by Schnyder and Borelli (1967). These two terms are still sometimes mentioned in some German reports, and in a few French works the term "eczéma constitutionnel" (Brocq 1927) or "prurigo Besnier" is used. Eczema ("to boil over"), which is used in the United Kingdom and sometimes in the United States, is a debatable definition, as has been revealed by discussion between leading dermatohistopathologists and clinicians (Ackerman and Ragaz 1984): the term was originally linked to spongiosis, but the latter is often absent in AD. Therefore the term coined by Sulzberger and co-workers, "atopic dermatitis," seems more appropriate. To quote Civatte (1984), "the term AD has wider acceptance because it includes all the cutaneous manifestations of atopy including those which never show spongiosis and which are not eczema". One example of confusion is when a statement such as the following may be read: "T lymphopenia occurs frequently in atopic disorders, e. g. in atopic eczema (Luckasen et al. 1974; McGeady and Buckley 1974), atopic dermatitis (Palacios et al. 1966) etc." (I have intentionally omitted the author of these lines.)

Atopic dermatitis is now the prevalent term in the United States and most other countries although it is open to criticism and not all dermatologists accept this term. It nevertheless appears to be the best name for the disease, and consequently is the name that the author has chosen to use in his book.

"Pure" AD (see Preface) is a frequently used term to characterize persons with skin but not respiratory AD.

Symptom-free skin it is term used by the present author for the macroscopically normal-looking skin of a person with AD. It seems more appropriate than "uninvolved" skin owing to observations that in apparently noninflammatory skin, structural and/or functional alterations such as barrier abnormality and low irritation threshold may be found (Al-Jaberi and Marks 1984). This means that in a subject with AD, the skin can generally be considered as altered and thus the possible site of a disease manifestation.

References

Ackerman AB, Ragaz A (1984) A plea to expunge the word "eczema" from the lexicon of dermatology and dermatopathology. Am J Dermatopathol 4: 315

Al-Jaberi H, Marks R (1984) Studies of the clinically uninvolved skin in patients with dermatitis. Br J Dermatol 111: 437

Besnier E (1892) Première note et observations preliminaires pour servir d'introduction à l'étude diathésiques. Ann Dermatol Syphiligr 4: 634

Brocq L (1927) Conception générale des dermatoses, nouvelle note sur leur classification. Ann Dermatol Syphilol 8: 65

Brocq L, Jacquet L (1891) Notes pour servir à l'histoire des névrodermites: du lichen circumscriptus des anciens auteurs, ou lichen simplex chronique de M le Dr E Vidal. Ann Dermatol Syphiligr 2: 97 and 193

Civatte J (1984) The term eczema should be better defined. Am J Dermatophatol 4: 333

Coca AF (1925) Zur Frage der Identität der anaphylaktischen und der atopischen Überempfindlichkeit. Med Klin 21: 57

Coca AF, Cooke RA (1923) On classification of the phenomena of hypersensitiveness. J Immunol 6: 63

Coca AF, Walzer M, Thommen AA (1931) Asthma and hay fever in theory and praxis. Thomas, Springfield

Hill LW, Sulzberger MG (1935) Evolution of atopic dermatitis. Arch Dermatol Syph 32: 451

Jacquet L (1904) In: Besnier E, Brocq L, Jacquet L (eds) La pratique dermatologique, vol 5. Masson, Paris, p 341

Korting GW (1954) Zur Pathogenese des endogenen Ekzems. Thieme, Stuttgart

Luckasen JR, Sabad A, Goltz RW, Kersey JH (1974) T and B lymphocytes in atopic eczema. Arch Dermatol 112: 1095

McGeady SJ, Buckley RH (1974) Depression of cell-mediated immunity in atopic eczema. J Allergy Clin Immunol 56: 393

Palacios J, Fuller EW, Blaylock WK (1966) Immunological capabilities with atopic dermatitis. J Invest Dermatol 47: 484

Pepys J (1975) Atopy. In: Gell PHG, Coombs RA, Lachmann PJ (eds) Clinical aspects of immunology. 3d Ed. Blackwell, Oxford London Edinburgh Melbourne, p 877

Rasch C (1903) Hudens sygdomme. Gyldendal, Copenhagen

Ring J (1985) Erstbeschreibung einer "atopischen Familienanamnese" im Julisch-Claudiuschen Kaiserhaus: Augustus, Claudius, Britannicus. Hautarzt 36: 470

Rost GA (1928) Über Erfahrungen der allergenfreien Kammer nach Storm van Leeuwen, insbesondere in der Spätperiode der exsudativen Diathese. Arch Dermatol Syph 155: 297

Rost GA, Marchionini A (1932) Asthma-Ekzem, Asthma-Prurigo und Neurodermitis als allergische Hautkrankheiten. Würzb Abh Gesamtgeb Prakt Med 27: 10

Schnyder UW, Borelli S (1967) Zur Nomenklatur der atopischen Dermatitis. Acta Derm Venereol 3: 75

von Hebra H (1884) Dermatomycosis diffusa flexorum. I. Die krankhaften Veränderungen der Haut und ihrer Anhangsgebilde mit ihren Beziehungen zu den Krankheiten des Gesamtorganismus. Wreden, Braunschweig

von Pirquet C (1906) Allergie. MMW 53: 1457

Willian R (1808) On cutaneous diseases. Johnson, London

Wise F, Sulzberger MB (1933) Editors' remarks. In: Yearbook of dermatology and syphilology. Year Book Medical Publishers, Chicago

2 Clinical Aspects

2.1 Prevalence

Regional statistics and records of hospital departments have provided most of the data on the prevalence of AD, but, as sources of accurate estimates, these are imperfect; statistical records, for example, make no sharp distinction between AD and other varieties of eczema. This is well instanced by the use of the heading "infantile eczema," under which some cases of seborrheic dermatitis are likely to be included. Thus, figures for the incidence of "infantile eczema," such as 3.1% (Walker and Warin 1956), are not necessarily precise estimates of the frequency of infantile AD. Furthermore, difficulty in differential diagnosis has led some authors to exclude cases of infantile AD from their series. The incidence of eczema in schoolchildren has been given as 1.1% by Brereton et al. (1959). Some reports have included the frequency both of AD and of other atopic manifestations. Even the incidence of atopy in the general population has been assessed by somewhat different methods and has been found to be as high as 20% (Carr et al. 1964). Further complexity has been added to the subject, for the author, studying monovular twins, found a significant disparity in the clinical course of their atopic manifestations (Rajka 1961), and this was quoted by Champion and Parish (1968) as an argument in favor of the concept of latent atopy. Therefore, only a few critical, selective statistics are available on the occurrence of AD in a large, normal population. They include those from Copenhagen, citing a frequency of 0.1% (Schwartz 1952), and those from Zürich, citing an incidence of 0.1%–0.5% (Schnyder 1960). The actual incidence may well be higher, and another source of error may be that incidence (new cases per unit time) and prevalence (sum of cases at the time of examination/estimation) are not differentiated in some reports. Moreover, some reports have included the frequency both of AD and of other atopic manifestations.

The most extensive statistics have come from the United States, based on the clinical examination of 20749 individuals between 1971 and 1974. The result was 0.69% and extrapolation to the United States' population gave an estimate of 1332 million persons with AD (Johnson and Roberts 1978). This percentage figure was higher than those cited by Schwartz and Schnyder (see above).

There is unanimous agreement that the prevalence of AD has increased in the last decade. The argument for this increase in prevalence comes from statistics concerning childhood AD (see Fig. 2.1). Similar numerical data emerge

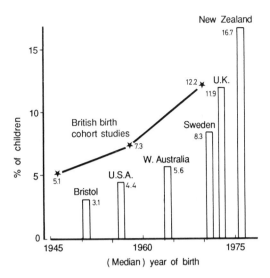

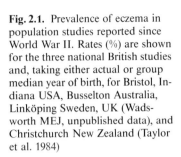

Fig. 2.1. Prevalence of eczema in population studies reported since World War II. Rates (%) are shown for the three national British studies and, taking either actual or group median year of birth, for Bristol, Indiana USA, Busselton Australia, Linköping Sweden, UK (Wadsworth MEJ, unpublished data), and Christchurch New Zealand (Taylor et al. 1984)

from Danish (Schultz-Larsen 1985) and Japanese (4.1%–14.7%, M. Uehara, personal communication) reports. Investigations of children thus show an increase from 3%–4% during the 1960s to 10% in the 1980s. The prevalence among teenagers is lower accoring to Swedish estimates: 2.3% for boys and 3.8% for girls (Larsson and Lidén 1980).

The prevalence of atopic diseases in the general population has been varyingly estimated due to differing methods of assessment (from questionaires to clinical examinations) and the different age categories investigated. It is probably about 10%–20% (Carr et al. 1964, Kjellman 1983, and others). This is, for example, reflected in outpatient attendance at Swedish pediatric clinics, which is 15%–20% (Kjellman and Pettersson 1980). Among the atopic diseases, atopic rhinitis is ten times, and asthma five times, more common than AD (Schnyder 1959). It is furthermore generally accepted that the prevalence of potential atopy in the population is higher than the occurrence of AD. There are indications that the prevalence of atopic diseases has also increased in the developing countries.

Among factors that may have contributed to the increase in atopic diseases, the most commonly mentioned are potent airborne allergens related to air pollution (including cigarette smoke and sulfur dioxide), microbial infection, and early exposure to allergenic foods (compared with earlier practices) (Johansson 1981; Foucard 1985). The month of birth, related to exposure during the first 6 months, e. g., to pollen or house dust mites, is also emphasized (Björksten and Suoniemi 1981), as is the frequent practice of keeping pets in the home (see p. 87). The fact that more people now have access to medical care, with improved diagnostic possibilities, may also be of significance.

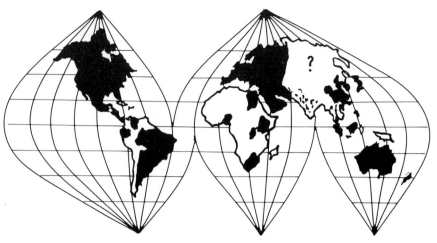

Fig. 2.2. Worldwide distribution of AD

2.1.1 Worldwide Distribution

In dermatological literature from European countries and North America there are a number of sets of data on the occurrence of AD and on certain factors which can influence it. In global terms, however, our knowledge is limited. The present author has carried out a study by questionnaires mailed to dermatologists associated with university departments or in private practice in Asia, Australia/New Zealand, Latin America, and Africa. According to the representative answers from 35 different countries, the incidence of AD is high in most countries in all continents, with some peaks (e. g., New Zealand) and some troughs (e. g., India and Thailand). There were no significant racial differences, although Caucasians most frequently suffered from AD. In countries with mixed races it seems that all races were involved. The conditions reported coincided well with a few literature reports (Lynch et al. 1984; Olumide 1986), with the author's experience, and with personal communications to him; they are depicted in Fig. 2.2.

The above-mentioned sources of information also attempted to elucidate factors that might be related to the frequency of influencing the course of AD in a given geographical area. Analysis of the collected data allowed the conclusion that several factors (see Chap. 9) were of likely importance. Among them, climatic and geographical factors were clearly predominant. Professional conditions and psychic stress also played an important role, whereas food items played only a minor one (Rajka 1986).

2.1.2 Sex Incidence

Several authors have stated, with certain reservations (Champion and Parish 1968), that women outnumber men in large series of cases of AD, and the reported ratios of females to males include 2:1 (Schnyder 1960) and 1.6:1 (Dorn 1961). Children with infantile AD are more often male.

2.2 Course

Although the course of the disease is intertwined with morphology, from the didactic point of view one can try to discuss these separately.

2.2.1 Onset, Phases, and Morphological Characteristics

The age at onset of the disease is frequently of interest. The author's statistics, in which account is taken of sex differences, are shown in Table 2.1, these being in agreement with most references (Nexmand 1948, Hellerström and Lidman 1956; Oddoze 1959; Wagner and Pürschel 1962). A still higher average age of onset was observed in a computerized study of 500 children with AD (Queille-Roussel et al. 1985).

2.2.1.1 Distribution of the First Lesions

The first single site to be affected differs with the age when the disease appears. It is usually the face (70%) in babies in their 1st year, and the flexures (44%) or the face (33%) in children between 1 and 5 years of age (de Graciansky 1966). Hands were a rather frequent (more than 4%) initial site of involvement in the statistics of Queille-Roussel et al. (1985).

Table 2.1. Age at onset of AD

Age at onset in years	Males	%	Females	%
– 1	328	60.2	360	55.0
1– 5	159	29.4	201	30.7
6–10	26	4.8	47	7.2
11–15	8	1.5	23	3.5
16–20	14	2.6	14	2.1
21–25	5	0.9	6	0.9
26–30	1	0.2	1	0.2
31–40	–	–	–	–
41–50	–	–	1	0.2
Uncertain	4	0.7	2	0.3
Total	545	100	655	100

2.2.2 Infantile Phase

Atopic dermatitis is a chronic disease of infants, children, and young adults ["maladie de jeunes gens" (Besnier 1892)], and its course is conveniently considered as it affects these age groups. The classification usually used (Hill and Sulzberger 1935) comprises:

Infantile phase: up to 2 years
Childhood phase: between 3 and 11 years
Adolescent and young adult phase: between 12 and 23 years.

It was previously thought that infantile AD begins usually in the 2nd or 3rd month. However, it can occur earlier, for the author and other workers (Bandmann 1965; Korting 1954) have undoubtedly seen several cases in which the disease has appeared during the 2nd or 3rd week after birth; nevertheless, the diagnosis should not be made lightly in those so young (Solomon and Esterly 1973). Several such cases may have been misdiagnosed in the past as seborrheic dermatitis. The age at onset is independent of the genetic predisposition to atopy (Schnyder 1960; Rajka 1960) and of whether the child was breast fed or artificially fed (Edgren 1943). Lesions first appear on the cheeks, forehead, and scalp (see Fig. 2.3), but may occur on the other recognized sites of predilection (see Fig. 2.4). In this age group, spread to the extremities or to the trunk occurs, and there may be involvement of the thumb (provoked possibly by thumb-sucking), of the anogenital region, or of the ear lobe (de Graciansky 1966). Oozing and crusted eczematous lesions characteristically predominate in these infants, in contrast with the less exudative eczematous changes of later phases of the disease; pyococcal infection is the usual cause of the crusting (see also complications). Scratching is not observed before the infant is 2 months old, by which time the necessary coordination is supposed to have fully developed, but thereafter it can be most intense and may result in crying, nocturnal restlessness, scratching crises, and so forth.

As the lesions of infantile AD are very eczematous in character, other varieties of eczema, such as seborrheic dermatitis, must be considered in differential diagnosis. A classical differential diagnostic procedure was described for distinguishing between infantile seborrheic dermatitis and AD (Sulzberger 1940). The present author found that the localization may often be the same (see Sect. 2.5.3 and Fig. 2.18) and there is little support for claims that the greasy red seborrheic lesions usually appear on the scalp in retroauricular and centrofacial areas, in axillae, and in napkin areas, whereas in AD the lesions appear on the lateral parts of the face, extensor surfaces of the limbs, and sometimes on the trunk.

Early onset characteristics for seborrheic dermatitis may also be found in AD cases; a major role should be attributed to familial/personal history in this respect. At the beginning of the twentieth century the overwhelming opinion was that infantile eczematous lesions are of seborrheic origin, but now the reverse view is held. Several authors doubt whether seborrheic dermatitis in infants really exists and speak of a seborrheic type (Vickers 1983) or clinical vari-

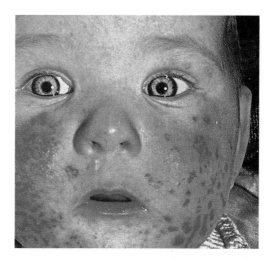

Fig. 2.3. Eczematous lesions on the face in infantile AD

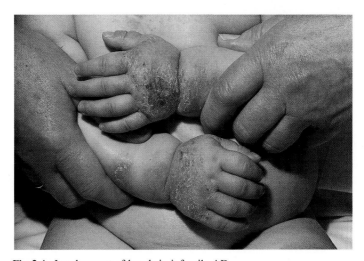

Fig. 2.4. Involvement of hands in infantile AD

ant (Podmore et al. 1986) of AD. In the author's opinion, seborrheic dermatitis does occur, but infrequently. Thorough follow-up shows that in at least one-third of seborrheic dermatitis cases, the disease later converts to typical AD. Others interpret these cases as chance occurence of seborrheic dermatitis in children with an inherited atopic tendency and cite a higher incidence of seborrheic dermatitis (Yates et al. 1983).

As the infant grows older, the distribution of the lesions my change, involvement of all surfaces of the limbs becoming common. The characteristic flexural involvement begins to appear at about 18 months of age, but becomes more

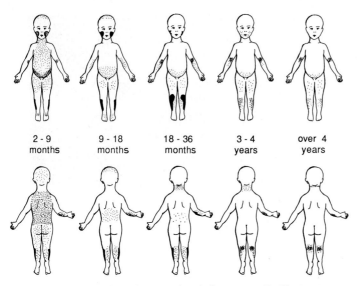

Fig. 2.5. Distribution of eczema in relation to age. (Sedlis 1965)

marked only in early childhood (see Fig. 2.5). By the end of the 2nd year of life, a considerable number of AD cases are definitely healed, while others continue into the childhood phase.

2.2.3 Childhood Phase

This is a phase of great importance, not least with regard to the onset of AD. The literature and the data of Table 2.1 indicate that, in about 86% of cases, the onset occurs before the child is 5 years old, and that not infrequently the childhood phase is a continuation of the infantile. As the child grows older the clinical picture usually bears an increasing resemblance to that seen in adolescents and adults. Flexural involvement becomes more marked and the face is less frequently affected by the age of 4 or 5 years. At the same time, the lesions become, in general, less acute, and are less often eczematous; lesions in childhood thus show the characteristics of AD which have already been discussed. In childhood, the hands not infrequently show lesions which are dry and chapped or are lichenified and eczematous; other varieties of hand eczema are relatively rare in this age group. Lip or perioral involvement is another feature of this phase, being manifested as a dry scaly eruption or as fissures at the corners of the mouth (see Fig. 2.6). Involvement of the backs of the thighs and of the buttocks can occur, to produce a picture resembling a toilet-seat dermatitis (Herzberg 1973). Severe pruritus produces intense scratching and a restless, anxious, hyperactive child.

Dryness of the fingertips is common, at least in Scandinavia, due to contact with snow and wet gloves.

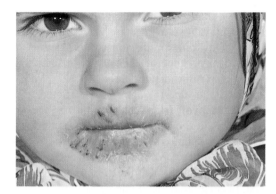

Fig. 2.6. Involvement of the lips in AD

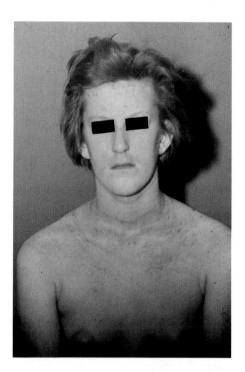

Fig. 2.7. Lesions on the neck and upper trunk in AD in the adolescent phase

School may be a source of difficulty for young AD patients because of concentration problems caused by itching, deterioration of the skin condition due to the disease, and so on.

2.2.4 Adolescent/Young Adult Phase

In the adolescent/young adult phase, pruritus and lichenification are the predominant lesions. The distribution of lesions is similar to that in the previous phase, mostly involving face, neck, flexures, and upper trunk (see Fig. 2.7).

During puberty, the numerous psychological difficulties and conflicts with authority may have a negative effect on the disease. This may be reflected in peaks of hospital admissions. The presence of respiratory atopy, particularly asthma, may sometimes negatively influence the course of the skin disease, but it may also run independently.

Women around the age of 20, particularly young mothers, frequently experience hand involvement as the only, or sometimes the first, sign of AD. Etiological factors in this connection will be mentioned later, but it is obvious that the differential diagnosis of other dermatitic conditions with hand involvement is a constant problem. The negative influence of psychological factors may be noted in young adults in connection with stress in marital selection, in military service, in pregnancy or in choice of career. Concerning occupational factors, see Sect 9.5.

2.2.5 Onset at Elder Age

The onset of the disease at an advanced age is very uncommon. In the author's material, patients more than 45 years old constituted only 2% of all cases (see Table 2.1). Due to the infrequent occurrence of elder subjects, differential diagnostic considerations are of importance, including, for instance, Hodgkin's disease and other conditions (see also Sect. 2.10.2).

2.3 Prognosis

2.3.1 Phases and Prognostic Problems

The disease may begin, relapse, or be absent in any phase, and, as it can thus take several courses, numerous variants may be recognized. Many cases heal in the infantile phase, improvement around puberty is common, and, after the second decade, there is a tendency to spontaneous healing, older patients rarely being seen (see also below): of the author's 1200 patients only 2% were over 45 years old. In most cases of AD the course is practically continuous, with no symptom-free intervals, as exemplified by those with early flexural lesions (Nexmand 1948), with early extensive lesions (Bandmann 1965), or with respiratory manifestations (Schnyder and Borelli 1965). Contrary to expectations, this does not apply to severe cases (Nexmand 1948). The author studied 50 "pure" AD patients from each of four age groups and found a continuous course with the following frequencies:

Under 6 years: 96%
Between 7 and 12 years: 82%
Between 13 and 18 years: 72%
Over 18 years (19–45 years): 48%

Osborne and Murray (1953) observed a somewhat more favorable course, with symptom-free periods, in 28% of their young patients. The duration of such remissions has received some attention. According to de Graciansky (1966) they last for 2–10 years in about 50% of cases, and for more than 10 years in about one-third; by contrast Nexmand (1948) reported that the average duration symptom-free intervals was approximately 6.5 years.

2.3.2 Cases Healed After the Infantile Phase

The rate of healing of infantile AD is one of the most hotly debated questions about this disease. The answer is clearly important, especially in relation to prognosis. A major difficulty in its evaluation is differentiation between atopic and nonatopic dermatitis in the infant. The duration of observation in some reports has been too brief to permit any conclusion as to whether the disease had definitely healed of whether it was merely quiescent. Figures published in the pediatric and the dermatological literature differ, the higher figures in the latter reflecting the inclusion of persistent adult cases. Reports based only on answers to questionnaires, the patients not being examined, are liable to contain more errors.

The relevant literature gives conflicting information on the healing rate (Osborne and Murray 1953; Heite 1961; Stifler 1965). It was therefore a significant achievement when Vickers (1980) published a large series consisting of 2000 children, with a thorough follow-up (in some cases up to 20 years). His results pointed to a much more optimistic prognosis than most clinicians had previously found, as his overall clearance rate was greater than 84%. Some data with long follow-up, including those of Vickers, are collected in Table 2.2, which reveals considerable divergence. Possible causes of this divergence, in addition to the above-mentioned sources of error seem to be differences in the patient material and diagnostic criteria and particularly the severity of skin lesions. The most often quoted factors giving unfavorable prognosis are severe/widespread infantile dermatitis, particularly on limbs and hands (see also Sect. 2.5.4), respiratory allergies and female sex. The importance of atopic familial history and early onset in this connection is not obvious in all these reports.

Early prognosis is difficult, and most clinicians consider familial history of importance here. It seems that high total cord IgE values have a predictive val-

Table 2.2. Results of some larger long-term follow-up studies in AD

Authors	No. of patients	Length of follow-up	Healing rate	Remarks
Purdy (1953)	93	16–22 years	72%	
Vowles et al. (1955)	84	13 years	45%	
Berlinghoff (1961)	234	8–22 years	66%	
Roth and Kierland (1964)	200	20 years	29%–40%	Mild or severe
Musgrove and Morgan (1976)	99	15 years	42%	
Vickers (1980)	2000 (1897)	5–20 years	84%	
Van Hecke and Leys (1981)	50	20 years	38%	
Wütrich and Schudel (1983)	212	15 years	37%	
Rystedt (1985a)	955	24–44 years	38%–60%	In- or outpatients

ue for the development of atopic disease (Kjellman 1976; Michel et al. 1980). Elevated phosphodiesterase levels at birth are also considered to have predictive value (Heskel et al. 1984).

The growth rate in AD may be impaired due to the application not only of systemic steroids, which is fortunately seldom, but also of potent topical steroids (Kristmundsdottir and David 1987).

2.3.3 Clearing of the Disease

In the late twenties, most AD cases tend to heal, the reason for which, despite all our knowledge of the disease, is a total mystery. Although in healed AD cases (Rajka, unpublished data), as in mild cases (Braathen 1985), a normalization of some immunological parameters, e.g., the helper/suppressor T cell ratio, can be registered, it is an open question as to whether this is a primary or only a secondary event. A more significant reduction of IgE in atiopc disease occurs only in age groups above 40 years (Stoy et al. 1981) while a decrease in IgE receptors follows the healing of AD (Spiegelberg 1986).

It is of the utmost importance in this connection that after successful bone marrow grafting (Parkman et al. 1978), the AD (and interestingly even the xerosis) dramatically cleared, without recurrence during a long follow-up period.

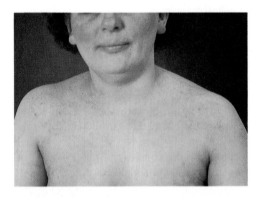

Fig. 2.8. Persisting AD in middle-aged woman

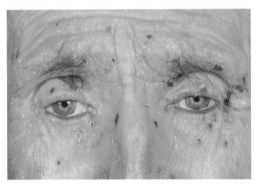

Fig. 2.9. Persisting AD in a man of 72 years of age

This is a strong agrument for the role of an immune disorder in the mechanism of AD (Saurat 1985); other mechanisms, e. g., enzymatic, may perhaps account for the xerosis).

2.3.3.1 Persistent Cases

Most cases of AD heal by the age of 30 or so years (Sulzberger 1940; Norrlind 1946), but very persistent cases have been reported; Schnyder and Borelli (1965), for example, claimed that the disease usually heals by the age of 50–60 years (see Fig. 2.8). The author has a few patients over 70 years of age with active disease, including food reactivity (see Fig. 2.9). Analyses of the data on the obstinate cases revealed no special etiological factors, although the majority had respiratory manifestations and generally produced several positive reactions on testing with inhalant and food allergens. Similar cases have shown ele-

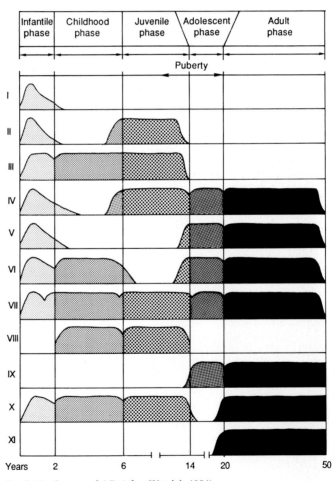

Fig. 2.10. Course of AD (after Wütrich 1981)

vated serum IgE levels, and psychological factors have seemed to play a striking role in some. However, these finding provide no explanation for the
prolonged nature of the skin disease in these patients.

Based on the above considerations it is evident that the disease may be long-
lasting. On the other hand, it may alternate between symptom-free intervals
(usually during the summer) and relapses. Many individual variations occur in
the course of AD, the more common ones being shown in Fig. 2.10. (Wütrich
and Schudel 1983).

2.4 Basic Clinical Features

The most important clinical features of AD are detailed below.

2.4.1 Primary Trait

The main symptom in AD is the characteristic itch which is elicited by the complex etiological factors. Any critical and simplified survey, which omits controversial aspects, should stress this feature at the outset. Jacquet (1904) was the
first to express this view clearly, and it has subsequently been stressed by,
among others, Haxthausen (1957) and the author (Rajka 1963, 1967, 1968). Details of the pruritus in AD are discussed in a separate chapter (Chap. 3).

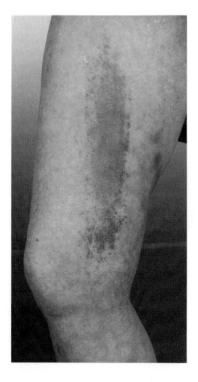

Fig. 2.11. Scratching marks in adult AD

Excoriations, consequent on the itch-provoked scratching, are a frequent manifestation in the disease (see Fig. 2.11.) Three other characteristic lesions may appear: prurigo papules, eczematous lesions, and lichenification. These four characteristic but nonspecific signs may be present in any combination, which can vary with time. The capricious aspect of the usually symmetrical eruption presents greater problems in diagnosis than are met with in monomorphic dermatoses. Attempts to separate this group of manifestations into "pure" types, such as those with and those without eczematous lesions, are defeated by this changeable nature. Consequently, the nonspecific morphology – "caractère absolument fondamental: aucune des lésions n'est pas spécifique" (Besnier 1892) – usually will not be diagnostic, and thus the diagnosis should be based on several criteria. The best morphological criterion is a combination of any of the four characteristic lesions, accompanied by pruritus and modified by scratching. Pruritus, therefore, is the basic symptom of AD, which also is characterized by itchy skin (Bickford 1938), and the vicious circle of pruritus and inflammatory lesions is commonly seen. (see chap. 3 and correlations between itch and AD, Sect. 3.2).

Major morphological patterns. As in several other skin diseases, the lesions in AD consist of a combination of nonspecific changes closely realted to itch. These are prurigo, lichenification, and eczematous lesions.

2.4.2 Prurigo

The morphological term "prurigo" signifies a small (0.5–1.5 mm in diameter), discrete, dome-shaped papule, usually with a vesicle at its summit (see Fig. 2.12). This lesion has no universally accepted definition and thus has a somewhat confused nomenclature. The acute form, known also as strophulus, is now believed to be a reaction to arthropod bites, whereas the chronic type is synonymous with prurigo nodularis of Hyde. It is the frequently encountered subacute variety which provokes the most discussion. It seems to have more than one cause, occurs in adults, shows variations in the number and distribution of lesions, and is associated clinically with eczematous lesions and with

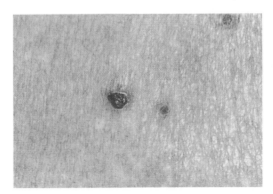

Fig. 2.12. The prurigo lesion

lichenification. Histological examination of a lesion shows marked acanthosis and moderate intercellular edema; the acanthosis, initially central to the lesion, produces the conical shape. This appearance differs only in degree from the typical spongiosis and vesicle formation in eczematous epidermis. The chronic scratching may provoke secondary lichenification, pigment changes (mostly hypopigmentation), sometimes scarring, and histologically observed secondary neural proliferation (Runne and Orfanos 1977). Prurigo, i.e., and intensely pruritic papule, is inevitably excoriated, producing an eroded, encrusted top, and is one of the most characteristic lesions of juvenile or adult AD ("prurigo Besnier"). Prurigo was considered by some earlier authors to be the primary event, but the author holds the contrary view, i.e., that itch is more likely to be the initial change, the epidermal reaction occurring secondarily; the chronological sequence of events in a positive provocation test in AD led him to this conclusion. Prurigo is by no means a specific lesion; it only reflects an underlying pruritic mechanism, such as may occur in response to arthropod bites (strophulus) and to several etiological factors, including diabetes, liver disease, hyperlipemia and gastrointestinal disturbances. It may be speculated that there is first an immediate and then a delayed response; the latter is due to persistence of proteins, e.g., insect proteins (the possible role of food proteins here is still unclear). Awaiting explanation is the inability of small children with AD to produce these subacute lesions despite their ability to develop prurigo after, for exampule, insect bites.

2.4.3 Lichenification

Lichenification can be characterized as poorly demarcated plaques in which grossly accentuated skin furrows separate slightly shiny rhomboid areas. This typically grayish or brownish thickening of the skin may be regarded as a dermal-epidermal reaction to persistent scratching, and thus appears most frequently around eczematous or prurigo lesions. Sites of predilection of lichenification are in and around the antecubital and the popliteal fossae (see Fig. 2.13), but it not uncommonly occurs diffusely on the face or as plaques on the backs of the hands or of the feet. Goldblum and Piper (1954) performed the basic study of this phenomenon by demonstrating experimentally that lichenification could be produced by scratching. They constructed a scratching machine to apply a "scratching" pressure of 75 g to the skin and, after 60–90 h of use, lichenification was reproduced – this was equivalent to scratching 140000 times. However, it is important to remember that early French authors assumed that persons with AD could be particularly predisposed to develop lichenification in response to trivial trauma. Presumably this predisposition only provides an illustration of the longstanding pruritus characteristic of AD.

Overlapping occurs between lichenification as a morphological pattern and lichen simplex chronicus (localized neurodermatitis), a variant of the eczematous inflammation group, when its major morphological expression, i.e., lichenification. On the other hand, lichen simplex chronicus may develop with-

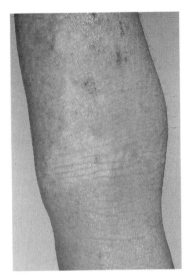

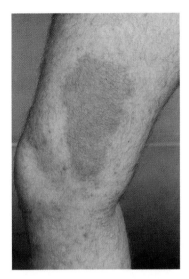

Fig. 2.13. Lichenification in the
antecubital fossa

Fig. 2.14. Nummular pattern in a
young adult with AD

out atopic signs (Hazell and Marks 1983), especially in older females and also
in the genital area (Grimmer 1979).

2.4.4 Eczematous Lesions

Eczematous lesions show an erythematous, papulous, scaly picture as an expression of polymorphous, intensely itching inflammation. They are less common than prurigo or lichenification but are undoubtedly an essential feature of
the disease in general, and are the most typical manifestation of infantile AD.
Histologically, however, the characteristic hallmark of eczema, spongiosis, may
be absent in AD, and therefore use of the term "eczema" is strongly criticized.
In this context it is advantageous to use the expression "eczematous lesions"
characterizing a dermoepidermal response (Russel Jones and MacDonald
1982), which can be used in a broader sense. One has to pay tribute to Sulzberger for introducing the term AD in place of "eczema" or "atopic eczema"
(see Sect. 1.2).

A nummular pattern (see Fig. 2.14) is not so infrequently observed in atopic
persons, and the question arises as to whether or not this represents a variant of
AD. Nummular eczematous dermatitis is an independent disease (Sirot 1983)
but according to the present author's experience, a nummular pattern may also
be observed in AD, particularly in children. The asteatosis (chapping), a predisposing factor in nummular eczematous inflammations and a feature of AD, is a
possible bridge between these conditions.

These clinical features are not specific to AD, and any can appear in combination with other lesions; consequently it can be difficult or even impossible to

make a sharp morphological distinction between this and several other dermatoses. Difficulties exist, therefore, in differential diagnosis and to a lesser degree in ascertaining the etiology and pathogenesis of the disease. It is important
to be aware that AD and the other skin diseases with prurigo or eczematous lesions may overlap to some degree or may perchance be concurrent in the same
patient (see also Sect. 2.16).

2.4.5 Correlations Between Itch and Major Features

The author considers the primary event of AD, the itch, to be strictly correlated
to the above morphological patterns (see Figs. 2.15, 2.16). Shelley, (1972) while
quoting the classical statement that "itch is the disease itself," adds: "All the

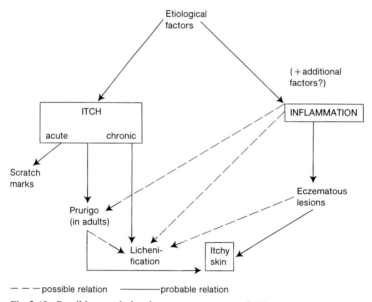

Fig. 2.15. Possible correlation between symptoms of AD

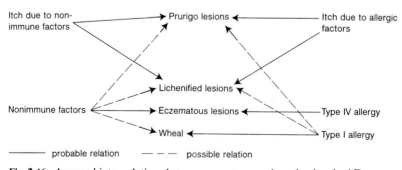

Fig. 2.16. Assumed inter-relations between symptoms and mechanism in AD

grossly visible signs, inflammation, lichenification, and excoriation, it must be realized, are sequential and secondary." This also fits well Ackerman's (1978) opinion on the histological changes of AD: "They are largely caused by rubbing and scratching. If the fingers of a patient with AD could be restrained, the skin lesions would disappear, although the itching would doubtless persist."

Itch, with its efferent reflex response, the scratching, constitutes a real vicious circle in AD that is one of the cardinal events in the disease. The fight against itch plays a tremendous role in the management of AD.

2.5 Morphology and Distribution

Although any of the cardinal lesions outlined above may involve most anatomical regions, common experience shows that certain morphological patterns are typical of particular areas. Examples include:

1. Flexures: lichenification, eczematous lesions, or both
2. Face: eczematous lesions, which may be of a seborrheic character
3. Hands and feet: eczematous lesions, lichenified plaques, or both. These examples do not run counter to the view that pruritus and prurigo are primary and essential signs; excoriations can occur on any site in AD.

2.5.1 Sites of Predilection

The principal sites of predilection of AD are the antecubital flexures, and rather less frequently the popiteal fossae. If infantile AD is included, the face and the flexures are affected with equal frequency. The hands and fingers (see below) and the front and sides of the neck are often involved; in addition, lesions on the body are not uncommon.

Involvement of the feet and the perigenital and perianal areas is less important statistically than it is in differential diagnosis. The sites of predilection are shown in Table 2.3 (Korting 1954) and are in agreement with the author's experiences, although somewhat different from the data of Schudel and Wütrich (1985).

Table 2.3. Sites of predilection in AD

Localization	Approx. % of AD cases
Antecubital	70
Neck	52
Popliteal	42
Face	40
Hands	32
Wrist	26
Extremities	14
Body	12

2.5.2 Head and Face

Dandruff or hyperkeratosis (cradle cap) on the scalp occur not uncommonly in infantile and also in child or adult AD (Heskel and Lobitz 1983; Lindmaier et al. 1987).

The face may show various changes in AD. In the majority of such cases a diffuse lichenification is noted, demonstrating a grayish white complexion (facial pallor). The pathological vascular reactivity in AD (compare with white dermographism) may also play a role here. On the other hand, facial erythema may prevail during active bouts of AD.

Eyelids sometimes show lichenification as an expression of AD (Svensson and Möller 1986; author's own clinical observations).

Thinning or absence of the lateral eyebrow (Hertoghe's sign) is frequently seen in AD but has also been described in hypothyroidism or trichorhinopharyngeal syndrome. Autonomic disturbances, selective rubbing, or both, have been assumed to play a part in its pathogenesis in AD, but due to absence of proof it is impossible to decide whether it is pertinent to or merely associated with the disease.

Morgan's crease (Dennis-Morgan fold) is a characteristic clinical sign, possibly in relation to lower eyelid dermatitis (Uehara 1981), and persists for long periods. Occasionally, a double fold is observed (see Fig. 2.17). Morgan's crease was found in 12% in a careful study, and there was no correlation with severity. Rubbing is often quoted as a cause, but this fails to explain why the majority do not have this sign (Meenan 1981).

Perioral dermatitis including perlèche and lip dermatitis is, as already mentioned, a frequent sign, particularly in childhood but also later on, as a dry, scaly, sometimes superinfected eruption with fissures. The upper lip is mostly involved (see also Fig. 2.6).

Hanifin (1983) mentions the furrowed mouth syndrome related to mouth breathing in patients with allergic rhinitis.

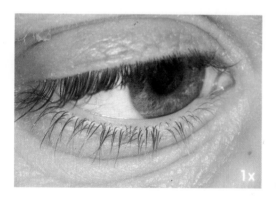

Fig. 2.17. Double Morgan fold in a adolescent with AD

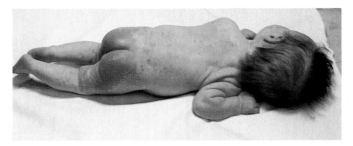

Fig. 2.18. Infantile AD on the napkin area

2.5.3 Body

The neck is often a site of predilection in AD. Anterior neck folds, i. e., horizontal creases, are present in many patients (Hanifin 1983). Anterolateral reticulate pigmentation, as found in other diseases, may appear in AD as a "dirty neck" (Colver et al. 1987).

Nipple dermatitis is an infrequent sign but may be present in young women with severe AD.

The napkin area has already been mentioned in connection with the infantile phase of AD. Napkin dermatitis (diaper rash) is a well-known clinical entity (see Fig. 2.18) with several causes, including (a) irritation due to ammoniacal fermentation, proteases in feces, or sweat ingredients, (b) rises in skin temperature through inhibited transpiration, (c) microbial (pyococci, candida) agents, and (d) irritation/sensitization to diaper material. On only the basis of the morphology it is not possible to state whether the skin disease in this localization corresponds to AD, seborrheic eczema, (napkin) psoriasis, true psoriasis, or candidal or pyococcal intertrigo. Helpful differential diagnostic signs favoring the diagnosis of AD are familial heredity, itch, high IgE, and food reactivity, whereas early onset of the disease is less characteristic.

2.5.3.1 Lower Gluteal/Posterior Femoral Area

This is also called toilet seat dermatitis (Toilettbrillendermatitis, Herzberg 1973). Here a skin inflammation develops in 7 to 8-year-old AD patients, possibly due to sweat retention caused by prolonged sitting when these predisposed individuals start school (Fredriksson and Færgemann 1981).

2.5.4 Hands

Special attention has to be paid to involvement of the hands, which are of such great importance, especially in the execution of many occupations and in social life (see Fig. 2.19). Differential diagnosis on clinical appearances alone can be very difficult, for example in women, when the dry plaques of housewives' dermatitis can be very closely simulated. Several clinicians have pointed out

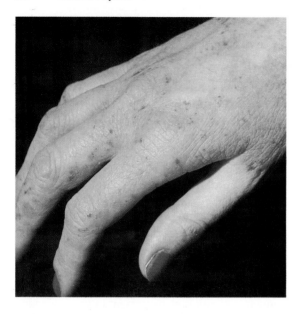

Fig. 2.19. Hand lesions in a young woman with AD

that the anatomical snuffbox and the surrounding area on the dorsum and the lateral aspect of the wrist are commonly involved in AD. Dry plaques on the volar surfaces of the fingers and recurrent hyperkeratosis with fissuring of their pulps (Temime et al. 1972) are very common in Scandinavia, but lichenified palmar plaques are also observed. Nail abnormality can result from involvement of the distal part of the fingers but the nails themselves may also be involved (Braun-Falco et al. 1981). Many cases of hand eczema follow a course which is typical of AD, indicating that in some this is the correct diagnosis. Serum levels of IgE are not helpful in differential diagnosis as they can be normal in AD (Johansson and Juhlin 1970). The quoted frequency with which hand eczema is due to AD has differed significantly in various statistical reports. Thus, Agrup (1969) analyzed 827 cases of hand eczema and, on the basis of strict criteria, classified 19% as AD, whereas Breit et al. (1972) reported that 69% of 130 patients with AD had hand eczema, and that of these, 24% were lichenified, 16% were eczematous, 10% were dyshidrotic, and the residue were of irritant or intermediate type. In a more extensive study of 1177 AD patients it was found that hand involvement was four to ten times more frequent in those who had earlier had AD. A relation to chemicals and other noxious factors was obvious (see Sect. 9.5) but in about 25% of atopics no hand dermatitis developed despite heavy exposure. Furthermore, involvement of the hands in childhood was a more important factor for development of adult hand dermatitis in AD patients than were exogenous factors (Rystedt 1985 a, b, c, d). A somewhat similar conclusion can be drawn form the results of Forsbeck et al. (1983), who found that contact allergy was equally common in AD patients with and AD patients without hand eczema. The hand dermatitis is usually more severe in atopics (Nilsson 1986). It should also be pointed out that hand involvement is quite frequent in children with AD. According to the author's statistics, almost half of the cases (45%) were children over 1 year of age with hand–finger–wrist lesions (Rajka, unpublished data) (see also Sect. 2.15.3.1).

2.5.5 Feet

The foot, particularly the plantar areas, is a site of predilection of AD, especially during the winter (Silvers and Glickman 1968; Möller 1972) (see Fig. 2.20). In differential diagnosis juvenile plantar dermatosis (MacKie and Husain 1976), which is a more frequent disease involving children and teenagers, has to be considered. This dermatosis appears mostly on the weight-bearing areas of the feet in wintertime or continuously as a nonitchy, sometimes painful, dry dermatosis. It seems to be a multifactorial entity due mainly to massive maceration, frictional trauma related to occlusive footwear, possibly during sporting activities. The role of disordered sweating is also discussed, but change of footwear only infrequently relieves the disease. In the majority no contact allergy can be found. Atopics are prone to this dermatosis (a common denominator might be dryness) but these persons do not usually have active AD, only a personal or a familial history of atopy. The rate of this latter group among juvenile plantar dermatosis patients is varyingly reported but in general it is stated to be more than 50%; perhaps one could speak of an atopy-associated and a non-atopic variant (Millard and Gould 1977; Verbov 1978; MacKie 1982; Young 1986; Ashton and Griffith 1986).

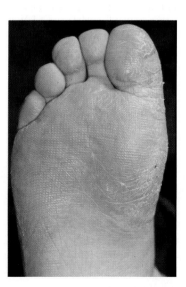

Fig. 2.20. Atopic winter feet in a young boy

2.6 Other Essential Features

2.6.1 Dry Skin

Dry skin is a characteristic although unspecific feature of the AD patient with obvious clinical significance. "Xerosis" (rough skin, Piérard 1987) is in general used in the clinical sense as a mild form of ichthyosis vulgaris (see Sect. 2.13) but would in fact be a more suitable synonym for dry skin. Terms used in this context include cracking, brittleness, chapping, and scale-forming (see Fig. 2.21), and the negative effect of winter, particularly due to cold and reduced humidity, is well recognized. In more expressed cases fissures may be seen (see Fig. 2.22). Clinicians often observe dryness of the fingers and fingertips (especially in children: Fig. 2.23) and hands (particularly in persons with occupational or home contact with defatting substances or strong detergents,

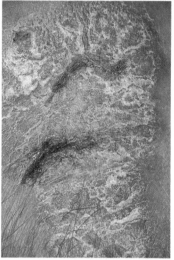

Fig. 2.21. Dry skin of a young girl during wintertime

Fig. 2.22. Fissures and dryness in adolescent AD ▷ during wintertime

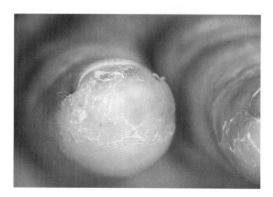

Fig. 2.23. Dryness of fingertips in a young boy during wintertime

see Table 2.4). The dryness is accentuated after bathing. Friction often aggravates this asteatotic condition, e. g., on the ankles and plantar areas (see Sect. 2.5.5).

While, according to the author's experience, dry skin often coexists with other signs of AD, e. g., eczematous lesions (cf. Uehara and Hayashi 1981; Finlay et al. 1980), or may sometimes be a forerunner to it (possibly by decreasing the threshold against irritative factors), it is principally *independent* of eczematous eruptions. On the basis of cohesional studies on corneocytes, this was proven by Finlay et al. (1980). These authors also remark that eczematous eruption does not occur at sites of maximal dryness (and in fact eczematous changes are also noted in symptom-free skin in AD, see p. 173). Dryness can only be evaluated by physiological parameters (see Chap. 7). The differential diagnostic problems are well expressed by Dahl (1986): "... patients with AD often have coexisting dry skin or ichthyosis vulgaris. But is the rough, scaling skin really dry skin or ichthyosis vulgaris, or is it a subtle manifestation of AD with epidermal acanthosis and scaling? Regardless of the answer, it is difficult to know what is involved skin, and what is uninvolved skin, in such individuals."

2.6.2 Photosensitivity

Up to 10% of AD patients deteriorate (during the summer) after solar exposure (see also Sect. 9.1). From personal experience, these cases should be carefully differentiated. The following points should be made in this respect:

1. The majority of cases seem to depend on the infrared effect of sunshine in leading to disturbances in the delivery of sweat.
2. UV-B phototoxicity plays a major role in AD patients with skin types I and II (prevalent in Scandinavia).
3. Coexistence of AD and polymorphous light eruption may be observed.
4. Summer prurigo (prurigo estivalis), considered in general as belonging to the polymorphous light eruption group, and similar clinical pictures mostly occurring in young girls (Frain-Bell and Scatchard 1971; Herzberg 1973) mimic AD.
5. Some AD cases that react clinically to sunlight despite a negative light sensitivity test may represent a nonspecific localizing effect of sunlight (Stevanovic 1960).
6. A few cases are elicited by photoallergy (Morison et al. 1978).
7. Some patients confuse absence of improvement after exposure to sun with sun-elicited symptoms.

For the above reasons it is important to perform light sensitivity testing in all patients who give a history of deterioration in sunlight.

2.7 Special Clinical Types

The complex clinical features and the resultant difficulties in differential diagnosis have been outlined and they help to explain why it may be almost impossible to distinguish between AD and certain other clinical pictures. Purely morphological criteria form an unfruitful basis for discussion; indeed, it is doubtful whether anything is to be gained by separating special clinical types (a minima variants, Herzberg 1973) from the AD group (see also Sect. 10.1).

2.7.1 Follicular Type

A follicular type localized particularly on the flanks is called juvenile papular dermatitis, or patchy pityriasiform lichenoid eczema (Kitamura 1966; Wütrich and Schnyder 1981). It seems to be a special form of AD given that some characteristics of the disease are present, but the differential diagnosis includes several diseases such as lichenoid variants, Gianotti-Crosti syndrome, and papulous id reaction.

Perifollicular accentuation of AD is a common feature among dark-skinned or oriental persons (Hanifin 1983).

2.7.2 Inhalative (Hand) Eczema

Rowe (1946) and Storck (1955) reported cases of inhalative eczema. Their observations can be confirmed by the present author, who has seen cases of inhalative AD on the hands; some of these cases followed exposure to birch (Rajka unpublished observations). The face, and especially the eyelids, may also be involved.

2.8 Correlations Between Distribution and Pathomechanism

Possible correlations between distribution of lesions and the pathomechanism of AD are shown in Table 2.4.

2.9 Complications Caused by Living Agents

Complications of AD, often difficult to differentiate from conditions associated with AD, are principally consequences of the disordered immune state, i. e., of decreased cell-mediated immunity [one of the basic features of AD, first described by the present author (Rajka 1963)] and of malfunctioning chemotaxis (Rogge and Hanifin 1976). Most symptoms are caused by living agents, including staphylococcal, viral, dermatophytic, scabies, and other infections, but other pathological conditions may also appear as a consequence of the immune al-

Table 2.4. Some examples of the correlation between distribution of skin lesions and etiological factors in AD

Localization of skin lesions	Some possible etiological factors[a]
Flexures	Foods Inhalants (pollens, animal hair, dust, mites, molds, foods) Hyperhidrosis (local) and inhibited sweat evaporation Hyperreactivity (local) to histamine
Hands (esp. fingers and palms) (incl. dyshidrosis)	Factors leading to dry skin + Lipid solvents, irritants, sensitizers, increase of *S. aureus* colonization
Face	Factors leading to dry skin + Airborne/contact irritants and sensitizers, increase of *S. aureus* colonization In some cases (additional) seborrheic dermatitis
Back Gluteal area Chest	Sweating, sweat-retentive textiles, sweat delivery disturbances
Plantar area	Factors leading to dry skin ("atopic winter feet") + Contact (mechanical) irritants/sensitizers (footwear, etc)

[a] These factors probably elicit itch with sequelae, as well as inflammatory lesions via immunological/biochemical pathways

terations. The decreased restistance to common infections was mentioned by Kaposi as long ago as 1887 and is well-known to clinicians.

Atopic dermatitis patients with a disordered immune state usually experience more frequently recurrent, more severe, more widespread, and/or more therapy-resistant infections than do nonatopic persons with intact cell-mediated immunity.

2.9.1 Staphylococcal Infections

Pyococci, in the overwhelming majority of cases *Staphylococcus aureus*, frequently infect lesions of AD, particularly those with excoriations and fissures. This complication, which is a principal cause of oozing or crusting or both, is usually seen in infants and children, but may be observed in adolescents and adults more frequently than some clinicians assume (see Fig. 2.24).

Regional lymphadenopathy is common, involving particularly the inguinal or axillary glands.

It is now proven that the occurrence of *Staphylococcus aureus* is more frequent and its main density higher on the skin of AD patients than on the skin of patients with other skin diseases or on normal skin. *Staphylococcus aureus* accounts for 91% of the total aerobic flora in lesional AD. The increased inci-

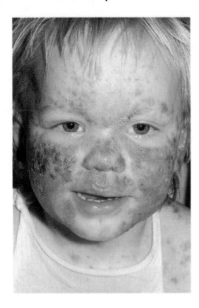

Fig. 2.24. Staphylococcal infection in a young boy with AD

dence is recorded not only in lesional but also on symptom-free skin and in the carriage rate of anterior nares (Bibel and Lovell 1976; Aly et al. 1977) (see Table 2.5, Aly 1980). Even when the lesions have not looked infected, *Staphylococcus aureus* has been recovered in huge numbers (Leyden et al. 1974; Kligman et al. 1976). It is assumed that a colonization of $1.0 \times 10^6/cm^2$ gives clinical symptoms. In lesional skin a count of $7.5 \times 10^4/cm^2$ was found, whereas on symptom-free skin $7.1 \times 10^3/cm^2$ was registered (Aly et al. 1977). Short-term occlusion, such as occurs in everday life, elevates the surface pH and elicits a considerable increase in the number of staphylococci (see Table 2.6, Rajka et al. 1981). Similar results after 3–4 days of occlusion were reported by Hartmann (1983).

The cause of the dominating staphylococcal colonization in AD may be complex, and several factors need to be considered. They include greater adherence to the corneocytes (Cole and Silverberg 1986), barrier disturbance in the functionally disturbed skin, decreased sebum production, inhibited sweat delivery (see Sects. 7.3.1, 7.3.2) with possible consequences for the bacterial flora of the skin surface, exudation, which perhaps constitutes a vicious circle with these organisms, and, last but not least, the immune defects.

Interestingly, deep pyogenic infections such as furuncles, cellulitis and erysipelas, despite frequent scratching, are less common than might be anticipated. As a hypothesis, an antibody-linked mechanism may compensate for the reduced delayed reactivity to pyococci.

The severe *Staphylococcus aureus* colonization on AD skin also has epidemiological significance as several outbreaks of staphylococcal infections as a result of dispersal from AD skin have been described (Hauser et al. 1985).

Table 2.5. Percent incidence of microorganism (39 atopics) (Aly 1980)

	Anterior nares	Lesions	Normal skin	Normal population (skin) %
Staphylococcus aureus	79	93	76	<10
Coagulase-negative staphylococci	77	79	82	80
Micrococci	2	13	25	40
Streptococci	2	0	2	0
Nonlipophilic diphtheroids	61	15	18	45
Lipophilic diphtheroids	20	0	2	47
Bacillus spp	10	15	20	20
Gram-negative rods	2	5	5	20
Yeasts	0	0	2	< 1

Table 2.6. Percent incidence of microorganisms in ten patients with atopic eczema before and after 24 h occlusion

Organism	Normal skin before occlusion	Normal skin after occlusion	Lesional skin before occlusion	Lesional skin after occlusion
Atopic eczema				
Staphylococcus aureus	63	75	80	80
Coagulase-negative staphylococci	100	88	90	70
Micrococci	63	0	20	0
Streptococci	0	0	0	0
Nonlipophilic diphtheroids	0	0	0	0
Lipophilic diphtheroids	13	25	10	20
Bacillus spp	38	13	30	10
Gram-negative rods	25	50	20	40
Yeasts	0	13	0	0

2.9.2 Viral Infections

2.9.2.1 Vaccinia

Early literature was dominated by observations of vaccinia virus in AD causing eczema vaccinatum (Kaposi's varicelliform eruption). The incidence of this, often serious, complication was shown to be between 1 in 25000 and 1 in 300000 after mass vaccinations (Waddington et al. 1964; Lancet 1970).

The probable mechanism of the susceptibility of AD patients to vaccinia was a decreased delayed reactivity to the virus. In order to avoid eczema vac-

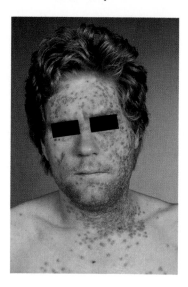

Fig. 2.25. Kaposi's varicelliform eruption due to herpes virus (with superinfection of *Staphylococcus aureus*) in a young adult with AD

cinatum, smallpox vaccination of children with AD was, in the past, rigidly prohibited or tried only very cautiously, e. g., by applying attenuated virus. Since smallpox has been globally eradicated, it is no longer necessary to give this vaccination and eczema vaccinatum has disappeared.

2.9.2.2 Herpes simplex

Herpes vaccinatum, elicited by herpes simplex virus I or II, is, in contrast to eczema vaccinatum, a highly relevant disease. It is also included in the clinical picture of Kaposi's varicelliform eruption (see Fig. 2.25), which can also be elicited by Coxsackie A 16 virus (Bonifazi et al. 1985).

After an initial incubation period of 5-12 days, a multiple, itchy, vesiculopustular eruption appears with umbilicated lesions, which tend to crop and often become hemorrhagic. A secondary bacterial infection, mostly due to the leading colonizer of the AD skin, i. e., *Staphylococcus aureus* – sometimes combined with beta-hemolytic streptococci – almost inevitably develops, giving an encrusted appearance.

A regional lymphadenopathy is most noticeable and the face may become edematous. Finally, scars are left. Sometimes, including in neonates, only local pustulosis is observed (Leyden and Baker 1979). High fever and constitutional symptoms are usually present.

The consequences of herpes infection in the course of AD are very significant, and an explosive deterioration in the dermatitis usually occurs. This is observed mostly in primary infections and in active cases, but sometimes even in quiescent phases of AD. More male than female children are affected. The most frequent transmission of the herpes virus to children is through kisses from herpes febrilis infected adults. The herpes virus can easily be demonstrated by electron microscopy and culture from the crusted lesions. (For mechanism see Sect. 5.7.6, and for treatment of the condition, Sect. 12.3.7.)

Other viral infections also occur more frequently or in a more widespread form, as most clinicians are aware. These infections include common warts [their incidence was twice as high among AD children (Currie et al. 1971; Bonifazi et al. 1985)], molluscum contagiosum (Solomon and Telner 1966), orf (Dupré et al. 1981), and chickenpox (Strannegård et al. 1985). By contrast, during measles, a beneficial effect may even be experienced due to changes in the immune conditions elicited by this virus.

2.9.3 Dermatophytosis and Candida

A higher incidence of dermatophytosis was, via trichophytin reactivity, shown in atopics, primarily in asthma patients (Jones et al. 1973); this was supposedly related to a diminished cell-mediated response. Lack of delayed reactivity was more frequently seen in chronic dermatophytosis, elicited by *Trichophyton rubrum*, approximately half of the cases being atopics (Hanifin et al. 1974; Hay and Brostoff 1977). Only those atopics with chronic dermatophytosis showed this hyporeactivity (Kaaman 1985).

Among 15-year-old Danish schoolchildren, the relative risk of contracting tinea pedis was three times higher among atopics (Svejgaard et al. 1983).

Atopic dermatitis, specifically, is more seldom mentioned in connection with long-lasting tinea infections than is atopy in general. However, the author's data, which first demonstrated reduced trichophytin reactivity in AD (Rajka 1963, 1967; Rajka and Barlinn 1979), and some other papers (Lobitz et al. 1972; Hanifin et al. 1974; Svejgaard et al. 1983; 1986) suggest a higher incidence of chronic dermatophytosis in this disease.

An increased susceptibility to *Candida* ssp in AD, as in other immunocompromised diseases, sometimes emerges from clinical reports, but as yet there is no convincing experimental evidence to support this possibility.

2.9.4 Scabies and House Dust Mite

A high incidence of atopy, including AD, was found in a series of 135 scabies patients. They also had elevated IgE concentrations and positive immediate skin tests and passive transfer reactions to scabies antigens. In persons with atopy, there was a more severe skin reaction following scabies (Falk and Bolle 1983 a, b). Clinical deterioration of AD may be observed after this infection (Heskel and Lobitz 1983). Furthermore, there might be differential diagnostic problems between two diseases.

Although less than in bronchial asthma, a pathological significance, supposedly based on hypersensitivity, can also be attributed to house dust mites (*Dermatophagoides pteronyssinus* and other spp) in AD, perhaps more by contact than by inhalation (see Sect. 5.2.6). Further, crossed immunoelectrophoresis revealed cross-reactivity to scabies antigens in sera from patients with *Dermatophagoides farinæ* allergy (Falk and Bolle 1983 a, b).

2.9.5 Pityrosporon Orbiculare

The yeast from *Malassezia furfur* was considered as a trigger for AD in the head-neck area of adults, and positive reactions were found by skintests in AD to this principally nonpathogenic saprophyte (Wærsted and Hjorth 1985, Young and Koers (1989) and also in RAST (Svejgaard et al. 1989). This concept was corroborated by improvement of AD after appropriate treatment (Clemmensen and Hjorth 1983). Thus, it may be speculated that this is a further example of the increased susceptibility to living agents in AD.

2.10 Complication of the Malfunctioning Immunomechanisms

2.10.1 Atopic Erythroderma

Infants (Hill 1956) and sometimes adults (Temime et al. 1972) with AD may develop generalized exfoliative dermatitis with affection of hairs and nails. AD accounted for 4.5% of a series of exfoliative dermatitis cases reported by Nicolis and Helwig (1973). On the other hand, reports of this complication in infants have been extremely rare in recent years.

2.10.2 Some Types of Cutaneous Lymphoma

Clinical evidence has indicated that some patients with Sézary's syndrome or Hodgkin's disease have previously had AD, and cases may even occur in which an exfoliative erythroderma due to AD evolves with Sézary's syndrome. In these groups high IgE levels are frequently registered (although patients with high IgE levels and without individual or familial atopic traits have also been reported). Thus it seems that the existence of AD/atopy may be a potentially aggravating or influencing factor in Sézary's syndrome and in Hodgkin's disease (Winkelmann and Rajka 1983; Rajka 1983). Although this phenomenon constitutes a rare event, it may have some clinical importance, e. g., in differentiation between the long-lasting or late onset AD and Hodgkin's disease.

2.10.3 Alopecia Areata and Vitiligo

It is known that patients with AD may develop alopecia areata (particularly in childhood) and/or vitiligo (Ikeda 1965; Penders 1968). There are, however, no comprehensive statistics comparing these patients and a normal population, with regard to the possible link between these conditions and AD. Furthermore, there are some indications that neither alopecia areata nor vitiligo is a homogeneous disease. Until these questions are to some extent resolved, the possible connection between these two diseases, which are claimed to be linked on an autoimmune basis, and AD is only speculative.

2.11 Other Complications

2.11.1 Atopic Cataract

A usually bilateral, rapidly developing anterior subscapular cataract (sometimes a type involving the posterior subscapular area) may appear in young AD patients – usually those with severe skin disease. The courses of skin and eye diseases may run parallel or independently, and there is no obvious relation between the atopic cataract and other clinical parameters of AD.

Statements regarding the frequency of the atopic cataract in AD diverge markedly. Earlier, high frequencies were mostly reported, e. g., 12% (Brunsting et al. 1955) and 17% (Ingram 1955). During recent decades, however, the incidence has generally been reported as low (Kornerup and Lodin 1959; Sprafke 1966; Christensen 1981; Vickers 1980), although Garrity and Liesegang (1984) and Uehara et al. (1985) found a frequency of 12%. Since systemic steroids may elicit posterior-subscapular cataracts, they are often suspected in the etiology of atopic cataracts too, and it may be difficult to distinguish between these types. Although the role of systemic steroids in the mechanism of atopic cataracts is not yet clear, it is necessary to consider the possibility of this side-effect.

2.12 Associated Conditions; Proven Correlations

The evidence that certain diseases are associated with AD is more convincing in some cases than in others. Therefore, these diseases are separated, in a somewhat scholarly fashion, into those with proven (2.12), probable (2.14), and possible (2.15) correlations.

2.12.1 Atopic correlations

This is the most important and obvious group and they could theoretically also be classified as complications of AD as they frequently appear on patients with AD. The reverse is also true, as AD commonly affects patients with bronchial asthma or allergic rhinitis or both. All three major atopic conditions show a similar hereditary background.

These were the primary reasons for separating AD from other eczemas. Only those features of asthma and of rhinitis which relate directly to AD will be discussed here. The frequency of respiratory allergic manifestations in AD patients has been reported as 50% (Sulzberger and Goodman 1936; Schnyder 1959; Rajka 1960), although somewhat lower figures have been recorded (Nexmand 1948; Bonnerie 1939; de Graciansky 1966). There is a preponderance of females.

The numerical results of a study of a large series of children up to 14 years of age (Bono and Levitt 1964) were expressed as a Venn diagram to emphasize that a combination of two atopic conditions is common but that coexistence of three is unusual. The numbers from an independent study of 200 atopic children and adults were also expressed as a Venn diagram, which showed that the coexistence of AD and respiratory allergy was more frequent than in the previous series (Hellerström and Rajka 1967) (see Fig. 2.26). Most of the difference between the two diagrams may be explained by the age at onset of atopic rhinitis (see below).

If skin and respiratory manifestations combine, the commonest pattern is that the patients initially get infantile AD and subsequently develop asthma and/or hay fever.

2.12.2 Bronchial Asthma

Bronchial asthma begins before the age of 5 years in about 60% of cases (Hellerström and Lidman 1956) (see Table 2.7), and its incidence in children with AD is higher if there is a family history of bronchial asthma, if the dermatitis started early in life, or if the skin lesions are severe. As atopic manifestations begin in the respiratory tract later than in the skin, age is a factor of considerable importance in patient surveys.

The courses of the two diseases may alternate – "alternance morbide" (Brocq 1927) – or they may flare up simultaneously in response, for example, to certain drugs or to inhaled allergens; these alternatives occur with about equal frequency.

Finally in a third of patients with AD and nonallergic (intrinsic: endogenous) asthma, the courses may be independent (Schnyder 1961). A latent predisposition to bronchial asthma in AD patients has been shown by several authors. In the first clear demonstration of this by using pulmonary function studies, Lutz and Korting (1958) found it in 60% of their cases, whereas experimental inhalation of different allergens provoked bronchoconstriction in 12 of 16 "pure" AD patients of Morsbach (1962). Studies of exercise-induced bronchoconstriction showed that a majority of 42 children with AD had a predisposition to develop asthma (Price et al. 1976).

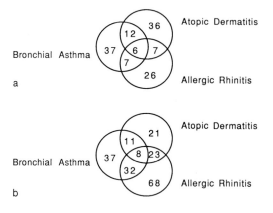

Fig. 2.26. a Venn diagram of distribution of AD, bronchial asthma, and allergic rhinitis in a series of children under 14 years of age (Bono and Levitt 1964). **b** Venn diagram of distribution of the same manifestations in a series of children as well as adults. (Since the onset of allergic rhinitis was mostly after 14 years of age, this explains the difference between the diagrams.) (Hellerström and Rajka 1967)

Table 2.7. Onset of bronchial asthma and atopic rhinitis in patients with AD (557 cases: 261 males, 296 females)

Onset in years	Bronchial asthma			Atopic rhinitis			Bronchial asthma + atopic rhinitis					
							Asthma			Rhinitis		
	Males	Females	Total	Males	Females	Total	Males	Females	Total	Males	Females	Total
- 1	3	7	10	14	6	20	4	6	10	4	8	12
1- 5	35	26	61	18	15	33	25	26	51	13	13	26
6-10	6	10	16	24	15	39	5	15	20	9	11	20
11-15	3	7	10	7	28	35	8	7	15	8	11	19
16-20	8	5	13	18	23	41	4	8	12	3	7	10
21-25	4	2	6	4	4	8	5	3	8	2	1	3
26-30	–	2	2	1	3	4	–	–	–	–	2	2
31-35	–	1	1	2	1	3	2	2	4	1	–	1
36-40	–	1	1	1	1	2	–	1	1	1	1	2
41-50	–	1	1	–	–	–	–	–	1	1	–	–
Sum	59	62	121	89	96	185	53	69	122	41	54	95
Unknown	13	10	23	34	45	79	13	14	27	25	29	54
Total	72	72	144	123	141	264	66	83	149	66	83	149

2.12.3 Atopic Rhinoconjunctivitis

The onset, in AD, of atopic rhinitis and of bronchial asthma are compared in Table 2.7. Hay fever, allergic rhinitis, and atopic rhinitis are terms generally used synonymously, whereas vasomotor rhinitis is grouped separately in various statistics. Schnyder (1960) has, however, shown that allergic and vasomotor rhinitis belong genetically to the group of atopic disorders. It is conceivable that, in the absence of clinical symptoms, the nasal mucosa of patients with AD could quite commonly have a latent predisposition to rhinitis. Indeed, the presence of changes in the nasal mucosa of such patients was stressed by Blamoutier et al. (1966). However, studies with larger numbers of controls will be necessary to confirm these observations. Those patients with respiratory atopic disease who have and those who have no AD show the same incidence of an allergic pathogenesis (Rajka 1960). On the other hand, studies of the prognosis in AD indicate that about 50% of cases presenting with that disease will develop respiratory atopic manifestations later in life (Roth and Kierland 1964; Stifler 1965, and others). However, the results of such studies are strongly influenced by several factors, including the patient's age and ability to answer questionnaires. Hypersensitivity to inhalants, such as pollens or animal hairs, frequently produces conjunctivitis and atopic rhinitis concomitantly. Such conjunctivitis has been assumed to be correlated with AD but no comprehensive relevant statistics have been published. Karel et al. (1965) expressed the view that atopic conjunctivitis comprises not only cases occurring in spring but also others with different courses, such as winter deterioration, and with different morphology.

Table 2.8. History of itching in reaction to foods in 95 of 1200 cases (a patient could have several reactions)

	No. of reactions
Itching of skin	151
Itching of the throat	23
Itching of lips	3
Perioral itching	20

In order of frequency, the main elicitors were:

Chocolate	Shellfish
Nuts	Almonds
Apples	Fish
Cheese	Berries
Oranges	Wine
Spices	Hips
Egg	

2.12.4 Oral Symptoms

The correlation of AD with lesions of the oral mucosa is, in the author's opinion, a neglected feature and occurs more frequently than is generally supposed. Provided they are sought by specific questioning or clinical investigation or both, oral symptoms are found in a fairly significant number of AD patients. Pruritus of the lips, of the mouth, or of the throat is experienced, despite both the denial by some authors that itch occurs in the mouth and the inability of Shelley and Arthur (1957) to produce oral pruritus by intramucosal injections of proteases or histamine. Other symptoms include oral aphthae and, less frequently, edema of the lips, of the oral mucosa, and possibly of the larynx. In the majority of cases these symptoms develop after ingesting common food allergens such as fish and shellfish, citrus fruits, almonds nuts, and eggs. Involvement of the corner of the mouth occasionally simulates herpes febrilis and oral symptoms may be confused with aphthous stomatitis, which indeed may be diagnosed if aphthous lesions appear. Table 2.8 summarizes the author's experience of cases responding only with itch. Hannuksela and Lahti (1977) also found itching and tingling of the lips, mouth, and tongue to be the most common complaints after eating raw fruits and vegetables. Oral itch with lip swelling and urticaria was also noted in the food allergy histories of AD patients (MacKie et al. 1979). Oral symptoms, therefore, may be characteristic of or associated with AD and should not be overlooked. Recent evidence has indicated that contact urticaria may also be added to this list (see p. 43).

2.12.5 Gastrointestinal Symptoms

As long ago as (1892) Besnier mentioned gastrointestinal symptoms in association with AD. They can undoubtedly occur, and include vomiting, abdominal pain, malaise, and bowel symptoms, particularly diarrhea or sometimes rectal itch. Foods or drugs are the usual eliciting agents. To prove an etiological correlation between an allergen and the symptoms, either oral or gastrointestinal provocation tests (Reimann et al. 1986) are necessary but as they can cause significant symptoms in these patients, they are rarely used. The true frequency of such symptoms in AD is thus unknown; they probably are quite common, especially in the infantile and childhood phases.

Inhaled allergens may subsequently appear and are excreted by the gastrointestinal tract (Wilson et al. 1973) but, of course, ingested food has greatest relevance here. In food allergic AD children the jejunum shows only moderate morphological changes (McCalla et al. 1980) even though, immunohistochemically, increases in IgM- and IgA-bearing cells were observed by the same group (Perkkio 1980). Braathen et al. (1979) also found only minor mucosal changes in the gut.

The permeability of the gut earlier demonstrated by the Walzer reaction (passive transfer elicited by food ingestion) and recently confirmed (Aoki et al. 1989), was investigated by absorption studies with differently sized polyethyleneglycol or metabolically inert saccharide molecules (rhamnose, lactulose, mannitol) and their excretion ratios. Most authors have registered increased intestinal passage in adult AD cases (Jackson et al. 1981; Zachary et al. 1982; Ukabam et al. 1984) but normal conditions have also been reported (Fairris et al. 1984; Bjarnason et al. 1985). Similarly, in children, increased (Pike et al. 1986) or normal (Du Mont et al. 1983; Fälth-Magnusson et al. 1984) values have been mentioned. Furthermore, the presence of some non-IgE antibodies was also assumed to indicate increased gut permeability (see Sect. 5.3).

Overall abnormal gut absorption was registered in most AD patients. Based on these observations, Atherton (1981, 1982) proposed a hypothesis that AD patients produce IgE and certain IgG antibodies early in life, and that food antigens entering the gastrointestinal tract lead to local IgE-mediated mast cell degranulation with subsequent enhanced antigen absorption. Thereafter circulating antigen/immunoglobulin-containing immune complexes produced in greater quantity in AD will not be rapidly cleared by the reticuloendothelial system but their deposition in the cutaneous microvasculature results in AD.

2.13 Xerosis-Ichthyosis Group

Ichthyosis vulgaris (cf Sect. 2.6.1 on "dry skin") and AD regularly affect the same patient. This frequently confirmed association has long been recognized and yet its true frequency is unknown because of the varied rigor with which the ichthyosis component has been diagnosed. Mild cases, in the form of xeroderma or keratosis pilaris (follicular keratosis), may have been excluded from some series, but, if all cases with keratosis pilaris are consistently taken into account, there is no doubt that the association is very common; about 50% of all AD patients were quoted as being affected by Hill and Sulzberger (1935). Furthermore, not only are AD and ichthyosis vulgaris associated (Table 2.9) but about 50% of autosomal dominant ichthyosis vulgaris cases show one or more atopic manifestations (Wells and Kerr 1966).

Table 2.9. Frequency of ichthyosis vulgaris (xeroderma) in AD

Frequency in patients	Percent	Source
6 of 100	6.0	Nexmand (1948)
8 of 330	2.4	Rost and Marchionini (1932)
5 of 308	1.6	Korting (1954)
3 of 117	2.4	Schnyder and Borelli (1965)
30 of 1200	2.5	Rajka (1961)
66 of 178	37.0	Uehara and Hayashi (1981)

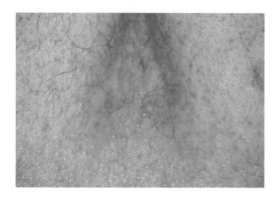

Fig. 2.27. Keratosis pilaris in a young girl with AD

One possible source of error in such statistics are the different criteria used to define atopy and AD.

Keratosis pilaris (see Fig. 2.27), which is not seen at birth, is very common from early childhood onwards, and is an early and frequent manifestation of ichthyosis vulgaris; its lesions are more prominent on the extensor surfaces of the limbs and on the buttocks. It may have an important bearing on the typical dryness of the skin in AD. The dry scaliness of classical ichthyosis vulgaris also is most pronounced on the extensor surfaces of the limbs, and is prominent on the back and face; localized hyperkeratosis on the knees and elbows and increased markings of the palms and soles are common. These markings have, for a long time, been a well-recognized sign which has recently been stressed in relation to atopic subjects, particularly those with AD. The sign is thus of importance in combined cases (Frost and Weinstein 1971; Leutgeb et al. 1972; Uehara and Hayashi 1981). The view has also been expressed that hyperlinear palms are a trait of AD per se (Höyer et al. 1981; Fartasch et al. 1987). By ultrastructural studies it was concluded that, whereas defective keratohyalin granules are a marker for autosomal dominant ichthyosis vulgaris, a reduced/absent granular layer does not always constitute a manifestation of this disorder and may occur in dry skin when AD alone is present. Thus ultrastructural studies seem to be necessary for the differentiation between these conditions in the future (Fartasch et al. 1987).

Netherton's syndrome, an autosomal recessive disease, is characterized by trichorrhexis invaginata of scalp and body hair, ichthyosis, and eczematous lesions in general corresponding to AD (Greene and Müller 1985).

Keratosis punctata palmaris et plantaris was also described, in 82% of cases, as being associated with familial or personal atopy, mostly AD (Anderson et al. 1984), but the nature of this relation is unknown.

2.14 Probable Correlations

2.14.1 Drug Reactions of the Immediate Type

Drug reactions and urticaria each have a similar relationship to AD. The relationship of AD to drug reactions as a whole is unconvincing; its relationship to immediate-type drug reactions could be proved, but no statistical support was found for a relationship to exanthematic, delayed-type drug reactions (Rajka and Skog 1965) (Table 2.10). The term "immediate drug reaction" includes all or some of the manifestations of anaphylactic shock, urticaria, and mucosal symptoms, the term "drug" is used in its widest sense and includes the administration of serum. Drugs capable of provoking systemic anaphylaxis should not be given to AD patients unless with great caution, in view of the serious complications which quite frequently ensue. However, it has also been pointed out that penicillin hypersensitivity, for example, is equally common in atopic and nonatopic persons (Rytel et al. 1963; Juhlin and Wide 1972).

2.14.2 Systemic Diseases (Related to Impaired Cell-Mediated Immunity)

Associations of AD to some systemic diseases have not infrequently been reported but, in general, further observations are needed before such correlations can be considered proven (Saurat 1987). Earlier it was not always clearly indicated whether AD or "eczematous lesions" were connected with systemic disease (Rostenberg and Solomon 1968), a distinction which the present author feels is of the utmost importance.

Table 2.10. Relation between 86 immediate drug reactions and atopic manifestations[a]

Urticaria	66
Respiratory symptoms	10
Shock	5
Pruritus	4
Flare up of AD	1
	86

[a] Of these patients, 32% had previously had atopic manifestations. (Of 57 delayed drug reactors, only 7% had previously had atopic manifestations.)

Further complexity is added because seborrheic dermatitis, for example, may be a symptom of the acquired immunodeficiency state (Mathes and Douglas 1985).

Wiskott-Aldrich syndrome is characterized by an impaired delayed hypersensitivity, a deficient cell-mediated immunity to herpesvirus hominis and to some other infecting agents with a consequent predisposition to frequent infections (Aldrich et al. 1954) (in our unpublished case also tinea infections), defective blood group agglutinins, and a dysgammaglobulinemia manifested as a frequently decreased IgM with a compensatory increase in IgA and particularly in IgE (Krivit and Good 1959; St Geme et al. 1965; de Graciansky and Schaison 1967; Berglund et al. 1968). As already mentioned, successful cases of bone marrow grafting lead to the clearing of skin lesions in this disease. In ataxia telangiectasia, the defect of delayed hypersensitivity (Eisen et al. 1965; Epstein et al. 1966) is similarly combined with a defect of humoral immunity. In some other conditions, such as IgA deficiency (Schwartz and Buckley 1971) or X-linked immunodeficiency with hyper – IgM (D. Vieluf, personal communication), some cases with AD are described. In some other diseases eczematous lesions are reported but the diagnosis of AD is unclear, as in chronic granulomatous disease ("perioral localized AD") or in the rare Shwachman syndrome with pancreatic insufficiency and bone marrow dysfunction (Shwachman et al. 1964). Similarly, although Peterson et al. (1962) reported AD in 4 of 23 children with X-linked agammaglobulinemia despite a lack of immediate reactivity, later descriptions only mention eczema (Rosen 1976).

Concerning hypergamaglobulinemia E/Job's syndrome, after an initial report mentioning AD (Paslin and Norman 1977), Buckley herself classified it as non-AD (Buckley 1983) and others agreed (Zachary and Atherton 1986). The two conditions may be differentiated on the basis of the presence of anti-*Staphylococcus aureus* IgE in hyperimmunoglobulinemia E (Dreskin et al. 1987). It may be speculated that the similarity to AD is based on an IgE-mediated histamine release with subsequent itching and its consequences.

In Table 2.11 the relations between the above-mentioned conditions and AD are summarized.

Table 2.11. AD versus eczematous lesions in some systemic conditions with predominant abnormalities of cell-mediated immunity (modified from Saurat 1985 and Saurat et al. 1985)

Immune alterations	Occurence of AD
Wiskott-Aldrich syndrome	Yes
Ataxia telangiectasia	Probable
X-linked hypogammaglobulinemia	Probable
Selective IgA deficiency	Probable
Chronic granulomatous disease	Possible
X-linked immunodeficiency with hyper-IgM	Possible
Shwachman syndrome	Possible

2.14.3 Certain Types of Urticaria

There is no doubt that urticaria, as a group, is not an atopic manifestation. Schnyder (1960) reported that most cases of urticaria have no genetic correlation with atopy. He also stressed the well-known opinion that only a small number of cases (5%–10% of the total) can be classified as allergic, reagin-bound urticaria. Champion et al. (1969) studied 554 patients with urticaria and found a past or a family history of atopic disorders with equal frequency in patients and in controls; the course was the same regardless of such a history. However, there is evidence for a certain relationship between AD and some types of urticaria:

1. *"Atopic" urticaria:* Patients with AD may react to allergens applied to the skin with a wheal and, after exposure to inhalant allergens, atopic patients often develop urticaria in addition to dermatitis, asthma, or rhinoconjunctivitis. Thus when there is a case history of exogenous allergen application plus a high IgE level and positive RAST and reliable skin tests, a variant of urticaria, tentatively called atopic urticaria, may be differentiated. This variant can be considered as associated to AD, or at least to those AD cases where an immediate-type mechanism is present.

2. *Cholinergic urticaria:* There is some evidence that cholinergic urticaria is found more frequently in atopics [including those with AD (Hanifin 1983)] than in the general population (Doeglas and Bleumink 1985; Hirschmann et al. 1987).

3. *Contact urticaria:* The immunologically mediated contact urticaria occurs not infrequently but not necessarily in atopics. Cases among AD patients were reported with regard to fish (Beck and Knudsen Nissen 1983), shrimps (Maibach 1986), and honey (Lombardi et al. 1983). Other examples include birch-reacting atopics who have cross-reactions to some fruits and vegetables (Hannuksela and Lahti 1977; Larkö et al. 1983). The basis of this correlation is unclear; it may involve coexistence (von Krogh and Maibach 1981) due to the increased permeability of inflamed skin to allergens. For instance, food allergens gave positive skin tests on inflamed but not on intact skin (Maibach 1976) (see also Sect. 2.15.3.2).

   The author is of the opinion that one could also speak of an association between immunological contact urticaria and AD, based on the known ability of AD patients to respond with type I reactivity to inhaled or ingested allergens. This ability may also relate to certain contact allergens such as foods. Food proteins are commonly registered as giving immediate reactions after contact with the oral mucosa (see Sect. 2.12.4). Langeland and Nyrud (1982) reported a 14-month-old, but still breast-fed, boy with AD who had positive skin, passive transfer, and exposure tests to wheat. He reacted with contact urticaria (on the skin) to wheat bran bath given as antipruritic treatment.

44 Clinical Aspects

Table 2.12. Some genetic disorders with eczematous lesions in relation to the occurrence of AD

Disorders	Occurrence of AD
Netherton's syndrome	Yes
Phenylketonuria	Probable
Anhidrotic ectodermal dysplasia	Probable
Histiocytosis X	No
Biotinidase deficiency	No
Hartnup disease	No
Acrodermatitis enteropathica	No

2.15 Possible Correlations

2.15.1 Some Genetic Disorders with Eczematous Lesions

According to a critical review of the available literature, there are some possible correlations between AD and genetic disorders which show different skin eruptions (see Table 2.12) but the mechanism is unknown (Vanselow et al. 1970; Levy 1977; Fisch et al. 1981, and others; for references, see, e. g., Irons and Levy 1986).

2.15.2 Adult Celiac Disease/Dermatitis Herpetiformis

A history of AD as well as of respiratory atopy was significantly more common in patients with adult celiac disease and in their first-degree relatives (Verkasalo et al. 1983). This was interpreted as reflecting a deficiency of local mucosal immunity due to abnormal IgA responses (Hodgson et al. 1976).

Similarly, some evidence supports a correlation between ulcerative colitis and AD (Roberts et al. 1978).

Davies et al. (1979) reported a correlation between AD/atopy and dermatitis herpetiformis, and this was confirmed by Buckley et al. (1983), who observed 2% familial and 6% personal atopy among their dermatitis herpetiformis patients. The present author has also seen several cases with a combination of AD and dermatitis herpetiformis (Rajka, unpublished observations).

2.15.3 Other Conditions

2.15.3.1 Dyshidrosis (Pompholyx)

Dyshidrosis (pompholyx) on the fingers and eczematous plaques on the back of hands and fingers commonly coexist (Young 1964; Oddoze and Témime 1968). An immediate type (and type IV) reaction is thought to play an etiological role in this condition (Schuppli 1954; Van Ketel et al. 1978) and should this prove to be the case, it would suggest a possible immunological relation to AD.

Generally speaking, it is possible that the dyshidrotic inflammation differs from AD only in its anatomical substrate and location (see Sect. 2.5.4).

2.15.3.2 Food Handlers' Hand Dermatitis

Investigating the not infrequent hand dermatitis in food handlers, Hjorth and Roed-Petersen (1976) demonstrated immediate and delayed hypersensitivity as well as irritative reactions. They called this condition protein contact dermatitis and their findings were later confirmed (Greig 1983; Cronin 1987). The common elicitors of the immediate-type reactions were fish, shellfish, fruits, vegetables, cheese, and meats (Hjorth and Roed-Petersen 1976; Greig 1983; Veien et al. 1983; Niinimæki 1987; Cronin 1987). Immediate tests were performed mostly as 20-min patch tests on scratched skin or on previously affected skin (Maibach 1976). Probably other proteins such as present in cow's hair (in veterinarians) and nonproteinous substances such as nickel or balsam of Peru also can elicit immediate, in addition to delayed, reactions. Delayed reactivity, assessed using the usual patch test technique and read after 2–4 days, was mostly found to be due to garlic or onions.

This clinical, mostly occupational condition occurred in variable frequency in atopics, including a few with AD, and in these patients there was a correlation with immediate-type food reactions (Cronin 1987).

2.15.3.3 Pityriasis Alba

Although the majority of authors believe that this condition presenting initial erythema and subsequent depigmented scaly areas, particularly on the face of children, is an independent disease with unknown etiology, there are claims that it is a special variant of AD (Watkins 1961; Leider 1961; Wolf et al. 1985). It is therefore included in the diagnostic list (see Table 10.1).

2.15.3.4 Miscellaneous

Insect stings: Local reactions and possibly anaphylactic symptoms may follow insect stings in many nonatopic subjects. It can be assumed that atopic patients, including those with dermatitis, are more prone to develop such reactions (see Sect. 5.4.3).

Migraine: At least some patients with migraine are atopic. A correlation with AD is therefore possible; such an association has been observed in individual cases and in statistical studies (Dorn 1961; Edfors-Lubs 1971).

Geographic tongue: This condition was mentioned as having a correlation with AD (Marks and Simons 1979; Ullmann 1981), but correlations with other skin diseases, including pustular psoriasis, have also been reported.

In conclusion, it may be added that several authors have shown an etiological relationship between certain diseases and AD, but it is the present author's opinion that correlations should be based on several criteria; this is a precaution particularly necessary in view of the polymorphic clinical picture of AD (see also Sect. 10.1). Furthermore, there exist numerous manifestations in the skin or other organs which have been thought, or known, to occur in association with atopy but not with AD.

2.16 Coexistence of AD with Common Skin Diseases

The primary lesions seen in AD include the prurigo papule, eczematous changes, and lichenification; each of these is also characteristic of other dermatoses, including the group of prurigos and eczemas. AD, therefore, cannot be clearly differentiated clinically from these diseases. On the other hand, coexistence of two common skin diseases is not infrequent. Allergic contact dermatitis has been mentioned in connection with AD and may provoke it (see Sect. 5.6.1). A combination between allergic (or possibly instant) contact dermatitis and AD has been termed "hybrid" by Malten (1968). Irritant contact dermatitis, often elicited by detergents and lipid solvents, may also be a complication of, or merely coexist with, AD. Seborrheic dermatitis may coexist with AD both in infants and in adults. The atopic seborrheic prurigo (Mali and Kuiper 1968) and some of the intertrigos in children (Grosshans et al. 1969) may be an expression of this. Other types of eczema may also sometimes appear with AD (see also Sect. 2.4.4).

References

Ackerman B (1978) Histologic diagnosis of inflammatory diseases. Lea and Febiger, Philadelphia
Aldrich RA, Steinberg AG, Campbell DC (1954) Pedigree demonstrating a sex-linked recessive condition characterized by draining ears, eczematoid dermatitis and bloody diarrhea. J Pediatr 13: 33
Agrup G (1969) Hand eczema and other hand dermatoses in South Sweden. Acta Derm Venereol (Stockh) 49 (Suppl 61)
Aly R (1980) Bacteriology of atopic dermatitis. Acta Derm Venereol [Suppl] (Stockh) 92: 16
Aly R, Maibach HI. Shinefield HR (1977) Bacterial flora of atopic dermatitis. Arch Dermatol 113: 780
Anderson WA, Elam MD, Lambert EC (1984) Keratosis punctata and atopy. Arch Dermatol 120: 884
Aoki T, Funai T, Kojima M, Adachi J, Okano M (1989) Antigen absorption by the gut observed by Walzer reaction. Acta Derm Venereol (Suppl 144) (Stockh) (in press)
Ashton RE, Griffith WAD (1986) Studies in sweating and bacterial ecology in juvenile plantar dermatosis: Br J Dermatol 11: 535
Atherton DJ (1981) Allergy and atopic eczema. II. Clin Exp Dermatol 6: 317
Atherton DJ (1982) Atopic exzema. In: Brostoff I, Challacombe SJ (eds) Food allergy, vol 2. Saunders, London, p 77
Bandmann HJ (1965) Ekzeme und ekzematoide Dermatitiden im frühen Kindesalter. In: Miescher G, Storck H (eds) Entzündliche Dermatosen. II. (Handbuch der Haut- und Geschlechtskrankheiten, vol II/1) Springer, Berlin Heidelberg New York, p 324
Beck HI, Knudsen Nissen B (1983) Contact urticaria to commercial fish in atopic persons. Acta Derm Venereol (Stockh) 63: 257

Berglund G, Finnström O, Johansson SGO, Möller KI (1968) Wiskott-Aldrich syndrome. Acta Pædiatr Scand 57: 89

Berlinghoff W (1961) Die Prognose des Säuglingsekzems. Dtsch Gesundheitswes 16: 110

Besnier E (1892) Première note et observation préliminaire pour servir l'introduction à l'étude des prurigos diathesiques. Ann Dermatol Syphiligr 4: 634

Bibel BJ, Lovell DJ (1976) Skin flora maps: a tool in the study of cutaneous ecology. J Invest Dermatol 67: 265

Bickford RG (1938) Experiments relating to itch sensation, its peripheral mechanism and central pathways. Clin Sci 3: 377

Bjarnason I, Goolamali SK, Levi AJ, Peters TJ (1985) Intestinal permeability in patients with atopic eczema. Br J Dermatol 112: 291

Björksten F, Suoniemi I (1981) Dependence of immediate hypersensitivity on the month of birth. Allergy 36: 263

Blamoutier J, Battistelli F, Denimal C, Barailles (1966) Renseignements fournis par l'examen des voies oto-rhinolaryngologiques dans l'eczéma atopique. In: Huriez C (ed) Actualités sur l'eczémas. Rev Med (Suppl) p 60

Bonifazi E, Garofalo L, Pisani V, Meneghini CL (1985) Role of some infectious agents in atopic dermatitis. Acta Derm Venereol [Suppl] (Stockh) 114: 98

Bonnevie P (1939) Dermatologi. Busck, Copenhagen/Barth, Leipzig

Bono J, Levitt P (1964) Relationship of infantile atopic dermatitis to asthma and other respiratory allergies. Ann Allergy 22: 72

Braathen LR (1985) T cell subsets in patients with mild and severe atopic dermatitis. Acta Derm Venereol [suppl] (Stockh) 114: 133

Braathen LR, Baklien K, Hovig T, Fausa O, Brandtzæg P (1979) Immunological, histological and electronmicroscopical investigations of the gut in atopic dermatitis. Acta Derm Venereol [Suppl] (Stockh) 92: 78

Braun-Falco O, Dorn M,, Neubert U, Plewig G (1981) Trachyonychie: 20-Nägel-Dystrophie. Hautarzt 32: 17

Breit R, Leutgeb C, Bandmann HJ (1972) Zum neurodermitischen Handekzem. Arch Dermatol Forsch 224: 353

Brereton EM, Carpenter RG, Rook AJ, Tyser PA (1959) The prevalence and prognosis of eczema and asthma in Cambridgeshire school children. Med Office Dec 18, p 317

Brocq L (1927) Conception générale des dermatoses, nouvelle note sur leur classification. Ann Dermatol Syphiligr 8: 65

Brunsting IA, Reed WB, Blair HL (1955) Occurrence of cataracts and keratoconus with atopic dermatitis. Arch Dermatol 72: 237

Buckley DB, English J, Molloy W, Doyle CT, Whelton MJ (1983) Dermatitis herpetiformis: a review of 119 cases. Clin Exp Dermatol 8: 477

Buckley RH (1983) Immunodeficiency. J Allergy Clin Immunol 72: 627

Carr RD, Berke M, Becker SW (1964) Incidence of atopy in patients with various neurodermatoses. Arch Dermatol Syph 89: 20

Champion RH, Parish WE (1968) Atopic dermatitis. In: Rook A, Wilkinson DS, Ebling FJG (eds) Textbook of dermatology, vol 1. Blackwell, Oxford, p 229

Champion RH, Roberts SOB, Carpenter RG, Roger JH (1969) Urticaria and angio-oedema. A review of 554 patients. Br J Dermatol 81: 588

Christensen JD (1981) Frequency of cataract in atopic dermatitis. Acta Derm Venereol (Stockh) 61: 76

Clemmensen OJ, Hjorth N (1983) Treatment of dermatitis of the head and neck with ketokonazole in patients with type I sensitivity to Pityrosporon orbiculare. Semin Dermatol 2: 26

Cole G, Silverberg NI (1986) The adherence of Staphylococcus areus to human corneocytes. Arch Dermatol 122: 166

Colver GB, Mortimer PS, Millard PR, Dawber PRP, Ryan TJ (1987) The "dirty neck" – a reticulate pigmentation in atopics. Clin Exp Dermatol 12: 1

Cronin E (1987) Dermatitis of the hands in caterers. Contact Dermatitis 17: 256

Currie JM, Wright RC, Miller OG (1971) The frequency of warts in atopic patients. Cutis 8: 243

Dahl MV (1986) Editorial reflex. Research on atopic dermatitis. Arch Dermatol 122: 265

Davies MG, Fifield R, Marks R (1979) Atopic disease and dermatitis herpetiformis. Br J Dermatol 101: 429

de Graciansky P (1966) Eczéma constitutionnel. Soc Med Hop Paris 117: 765

de Graciansky P, Schaison G (1967) Le syndrome d'Aldrich. Ann Dermatol Syphiligr 94: 255

Doeglas HMG, Bleumink E (1985) Plasma protease inhibitors in chronic urticaria. In: Champion RH, Greaves MC et al. (eds) The urticarias. Churchill Livingstone, Edinburgh, p 59

Dorn H (1961) Neurodermitis vom humangenetischen Standpunkt. Acta Allergol 16: 451

Dreskin SC, Kaliner MA, Gallin JI (1987) Elevated urinary histamine in the hyperimmuno-globulin E and recurrent infection (Job's) syndrome: association with eczematoid dermatitis and not with infection. J Allergy Clin Immunol 79: 515

Du Mont GCL, Beach RC, Menzies IS (1983) Gastrointestinal permeability in food-allergic eczematous children. Clin Allergy 14: 55

Dupré AS, Christol B, Lassère J (1981) Dermatite atopique et superinfection avec poxvirus. Ann Dermatol Venereol 108: 829

Edfors-Lubs ML (1971) Allergy in 700 twin pairs. Acta Allergol 26: 249

Edgren C (1943) Prognose und Erblichkeitsmomente bei Ekzema infantum. Acta Pædiatr Scand 30 (Suppl 2)

Eisen AH, Karpati G, Laszlo T, Andermann F, Robb JP, Bacal HL (1965) Delayed hypersensitivity in ataxia teleangiectasia. N Engl J Med 272: 18

Epstein WL, Fudenberg HH, Reed WB, Boder E, Sedgwick RP (1966) Immunologic studies in ataxia telangiectasia. I. Delayed hypersensitivity and serum immune globuline levels in probands and first degree relatives. Int Arch Allergy 30: 15

Fairris GM, Hamilton I, Cunliffe WJ, Axon ATR (1984) Intestinal permeability in adults with atopic eczema (abstract). Br J Dermatol 111: 7111

Falk E, Bolle R (1983a) IgE antibodies to house dust mite in patients with scabies. Br J Dermatol 102: 283

Falk E, Bolle R (1983b) In vivo demonstration of specific immediate hypersensitivity to scabies mite. Br J Dermatol 103: 367

Fälth-Magnusson K, Kjelman NIM, Magnusson KE, Sundqvist T (1984) Intestinal permeability in healthy and allergic children before and after sodiumcromoglycate treatment assessed with different-sized polyethyleneglycols (PEG 400 and PEG 1000). Clin Allergy 14: 277

Fartasch M, Hanke E, Anton-Lamprecht I (1987) Ultrastructural study of the occurrence of autosomal dominant ichthyosis vulgaris in atopic eczema. Arch Dermatol Res 279: 270

Finlay A, Nicholls S, King CS, Marks RA (1980) The "dry" noneczematous skin associated with atopic eczema. Br J Dermatol 102: 249

Fisch RO, Tsai MY, Gentry WC (1981) Studies in phenylketonuria with dermatitis. J Am Acad Dermatol 4: 284

Forsbeck M, Skog E, Åsbrink E (1983) Atopic hand dermatitis: a comparison with atopic dermatitis without hand involvement, especially with respect to influence of work and development of contact sensitization. Acta Derm Venereol (Stockh) 63: 9

Foucard T (1985) The epidemiology of allergic diseases in childhood. Proceedings of European Academy of Allergology, Stockholm, p 105

Frain-Bell W, Scatchard M (1971) The association of photosensitivity and atopy in the child. Br J Dermatol 85: 105

Fredriksson T, Færgemann J (1981) The atopic thigh: a "starting-school" symptom? Acta Derm Venereol (Stockh) 61: 452

Frost J, Weinstein GD (1971) Ichthyosiform dermatoses. In: Fitzpatrick TB, Arndt K et al. (eds) Dermatology in general medicine. McGraw-Hill, New York, p 249

Garrity JA, Liesegang TJ (1984) Ocular complications of atopic dermatitis. Can J Ophthalmol 19: 21

Goldblum RW, Piper WN (1954) Artificial lichenification produced by a scratching machine. J Invest Dermatol 22: 405

Greene SL, Muller SA (1985) Netherton's syndrome. J Am Acad Dermatol 13: 329

Greig D (1983) Dermatitis in catering workers. Thesis, University of Auckland

Grimmer H (1979) Lichen simplex chronicus der Vulva. Hautarzt 30: 55

Grosshans E, Basset A, Dakhel R (1969) Les tests vaso-moteur en dermatologie. Dermatologica 138: 391

Hanifin JM (1983) Clinical and basic aspects of atopic dermatitis. Semin Dermatol 2: 5

Hanifin JM, Ray LF, Lobitz WC (1974) Immunologic reactivity in dermatophytosis. Br J Dermatol 90: 1

Hannuksela M, Lahti A (1977) Immediate reactions to fruit and vegetables. Contact Dermatitis 3: 79

Hartmann AA (1983) Effects of occlusion on resident flora, skin moisture and skin-pH. Arch Dermatol Res 275: 251

Hauser C, Wütrich B, Matter L, Wilhelm JA, Sonnabend W, Schopfer K (1985) *Staphylococcus aureus* skin colonisation in atopic dermatitis. Dermatologica 170: 35

Haxthausen H (1957) Interpretation and value of skin tests in atopic dermatitis. Acta Derm Venereol (Stockh) 3: 6

Hay RJ, Brostoff J (1977) Immune responses in patients with chronic *Trichophyton rubrum* infections. Clin Exp Dermatol 2: 373

Hazell M, Marks R (1983) Lichen simplex chronicus and atopy (abstract). Br J Dermatol 108: 722

Heite HJ (1961) Katamnestische Erhebungen, klinische Untersuchungen und Testungen zur Spätprognose der Eczema infantum. Arch Klin Exp Dermatol 213: 460

Hellerström S, Lidman H (1956) Studies of Besnier's prurigo (atopic dermatitis). Acta Derm Venereol (Stockh) 36: 11

Hellerström S, Rajka G (1967) Clinical aspects of atopic dermatitis. Acta Derm Venereol (Stockh) 47: 75

Herzberg J (1973) Wenig bekannte Formen der Neurodermitis. Hautarzt 24: 47

Heskel N, Lobitz WC (1984) Atopic dermatitis in children: clinical features and management. Semin Dermatol 102: 134

Heskel N, Chan SC, Thiel ML, Stevens SR, Casperson LS, Hanifin JM (1984) Elevated umbilical cord blood leukocyte cyclic adenosine monophosphate-phosphodiesterase activity in children with atopic parents. J Am Acad Dermatol 11: 422

Hill LW (1956) The treatment of eczema in infants and children. Mosby, St. Louis

Hill LW, Sulzberger MB (1935) Evolution of atopic dermatitis. Arch Dermatol Syph 32: 451

Hirschmann JW, Lawler F, English JSC, Lonback JB, Winkelmann RH, Greaves MC (1987) Cholinergic urticaria. A clinical and histologic study. Arch Dermatol 123: 462

Hjorth N, Roed-Petersen J (1976) Occupational protein contact dermatitis in food handlers. Contact Dermatitis 2: 28

Hodgson HJ, Davies RJ, Gent AE, Hodson ME (1976) Atopic disorders and adult coeliac disease. Lancet I: 115

Höyer H, Agdal N, Munkvad M (1981) Palmar hyperlinearity in atopic dermatitis. Acta Derm Venereol (Stockh) 62: 436

Ikeda T (1965) A new classification of alopecia areata. Dermatologica 131: 421

Ingram JT (1955) Besnier's prurigo: an ectodermal defect. Br J Dermatol 67: 43

Irons M, Levy HL (1986) Metabolic syndromes with dermatologic manifestations. Clin Rec Allergy 4: 101

Jackson PG, Lessoff MH, Baker RW, Ferrett J, MacDonald DM (1981) Intestinal permeability in patients with eczema and food allergy. Lancet I: 1285

Jacquet L (1904) In: Besnier E, Brocq L, Jacquet L (eds) La pratique dermatologique, vol 5. Masson, Paris

Johansson SGO (1981) The clinical significance of IgE. In: Franklin EC (ed) Clinical immunology update. New York, p 123

Johansson SGO, Juhlin L (1970) Immunoglobulin E in healed atopic dermatitis and after treatment with corticosteroids and azathioprine. Br J Dermatol 82: 10

Johnson ML, Roberts J (1978) Skin conditions and related needs for medical care among persons 1–74 years, United states 1971–1974. US Dept of Health, Education and Welfare, Publ No (PHS) 79–1660, p 1

Jones HE, Reinhardt JH, Rinaldi MG (1973) A clinical, mycological and immunological survey for dermatophytosis. Arch Dermatol 108: 61

Juhlin L, Wide L (1972) IgE antibodies and penicillin allergy. In: Dash CH, Jones HEH (eds) Mechanisms in drug allergy. Churchill Livingstone, Edinburgh, p 139

Kaaman T (1985) Skin reactivity in atopic patients with dermatophytosis. Mykosen 28: 183

Kaposi M (1887) Pathologie und Therapie der Hautkrankheiten. Urban und Schwarzenberg, Berlin, p 483

Karel I, Myska V, Kvicalova E (1965) Ophthalmological changes in atopic dermatitis. Acta Derm Venereol (Stockh) 45: 381

Kitamura K (1966) Zur Frage des Kinderekzems. Hautarzt 17: 53

Kjellman B, Pettersson R (1980) Atopic disease and pediatric ambulatory care. Allergy 35: 531

Kjellman NIM (1976) Predictive value of high IgE levels in children. Acta Pædiatr Scand 65: 465

Kjellman NIM (1983) Serum IgE and the predictive value of IgE determination. In: Buscinco L (ed) Advances in pediatric allergy, vol 69. Excerpta Medica, Amsterdam

Kligman AM, Leyden JJ, McGinley KJ (1976) Bacteriology. J Invest Dermatol 67: 160

Kornerup T, Lodin A (1959) Ocular changes in 100 cases of Besnier's prurigo (atopic dermatitis). Acta Ophthalmol 37: 508

Korting GW (1954) Zur Pathogenese des endogenen Ekzems. Thieme, Stuttgart

Kristmundsdottir F, David TJ (1987) Growth impairment in children with atopic eczema. J R Soc Med 80: 9

Krivit W, Good RA (1959) Aldrich syndrome. Am J Dis Child 98: 579

Lancet (Editorial) (1970) Routine small vaccination: a dilemma. Lancet I: 1270

Langeland T, Nyrud M (1982) Contact urticaria to wheat bran bath: a case report. Acta Derm Venereol (Stockh) 62: 82

Larkö O, Lindstedt G, Lundberg PA, Mobacken H (1983) Biochemical and clinical studies in a case of contact urticaria to potato. Contact Dermatitis 9: 108

Larsson PÅ, Lidén S (1980) Prevalence of skin diseases among adolescents 12–16 years of age. Acta Derm Venereol (Stockh) 60: 415

Leider ML (1961) Practical pediatric dermatology. Mosby, St. Louis

Leutgeb C, Bandmann HJ, Breit R (1972) Handlinienmuster, Ichthyosis vulgaris und Dermatitis atopica. Arch Dermatol Forsch 244: 354

Levy HL (1977) Hartnup disease. In: Goldensohn ES, Appel SH (eds) Scientific approaches to clinical neurology. Lea and Febiger, Philadelphia, p 75

Leyden JJ, Baker DA (1979) Localized herpes simplex infections in atopic dermatitis. Arch Dermatol 115: 311

Leyden JJ, Marples RR, Kligman AM (1974) *Staphylococcus aureus* in the lesions of atopic dermatitis. Br J Dermatol 90: 525

Lindmaier A, Lindemayr H, Schmidt JB (1987) Kopfschuppen – ein atopisches Stigma? Hautarzt 38: 138

Lobitz WC, Honeyman JF, Winkler NW (1972) Suppressed cell mediated immunity in two adults with atopic dermatitis. Br J Dermatol 86: 317

Lombardi P, Campolmi P, Giorgini S, Spallanzani P, Sertoli A (1983) Contact urticaria from fish, honey and peach skin. Contact Dermatitis 9: 422

Lutz E, Korting GW (1958) Zur Lungenfunktion des endogenen Ekzematikers. Arch Klin Exp Dermatol 205: 597

Lynch NR, Medouze LBS, di Prisco Fuenmayor MC et al. (1984) Incidence of atopic disease in a tropical environment: partial independence from intestinal helminthiasis. J Allergy Clin Immunol 73: 229

MacKie RM (1982) Juvenile plantar dermatosis. Semin Dermatol 1: 67

MacKie RM, Husain SL (1976) Juvenile plantar dermatosis. A new entity? Clin Exp Dermatol 2: 253

MacKie RM, Cobb SJ, Cochran REI, Thomson J (1979) Total and specific IgE levels in patients with atopic dermatitis. The correlation between prick testing clinical history of allergy, in vitro quantification of IgE during clinical exacerbation and remission. Clin Exp Dermatol 4: 187

Maibach HI (1976) Immediate hypersensitivity in hand dermatitis. Role of food-contact dermatitis. Arch Dermatol 112: 1289

Maibach HL (1986) Regional variation in elicitation of contact urticaria-syndrome (Immediate hypersensitivity syndrome): shrimp. Contact Dermatitis 15: 100

Mali JW, Kuiper JP (1968) Atopic seborrheic prurigo. Dermatologica 136: 400

Malten KE (1968) The occurrence of hybrids between contact allergic eczema and atopic dermatitis (and vice versa) and their significance. Dermatologica 136: 395

Marks R, Simons MJ (1979) Geographic tongue – a manifestation of atopy. Br J Dermatol 101: 159

Mathes BM, Douglas MC (1985) Seborrheic dermatitis in patients with acquired immunodeficiency syndrome. J Am Acad Dermatol 13: 947

McCalla R, Savilahti E, Perkkio M, Kuitunen P, Backman A (1980) Morphology of the jejunum in children with eczema due to food allergy. Allergy 35: 536

Meenan FOC (1981) Further observations of the Dennie-Morgan fold. Ir J Med Sci 150: 89

Michel FB, Bousquet J, Greillier P, Robinet-Levy M, Coulomb SY (1980) Comparison of cord blood immunoglobulin E concentrations and maternal allergy for prediction of atopic diseases in infancy. J Allergy Clin Immunol 65: 422

Millard LG, Gould DJ (1977) Juvenile plantar dermatosis. Clin Exp Dermatol 2: 186

Möller H (1972) Atopic winter feet in children. Acta Derm Venereol (Stockh) 52: 401

Morison WW, Parrish JA, Fitzpatrich TB (1978) Oral photochemotherapy of atopic eczema. Br J Dermatol 98: 25

Morsbach P (1962) Über inhalative Provokationstests bei Atopie. Inaugural disseration, Juris, Zürich

Musgrove K, Morgan JK (1976) Infantile eczema. A long term follow-up study. Br J Dermatol 95: 365

Nexmand PH (1948) Clinical studies of prurigo Besnier. Rosenkilde and Bagger, Copenhagen

Nicolis GD, Helwig EB (1973) Exfoliative dermatitis. Arch Dermatol 108: 788

Niinimæki A (1987) Scratch-chamber test in food handler dermatitis. Contact Dermatitis 16: 11

Nilsson E (1986) Individual and environmental risk factor for hand eczema in hospital workers. Thesis, Umeà University

Norrlind R (1946) Prurigo Besnier (atopic dermatitis). Acta Derm Venereol [Suppl 13] (Stockh)

Oddoze L (1959) Notre statistique sur l'étiologie du prurigo de Besnier en France. Acta Allergol 13: 410

Oddoze L, Témime P (1968) Dysidrose et atopie: le terrain atopique dans les dysidroses. Bull Soc Fr Dermatol Syphiligr 75: 368

Olumide YM (1986) The incidence of atopic dermatitis in Nigeria. Int J Dermatol 25: 367

Osborne ED, Murray PF (1953) Atopic dermatitis. A study of its natural course and of wool as a dominant allergenic factor. Arch Dermatol Syphilol 68: 619

Parkman R, Rappeport D, Geha RS, Cassady E et al. (1978) Complete correction of the Wiscott-Aldrich syndrome by allogeneic bone marrow transplantation. N Engl J Med 298: 921

Paslin D, Norman HE (1977) Atopic dermatitis and impaired neutrophil chemotaxis in Job's syndrome. Arch Dermatol 113: 408

Penders AJM (1968) Alopecia areata and atopy. Dermatologica 136: 395

Perkkio M (1980) Immunohistochemical study of intestinal biopsies from children with atopic eczema due to food allergy. Allergy 35: 573

Peterson RDA, Page AR, Good RA (1962) Wheal and erythema allergy in patients with agammaglobulinaemia. J Allergy 33: 406

Piérard GE (1987) What does "dry skin" mean? Int J Dermatol 26: 167

Pike MG, Haddle RJ, Boulton P, Turner MW, Atherton DJ (1986) Increased intestinal permeability in atopic eczema. J Invest Dermatol 86: 101

Podmore O, Burrows D, Eedy DJ, Stanford CF (1986) Seborrhoic eczema – a disease entity or a clinical variant of atopic eczema? Br J Dermatol 115: 341

Price JF, Cogswell JJ, Joseph MC, Cochrane GM (1976) Exercise-induced bronchoconstriction, skin sensitivity and serum IgE in children with eczema. Arch Dis Child 51: 912

Purdy MJ (1953) The long-term prognosis in infantile eczema. Br Med J II: 1366

Queille-Roussel C, Raynaud F, Saurat HJ (1985) A prospective computerized study of 500 cases of atopic dermatitis in childhood. I. Initial analysis of 250 parameters. Acta Derm Venereol [Suppl] (Stockh) 114: 87

Rajka G (1960) Prurigo Besnier (atopic dermatitis) with special reference to the role of allergic factors. I. The influence of atopic hereditary factors. Acta Derm Venereol (Stockh) 40: 285

Rajka G (1961) Prurigo Besnier (atopic dermatitis) with special reference to the role of allergic factors. II. The evaluation of the results of skin reactions. Acta Derm Venereol (Stockh) 41: 1

Rajka G (1963) Studies in hypersensitivity to molds and staphylococci in prurigo Besnier (atopic dermatitis). Acta Derm Venereol (Stockh) 43 (Suppl 54)

Rajka G (1967) Itch duration in the involved skin of atopic dermatitis (prurigo Besnier). Acta Derm Venereol (Stockh) 47: 154

Rajka G (1968) Itch duration in the uninvolved skin of atopic dermatitis (prurigo Besnier). Acta Derm Venereol (Stockh) 48: 320

Rajka G (1983) Atopic dermatitis and Hodgkin's disease. Acta Derm Venereol (Stockh) 63: 176

Rajka G (1986) Atopic dermatitis. Correlation of environmental factors with frequency. Int J Dermatol 25: 301

Rajka G, Barlinn C (1979) On the significance of the trichophytin reactivity in atopic dermatitis. Acta Derm Venereol (Stockh) 59: 45

Rajka G, Skog E (1965) On the relation between drug allergy and atopy. Acta Allergol 20: 387

Rajka G, Aly R, Bayles C, Tang Y, Maibach H (1981) The effect of short-term occlusion on the cutaneous flora in atopic dermatitis and psoriasis. Acta Derm Venereol (Stockh) 61: 160

Reimann HJ, Schmidt U, Lewin J, Zellmer A, Ring J (1986) Intragastric provocation under endoscopic control. In: Ring J, Burg G (eds) New trends in allergy. II. Springer, Berlin Heidelberg New York, p 146

Roberts DL, Rhodes J, Heathley RV, Newcombe RG (1978) Atopic features in ulcerative colitis. Lancet I: 1262

Rogge JL, Hanifin JM (1976) Immunodeficiencies in severe atopic dermatitis. Arch Dermatol 112: 1391

Rosen FS (1976) The primary immunodeficiencies: dermatologic manifestations. J Invest Dermatol 67: 402

Rost GA, Marchionini A (1932) Asthma-eksem, Asthma-prurigo und Neurodermitis als allergische Hautkrankheiten. Würz Abh Gesamtgeb prakt Med 27: 10

Rostenberg A jr, Solomon LM (1968) Infantile eczema and systemic disease. Arch Dermatol 98: 41

Roth HL, Kierland RR (1964) The natural history of atopic dermatitis. Arch Dermatol 89: 209

Rowe AH (1946) Dermatitis of the hands due to atopic allergy to pollen. Arch Dermatol Syph 53: 437

Runne O, Orfanos CE (1977) Cutaneous neural proliferation in highly pruritic lesions of chronic prurigo. Arch Dermatol 113: 787

Russel Jones R, MacDonald DM (1982) Eczema. Immunopathogenesis and histogenesis. Am J Dermatopathol 4: 335

Rystedt I (1985a) Long term follow-up in atopic dermatitis. Acta Derm Venereol [Suppl] (Stockh) 114: 117

Rystedt I (1985b) Work-related hand eczema in atopics. Contact Dermatitis 12: 164

Rystedt I (1985c) Factors influencing the occurrence of hand eczema in adults with a history of atopic dermatitis in childhood. Contact Dermatitis 12: 185

Rystedt I (1985d) Prognostic factors in atopic dermatitis. Acta Derm Venereol (Stockh) 65: 206

Rystedt I, Strannegård IL, Strannegård Ö (1986) Recurrent viral infections in patients with past or present atopic dermatitis. Br J Dermatol 114: 575

Rytel MW, Klion FM, Arlander TR, Miller LF (1963) Detection of penicillin hypersensitivity with penicilloyl-polylysine. JAMA 186: 894

Saurat JH (1985) Eczema in primary immuno-deficiencies. Acta Derm Venereol [Suppl] (Stockh) 114: 125

Saurat JH (1987) Atopic dermatitis-like eruptions in primary immunodeficiencies. In: Happle R, Grosshans E (eds) Pediatric dermatology. Springer, Berlin Heidelberg New York, p 96

Saurat JH, Woodley H, Helfer N (1985) Cutaneous symptoms in primary immunodeficiencies. In: Orfanos CE (ed) Current problems in dermatology, vol 13: Recent developments in clinical research. Karger, Basel, p 50

Schnyder UW (1959) Konstitutionelle Neurodermitis-atopic dermatitis-Prurigo Besnier. In: Schuppli R (ed) Aktuelle Probleme der Dermatologie, vol 1. Karger, Basel, p 216

Schnyder UW (1960) Neurodermitis-Asthma-Rhinitis. Karger, Basel

Schnyder UW (1961) Neurodermitis vom klinischen-dermatologischen Standpunkt. Acta Allergol 16: 463

Schnyder UW, Borelli S (1965) Neurodermitis constitutionalis sive atopica. In: Miescher G, Storck H (eds) Entzündliche Dermatosen. II. Springer, Berlin Heidelberg New York, p 228 (Handbuch der Haut- und Geschlechtskrankheiten, vol II/1)

Schudel P, Wütrich B (1985) Klinische Verlaufsbeobachtungen bei Neurodermitis atopica nach dem Kleinkindesalter. Eine katamnestische Untersuchung anhand von 121 Fällen. Z Hautkr 60: 479

Schultz-Larsen F (1985) Atopic dermatitis. Etiological studies based on a twin population. Thesis, Legeforeningens, Copenhagen

Schuppli R (1954) Zur Aetiologie der Dyshidrosis. Dermatologica 108: 393

Schwartz D, Buckley RH (1971) Serum IgE concentrations and skin reactivity to anti-IgE antibody in IgA-deficient patients. N Engl J Med 284: 513

Schwartz M (1952) The heredity in bronchial asthma. Acta Allergol [Suppl 2]

Sedlis E (1965) Some challenge studies with foods. J Pediatr 66 (2): 235

Shelley WB (1972) Consultations in dermatology. Saunders, Philadelphia, p 36

Shelley WB, Arthur RP (1957) The neurohistology and neurophysiology of the itch sensation in man. Arch Dermatol 76: 296

Shwachman H, Diamond LK, Oski FA, Khaw KT (1964) The syndrome of pancreatic insufficiency and bone marrow dysfunction. J Pediatr 65: 645

Silvers SH, Glickman FS (1968) Atopy and eczema of the feet in children. Am J Dis Child 116: 400

Sirot G (1983) Nummular eczema. Semin Dermatol 2: 68

Solomon LM, Esterly NB (1973) Neonatal dermatology. Major problems in clinical dermatology. IX. Saunders, Philadelphia, p 125

Solomon LM, Telner P (1966) Eruptive molluscum contagiosum in atopic dermatitis. Can Med Assoc J 95: 978

Spiegelberg HL (1986) IgE receptors on lymphocytes. In: Ring J, Burg G (eds) New trends in allergy. II. Springer, Berlin Heidelberg New York, p 33

Sprafke H (1966) Cataracta juvenilis syndermotica. Dermatol Wochenschr 152: 928

Stevanovic DV (1960) Apparent light sensibility in atopic subjects. Acta Derm Venereol (Stockh) 40: 220

St Geme JW, Prince JT, Burke BA. Good RA, Krivit W (1965) Impaired cellular resistance to herpes simplex virus in Wiskott-Aldrich syndrome. N Engl J Med 273: 229

Stifler WC (1965) A 21 year follow-up of infantile eczema. J Pediatr 66 (2): 166

Storck H (1955) Ekzem durch Inhalation. Schweiz Med Wochenschr 85: 608

Stoy, PJ, Roitman-Johnson B, Walsh G, Gleich GJ, Mendell N, Yunis E, Blumenthal MN (1981) Aging and serum immunoglobulin E levels, immediate skin tests and RAST. J Allergy Clin Immunol 68: 421

Strannegård Ö, Strannegård IL, Rystedt I (1985) Viral infections in atopic dermatitis. Acta Derm Venereol [Suppl] (Stockh) 114: 121

Sulzberger MB (1940) Dermatologic allergy. Thomas, Springfield

Sulzberger MB, Goodman J (1936) The relative importance of specific hypersensitivity in adult atopic dermatitis. JAMA 106: 1000

Svejgaard E, Albrectsen B, Baastrup N (1983) The occurrence of tinea of the feet in 15-year-old school children. Mykosen 26: 450

Svejgaard E, Christophersen J, Jelsdorf HM (1986) Tinea pedis and erythrasma in Danish recruits. J Am Acad Dermatol 14: 993

Svejgaard E, Kieffer M, Færgemann J, Jemec G, Ottevanger V (1989) Fungal skin infection and atopic dermatitis. Acta Derm Venereol (Suppl 144) (Stockh) (in press)

Svensson A, Möller H (1986) Eyelid dermatitis: the role of atopy and contact allergy. Contact Dermatitis 15: 178

Taylor B, Wadworth M, Wadworth J, Peckham C (1984) Changes in the reported prevalence in childhood eczema since the 1939-1945 war. Lancet I: 1255

Témime P, Bazex A, Graciansky P de, Marchand JP, Taieb M (1972) The atypical cutaneous manifestations of atopy. In: Charpin J, Boutin C, Aubert J, Frankland W (eds) Allergology. Proceedings 8th European Congress of Allergology. Excerpta Medica, Amsterdam, p 147

Uehara M (1981) Intra-orbital fold in atopic dermatitis. Arch Dermatol 117: 627

Uehara M, Hayashi S (1981) Hyperlinear palms, association with ichthyosis and atopic dermatitis. Arch Dermatol 117: 490

Uehara M, Amemiya T, Arai M (1985) Atopic cataract in a Japanese population. Dermatologica 170: 180

Ukabam SO, Mann RJ, Cooper BT (1984) Small intestine permeability to sugars in patients with atopic eczema. Br J Dermatol 110: 649

Ullmann W (1981) Korrelationen zwischen Exfoliatio linguae areata und Atopie. Hautarzt 32: 629

Van Hecke E, Leys G (1981) Evolution of atopic dermatitis. Dermatologica 163: 370

Van Ketel WG, Alberse RC, Reerink-Brongers E, Woerdeman-Evenhuis JT (1978) Comparative examination of the results of the RAST and intracutaneous tests in eczema dyshidroticum. Dermatologica 156: 304

Vanselow N, Yamate M, Adams MS, Callies O (1970) The increased prevalence of atopic diseases in anhidrotic congenital ectodermal dysplasia. J Allergy 45: 302

Veien NK, Hattel T, Justesen O, Norrholm A (1983) Causes of eczema in the food industry. Derma Beruf Umwelt 31: 84

Verbov JL (1978) Atopic eczema localized to the forefoot. An unrecognized entity. Practitioner 220: 465

Verkasalo M, Tillikainen A, Kuitunen P, Savilahti E, Backman A (1983) HLA antigens and atopy in children with coeliac disease. Gut 24: 306

Vickers CHF (1980) The natural history of atopic eczema. Acta Derm Venereol [Suppl] (Stockh) 92: 113

Vickers CHF (1983) Infantile seborrheic dermatitis. Discussion to Yates et al. Br J Dermatol 108: 722

Von Krogh G, Maibach HI (1981) The contact urticaria syndrome – an updated review. J Am Acad Dermatol 5: 328

Vowles M, Warin RP, Apley J (1955) Infantile eczema: observations on natural history and prognosis. Br J Dermatol 67: 53

Waddington E, Bray PT, Evans AD, Richards IDG (1964) Cutaneous complications of mass vaccination against smallpox in South Wales 1962. Trans St Johns Hosp Dermatol Soc 50: 22

Waersted A, Hjorth N (1985) Pityrosporon orbiculare – a pathogenic factor in atopic dermatitis of the face, scalp and neck? Acta Derm Venereol [Suppl] (Stockh) 114: 146

Wagner G, Pürschel W (1962) Klinisch-analytische Studie zum Neurodermitisproblem. Dermatologica 125: 1

Walker RB, Warin RP (1956) The incidence of eczema in early childhood. Br J Dermatol 68: 182

Watkins D (1961) Pityriasis alba, a form of atopic dermatitis. Arch Dermatol 83: 915

Wells RS, Kerr CI (1966) Clinical features of autosomal dominant and sex-linked ichthyosis in English population. Br Med J I: 947

Wilson AF, Novey HS, Berke RA, Syprenant EL (1973) Deposition of inhaled pollen and pollen extract in human airways. N Engl J Med 288: 1056

Winkelmann RK, Rajka G (1983) Atopic dermatitis and Hodgkin's disease. Acta Derm Venereol (Stockh) 63: 176

Wolf R, Sandbank M, Krakowski A (1985) Extensive pityriasis alba and atopic dermatitis. Br J
Dermatol 112: 247

Wütrich B (1973) IgE-Bestimmungen bei Neurodermitis und anderen Dermatosen. Hautarzt
24: 381

Wütrich B (1983) Atopische Dermatitis. Aktuelles zu Klinik, Pathogenese und Therapie. Aktuel Dermatol 7: 85

Wütrich B, Schnyder UW (1981) Eine wenig bekannte Ausdrucksform des Neurodermitis
atopica im Kindesalter: das patchy pityriasiform lichenoid eczema ("Kitamura-Takahashi-
Sasagawa"). Aktuel Dermatol 7: 85

Wütrich B, Schudel P (1983) Die Neurodermitis atopica nach dem Kleinkindesalter. Eine
katamnestische Untersuchung anhand von 121 Fällen. Z Hautkr 58: 1013

Yates VM; Kerr EIR, MacKie RM (1983) Early diagnosis of infantile seberrhoic dermatitis
and atopic dermatitis - clinical features. Br J Dermatol 108: 633

Young E (1964) Dyshidrotic (endogenous) eczema. Dermatologica 129: 306

Young E (1986) Forefoot eczema - further studies and a review. Clin Exp Dermatol 11: 523

Young E, Koers WJ (1989) Intracutaneous tests with pityrosporon extracts in atopic dermatitis. Acta Derm Venereol (Suppl 144) (Stockh) (in press)

Zachary CB, Atherton DJ (1986) Hyper IgE syndrome - case history. Clin Exp Dermatol 11:
403

Zachary CB, Baker RW, Lessoff MH, MacDonalds DM (1982) Increased intestinal permeability in atopic eczema - polyethylene glycol used as a probe molecule. Br J Dermatol
(Suppl 22): 14

3 Itch

3.1 Short Survey

The central role played by pruritus in AD was stressed in Chap. 2 and it is apposite to present a short survey of itch in general.

Tissue injury, or an immune reaction, produces an initial chemical stimulus which, possibly by kinase production and proenzyme activation (Cormia et al. 1957), liberates proteolytic enzymes. The latter are either mediators of itch or liberate such mediators - primarily histamine (Rocha de Silva 1940; Craps and Inderbitzin 1957). In ordinary skin inflammation, for instance allergic reactions (Ungar and Hayashi 1958), proteinases are released from the epidermis, blood, and cellular infiltrates, or from the bacteria and fungi. The activity of these proteinases (endopeptidases) in tissues is complex, as it may be dependent on several factors, including inhibitors (Arthur and Shelley 1958).

These chemical mediators, in analogy to mechanical, electrical, and chemical stimuli, act on the itch receptors. These are free unmyelinated penicillate nerve endings adherent to the dermoepidermal junction (or terminating in the epidermis; Arthur and Shelley 1959; Cauna 1976). They are limited to the skin, mucous membranes, and cornea. It is still undecided whether they are identical to, or differ from, the polynodal nocireceptors, i. e., pain receptors reacting to different stimuli. The nocireceptor units are supplied by C and A delta fibers. The afferent pathway for pruritus from the itch receptors comprises three sets of neurons. Thin, unmyelinated, slowly conducting (2 m/s) C fibers (Zotterman 1939), which may vary in number in the different cutaneous nerves (Tomash and Britton 1956), extend from the receptors to the posterior root ganglia. From synapses there, fibers pass up to the thalamus by way of the spinothalamic tracts. The final groups of neurons connect the thalamic ganglia to the somatesthetic area of posterior central gyrus in the cerebral cortex. Probably (though this has not been convincingly demonstrated), small myelinated A delta fibers also transmit itch.

Itch perception is initiated by persistent low-grade stimulation of the pathway and is identified in the cortex as the itch sensation, which has the following characteristics: its localization is imprecise, its intensity is imperfectly quantifiable, it persists after the stimulation has ceased, it can cause prolonged discomfort, and it may be influenced by emotional factors (Rothman 1922, 1954, 1960) which may themselves be engendered by visual or auditory perceptions.

The A delta fibers transmit a sharp pricking itch quality. The efferent limb of the reflex arch carries motor stimuli to produce scratching. It is by no means clear how scratching relieves pruritus. Zotterman (1959) thought that it mechanically damages or deranges the most superficial nerve endings, and that itch cannot recur until these minute fibers have regrown, which, however, they do rapidly. Others suggested that pain caused by scratching replaces itch or that depots of itch-transmitting chemicals are exhausted.

3.1.1 Itch and Pain

Itch shares many features and pathways with pain. Both are warning signals induced by noxious stimuli, transmitted to the spinal cord by the same nerve fibers. Some stimuli which at low intensity may induce itch, at higher intensity cause pain.

In areas insensitive to pain, itch does not occur. Some substances, like prostaglandins, enhance both itch and pain. However, there are several differences between them. Pruritus is a more superficial sensation; removal of epidermis and superficial dermis abolishes itch, but not pain. Diminishing low intensity pain never goes over to itch. Heating skin to 41 °C blocks itch but increases pain. Opiates alleviate pain but induce itch. Thus itch and pain should be considered as distinct sensations.

3.1.2 Mediator of Itch

Our knowledge of pruritus, including mediators of itch, derives mostly from experimental studies. Production of itch by inserting spicules of *Mucuna pruriens* (cowhage) into the skin was first undertaken by Török (1907) and subsequently by several other authors.

Later it was demonstrated that histamine produces itch (Cormia 1952; Cormia and Kuykendall 1953), as can be shown by injecting it intracutaneously in concentrations as low as 10^{-4}M. However, as whealing is produced by concentrations as low as 10^{-3}M, it is felt that pruritus is independent of any overt vasodilatory reaction, despite a possible connection between itch and the initial phase of vasodilatation, especially in clinical situations and in diurnal variations (Graham et al. 1957; Chapman et al. 1960). Fine nerve fibers running close to vessels are assumed to have a role here (Wedell et al. 1959).

Histamine-elicited itch involves H_1 receptors, while the role of H_2 receptors, (Davies and Greaves 1981) is strongly disputed. Arthur and Shelley (1955), using cowhage spicules, discovered an endopeptidase (the pruritogen is a thermolabile protein of molecule weight 40000, Denman and Wuepper 1982) and induced itch with this proteinase (see above). Trypsin, acting in part as a histamine liberator, and papain, which acts without liberating histamine (see below), are the two best studied representative substances (Arthur and Shelley 1955, 1958; Rajka 1967, 1968); furthermore, chymase (Hägermark et al. 1972) has been investigated.

Several new substances have recently been investigated for a putative itch-inducing effect. It was found that PGE$_2$ (Hägermark and Strandberg 1977) has a weak pruritogenic effect, and PGE$_1$ (Greaves and McDonald-Gibson 1973) also influences the papain-induced itch (Lovell et al. 1976). PGH$_2$ and a stable endoperoxide analogue (Hägermark et al. 1977) had similar effects.

Of still more interest were, from the point of view of pruritus, peptides having a neurotransmitter role. Substance P (Hägermark et al. 1978) and vasoactive intestinal polypeptide (VIP) had an itch-inducing effect at a concentration of 10^{-6} M, whereas neurotensin, Gln^4-neurotensin, and secretin were pruritogenic only at higher concentrations (Fjellner and Hägermark 1981). In addition, endogenous opioid peptides, which also have neurotransmitter function and in general are analgesics, were investigated. Of them, morphine had long been recognized as an itch inducer. The morphine antagonist naloxone (Bernstein et al. 1982), when given systemically – though not when given locally – reduced itch and increased the itch treshold; similar effects were demonstrated with N-allylnoroxymorphone. (Whitney and Bernstein 1984). Pruritogenic effects were rpeorted of the opioid peptides methionine-encephalin (and its stable analogue FK 33.824), leucine-encephalin, and β-endorphin (Fjellner 1981). A nonopioid neuropeptide, bombesin, given, for example, intrathecally to rats, elicited scratching (Gmerek and Cowan 1983). Seortonin induced itch in healthy volunteers and together with PGE$_2$ may have a role in the itch of polycythemia vera, where the role of histamine seems negligible (Fjellner and Hägermark 1979).

Platelet activating factor [PAF-acether], a lipid substance, also elicited itch in experimental studies (Fjellner and Hägermark 1985).

Table 3.1 summarizes these investigative findings. In most cases there is a well-established distinction between those substances supposed to cause, and those supposed not to cause, release of histamine from mast cells; exceptions are papain (see above) and kallikrein (Hägermark 1974), where no triple response-like skin changes are observed [which is also the case in aquagenic pruritus despite high histamine blood levels (Greaves et al. 1981)] and which perhaps affect the itch receptors directly (Fjellner 1981). The other groups of itch

Table 3.1. Itch-inducing Substances (see also text)

I.*Direct itch inducers*	
a) Histamine	Trypsin, papain, chymase (bradykinin,
b) Histamine releasers:	kallikrein
Endopeptidases	
Neurotransmitter peptides	Substance P, VIP (neurotensin, secretin)
Lipids	PAF-acether
II. *Substances potentiating*	
(histamine-elicited)	
itch via other mechanisms:	
Lipids	PGE$_2$ (and some other prostaglandins)
Opioid peptide neurotransmitters	Morphine, Met-enkephalin/FK 33-824,
	Leu-enkephalin, β-endorphin
Other neuropeptides	Serotonin, bombesin (?)

Table 3.2. Itch duration values for involved skin, obtained by repeated tests

Compared with initial value	Congruity in the patients investigated (%)
After 1 day	76
After 2 days	74
After 1 week	79
After 2 weeks	75
After 1–4 months	76

modulating substances potentiated the histamine-induced itch (e. g., when in-jected in a mixture with histamine) by unknown mechanisms; pretreatment with antihistaminics or compound 48/80 did not influence this effect. Here, an influence on the adenylate cyclase system or on other (than the ordinary) opi-ate receptors for the opiate neurotransmitters is suspected.

It is important to stress that these chemical substances provoke itch in the majority of, but not all, persons investigated. Pruritus may take as long as 10–15 s to develop after an intracutaneous injection of endopeptidase or hista-mine, suggesting that they may not have a direct action.

Special techniques have also been used in which, for instance, the stimuli are applied to a cantharidin blister base (Keele and Armstrong 1964) or epicu-taneously (Stüttgen et al. 1965). By all these experimental methods the latency, duration, and threshold of itch were estimated. Using trypsin in such experi-ments, it was shown that an individual's estimated itch threshold was constant in the majority of cases studied (Rajka 1967) (Table 3.2). Cormia (1952), using histamine for consecutive daily and weekly testing, recorded similar findings, but later also reported that the itch threshold is lower during the night, after psychic trauma, and after elevation of skin temperature (Cormia and Kuyken-dall 1953). Several studies have observed that the itch threshold shows signifi-cant regional differences but that in symmetrical sites it is generally uniform.

3.1.3 Nonchemical Stimuli

Experimental studies were undertaken by the use of mechanical (vibratory), electrical, or thermal stimuli. These elicit pruritus within a few seconds and supposedly act directly on the itch receptors. By applying mechanical stimuli to an area of skin in which the itch threshold was lowest, and which was innervat-ed by an aggregate of unmyelinated nerve fibers and endings, the concept of itch points was evolved (von Frey 1910; Shelley and Arthur 1957).

Experimentally induced mental stress, via color–word conflict and arithme-tic tests, influences the responsiveness of skin. The latter seems to depend on the individual psychosomatic state and on psychosocial factors, partly related to the urinary adrenaline response pattern, i. e., adrenaline depressed the itch (Fjellner et al. 1985; Fjellner and Arnatz 1985).

According to Trotter and Wilkin (1986), reduction of blood circulation in the finger due to stress unrelated to mental activity can lead to a lowered itch threshold.

More recent and up-to-date summaries of the pathophysiology and mechanism of itching, which bear an obvious relation to pruritus in AD, are given by Savin (1980), by the author (Rajka 1980 b), and in the thesis of Fjellner (1981). Savin's overview also discusses the important psychological aspects, and this same topic was elaborated by Whitlock (1976).

The longer duration of itch in AD patients was emphasized by Harnack (1980) even if this feature is not sufficiently specific for differential diagnosis. Similarly, nocturnal scratching, evaluated by computer analysis, was about equal in AD and in another itchy condition, i. e. generalized eczema (Aoki et al. 1980). A correlation was demonstrated between serum IgE level and experimental pruritus (Rajka 1980 a), but no such correlation existed with the duration of nocturnal scratching (Aoki et al. 1980). Attention was recently drawn to the characteristics of the scratching rather than the quality and quantity of pruritus. Thus Savin et al. (1973, 1975), using a sensitive movement detector and vibration transducer, registered a certain pattern of bouts of scratching during different stages of sleep which is characteristic of itching conditions, including AD. Similar experiments were performed by Felix and Shuster (1975). This new and fruitful approach has greatly broadened our capacity to evaluate pruritus and expecially its consequences, but has the drawback of recording not only scratching but also limb movement due to anxiety, nervousness, or sleeplessness; in this context it should nevertheless be noted that Summerfield and Welch (1980) interpreted a marked increase of arm movements as due to scratching. Otherwise, for therapeutic evaluations the visual analogue scale (VAS) is used in the majority of reports.

3.1.4 Itch and Late Cutaneous Reactions

In clinical situations as well as in experimental itch studies (Rajka 1963) itching not only appears 15 min after allergenic (or nonimmunological) challenge; rather new waves of itching occur after 4–6 h and can last up to 24 h, e. g., after challenge with egg (Brostoff et al. 1979). Itching is frequently combined with other inflammatory phenomena, as was excellently described by Solley et al. (1976) in respect of passive sensitization experiments: "At about 4–6 hours a mild pruritus heralded an exacerbation of inflammation which peaked at 6–12 hours. At the height of the response the lesion was characterized by erythema, warmth, pruritus and/or tenderness, much more extensive in area and producing greater discomfort than the initial wheal and flare response." This phenomenon, which is attracting growing interest, is termed the late cutaneous reaction and is based on the release of mediators from the surface of mast cells or basophils during an IgE–anti-IgE reaction (Dolovitch et al. 1973). It is also called the late phase of immediate-type reaction.

This reaction seems to be mediated not by histamine but by chemotactic mediators from mast cells and basophils (Solley et al. 1976; Wasserman 1980). In this context it is of interest that pretreatment with oral sodium cromoglycate, which inhibits mast cell degranulation, prevented itching from occurring both 30 min and 6 h after egg challenge (Brostoff et al. 1979; Paganelli et al. 1979). The author has similar experience of the effect of cromoglycate on itching after challenge in food-allergic patients, though in some cases no inhibition could be shown (Rajka, unpublished observations). Furthermore, oral disodium cromoglycate improved pruritus markedly in patients with mastocytosis (Czarnetzki and Behrendt 1981). Based on all these observations, the author suggests that itching occurring 4–6 h after challenge is a manifestation of late cutaneous response. This hypothesis has obvious clinical implications. On the other hand, it has not as yet been established which mediator is responsible for this type of pruritus, and as in most other pruritic phenomena, the role of histamine is a possibility. Perhaps several agents are concerned, including histamine and mast cell mediators.

3.2 Role of Itch in AD

Two types of pruritus can be distinguished in AD. The first is *itch* in its strict sense, which is provoked by various immunological or nonimmunological stimuli and which is supposed to be the primary and dominant symptom of AD (see Chap. 2 and below). The second type is *itchy skin* (Bickford 1938). It has been postulated that in some clinical conditions, primarily in prurigo papules, in lichenification, and in eczematous lesions, there is partial damage to the multisensory innervation, which leads to an increased reactivity to itch, i. e., itchy skin. In this condition there is a lowering of itch threshold for chemical, thermal, and mechanical stimuli, which is exemplified commonly as intolerance to woollen garments.

The pruritus may be either generalized or localized to certain areas where there is a high density of itch points. The reason for the itchiness of the dry skin of AD patients is not clearly understood; suggestions have included (a) reduction in skin surface lipid leading to impaired resistance to injury and to sensory stimuli, and (b) increased skin electrostatic charge (Davis and Moursund 1955). Of interest in this context is the fact that urea not only improves the dry skin of AD patients but also has an antipruritic effect (Swanbeck and Rajka 1970; see also Chap. 7 and 12). A well-known feature of the pruritus in AD (though it is not peculiar to AD) is its intermittent character – it is most severe in the evening (Borelli et al. 1966; Serowy and Klinker 1971) and during the night. This is usually attributed to the higher body temperature and the capillary dilatation in the evening, to the absence of distraction by daily activities, and to increased skin temperature in bed. It is commonly observed that emotional tension provokes scratching in AD patients, and such tension may also lead to a conditioned scratch response differing both clinically and experimentally from that in controls (Jordan and Whitlock 1972).

The role of itch in AD has been illustrated by studies on pruritus induced *experimentally* in the macroscopically intact and the involved skin of these patients. Early investigators demonstrated a lowered itch threshold in the macroscopically normal skin in AD; stimuli used were intracutaneous histamine (Cormia 1952) and trypsin (Arthur and Shelley 1958). When spicules of *Mucuna pruriens* were inserted in the antecubital fossa of five AD patients, it was found that the resultant pruritus lasted significantly longer than in controls. The author has used a fresh solution of crystalline trypsin (25 Anson E/g), stabilized with 4% calcium chloride and diluted with physiological saline (Trypure Novo); this he injected superficially into the skin in amounts of 2–3 mg. A placebo was administered in these studies to patients investigated and to controls; selection was by a simple blind technique. In earlier studies trypsin was injected into the forearm, but in later ones it was injected into at least two areas of the involved or uninvolved skin on the dorsal or volar surfaces of the arms. Pruritus was elicited in the majority of patients investigated, and it was found that not only skin on the dorsal surface of the arm but also symptom-free skin was somewhat more reactive. The facet of particular interest was the duration of the pruritus; this was longer in AD patients than in controls – including persons with atopic rhinitis (Rajka 1967, 1968) (Tables 3.3, 3.4).

The lower itch threshold in *symptom-free* AD skin shown by the author corresponds well with earlier findings (Cormia 1952; Arthur and Shelley 1958), pointing to a characteristic quality of AD skin analogous to its other morphological and functional alterations (see Chap. 7). A satisfactory explanation cannot at the moment be given for the higher responsiveness of symptom-free AD skin to pruritogenic stimuli. The increased releasability of histamine (see Chap. 6) or a similar mechanism may perhaps play a role.

Table 3.3. Itch duration tests in patients with AD, various eczematous lesions, and psoriasis (involved skin)

Itch duration	I. AD	II. Various eczematous patients	III. Psoriasis
a) Over 2 min	23	1	1
b) Between 1 and 2 min	2	20	17
c) Less than 1 min	–	4	7
Total	25	25	25

χ test and significance I to II for a: $P < 0.1\%$

Table 3.4. Duration of itch in symptom-free skin of patients with AD and some other diseases

Itch duration	I. AD	II. Various eczemas	III. Psoriasis	IV. Atopic rhinitis	V. Atopic rhinitis with previous AD
a) Over 2 min	26	1	0	2	5
b) Under 2 min	14	19	20	18	–
Total	40	20	20	20	5

χ test and significance I to II, III, IV, V for a: $P < 0.1\%$

3.2.1 Itch as the Essential Symptom of AD

The concept of the basic role of itch in AD is by no means new; it is in agreement with the view of the earliest observers of the disease, and in this respect the *etiological* role that pruritus plays received early mention by, for example, Haxthausen (1957). To insist that an exposure experiment should provoke the typical skin changes would be unreasonable. However, that it should produce distinct attacks of pruritus is a logical requirement, and in fact a specific challenge is seen much more commonly to elicit itch than to produce new lesions. Obviously the increase in pruritus exacerbates the inflammatory change in the areas of dermatitis and this in turn aggravates the itching to establish a vicious circle. Despite the clinical difficulties of recording and evaluating itch after challenge, reports in the literature very frequently refer to pruritus following provocation tests or spontaneous exposure to an allergen (for example, Engman et al. 1936; Zakon and Taub 1938; Bonnevie 1939; Nexmand 1948; Tuft 1949; O'Leary 1953; Rostenberg 1955; Storck 1961). Eliciting itch after provocation may include pruritus during hyposensitization or skin testing (Di Prisco Fuenmayor and Champion 1979) and may be extended to peroral provocation of chrome sensitivity (Kaaber and Veien 1977). Furthermore, itch "is the first and most persistent symptom of IgE-mediated reactions in the skin following direct skin testing or passive transfer" ad modum Prausnitz-Küstner (Aas 1979). The hypothesis of the significance of itch, has been tested by the author as follows. The itch threshold was estimated by administering a range of concentrations of trypsin solution intradermally in the left arm. One hour later, the control solution and the relevant allergen were administered in sequence by an inhaler; the allergen was one to which the AD patient had previously been shown to be skin-sensitive (on allergens, see Chap. 5). After intervals of 15 min and 4 h, the itch threshold was reestimated on the right arm. Patients with AD who did not react to skin testing with the relevant inhalant allergens were also investigated by this technique. The results, excluding one patient who also reacted to the control solution, are summarized in Table 3.5. Lowering of the itch threshold was observed in five patients at 4 h after inhalation exposure to an allergen; furthermore three of these patients developed a focal reaction in the skin. When the same test was performed on 20 patients with non atopic eczema, of whom two had reacted to molds, a reduced itch threshold but no other change in the skin was produced.

These rapid changes in itch threshold have their counterpart in observations by Morsbach (1962) during an investigation of "pure" AD patients who were exposed to the allergen by inhalation. Between 10 and 30 min later, a specific bronchoconstriction usually occurred, and this was followed by itching in four of 16 patients. The reason why some but not all AD patients react with pruritus or an exacerbation of their dermatitis or both is unknown; differences in the itch threshold or in the severity of the skin lesions may be relevant.

The interval between inhalation of the allergen and the development of clinical manifestations, such as generalized pruritus or exacerbation of the dermatitis, was usually 3-6 h, but was shorter in certain cases. With regard to the inges-

Table 3.5. Changes in itch threshold in AD patients after inhalation of allergen (mold, pollen, dust)

Hypersensitive AD patients	Allergen	Conc. in %	Changes in itch threshold		Subsequent focal reaction	'Nonallergic' AD patients	Substance	Conc. in %	Changes in itch threshold		Subsequent focal reaction
			At 15 min	At 4 h					At 15 min	At 4 h	
NB	Mold[a]	10	Unchanged	Unchanged	–	NL	Birch	0.1	Unchanged	Unchanged	–
FJ	Mold	0.1	Unchanged	Unchanged	–	DH	Birch	0.1	Lowered	Unchanged	–
RS	Mold	10	Lowered	Lowered	+	MK	Mold	10	Unchanged	Unchanged	–
SC	Dust	10	Lowered	Unchanged	+	RV	Birch	0.1	Unchanged	Unchanged	–
AH	Mold	0.1	Unchanged	Lowered	–	GS	Timothy	0.1	Unchanged	Unchanged	–
EA	Mold	10	Unchanged	Lowered	+	LG	Mold	10	Unchanged	Unchanged	–
NL	Mold	10	Unchanged	Unchanged	–	EB	Birch	0.1	Unchanged	Unchanged	–
GC	Mold	10	Unchanged	Unchanged	–	HA	Mold	10	Unchanged	Unchanged	–
HK	Mold	10	Unchanged	Unchanged	–	WR	Mold	10	Unchanged	Unchanged	–
JU	Birch	0.1	Unchanged	Unchanged	–	VB	Timothy	0.1	Lowered	Lowered	–
SPO	Dust	0.1	Unchanged	Unchanged	–	JC	Birch	0.1	Unchanged	Unchanged	–
SPO	Birch	0.1	Unchanged	Unchanged	–	JC	Timothy	0.1	Unchanged	Unchanged	–
RV	Mold	0.1	Unchanged	Unchanged	–	NM	Mold	0.1	Lowered	Lowered	+
JB	Birch	0.1	Lowered	Lowered	+	NM	Timothy	0.1	Unchanged	Unchanged	–
JB	Mold	0.1	Lowered	Lowered	–	NM	Birch	0.1	Unchanged	Unchanged	–
LA	Mold	10	Unchanged	Unchanged	–	SE	Timothy	0.1	Unchanged	Unchanged	–
JC	Mold	10	Unchanged	Unchanged	–	SE	Dog-daisy[b]	0.1	Lowered	Unchanged	–
SC	Birch	0.1	Unchanged	Unchanged	–	LAM	Timothy	0.1	Unchanged	Unchanged	–
ÖB	Birch	0.1	Lowered	Not done	–	LC	Mold	10	Unchanged	Unchanged	–
WM	Mold	0.1	Unchanged	Not done	–	LC	Timothy	0.1	Unchanged	Unchanged	–
20			5 lowered	5 lowered	4	20			4 lowered	2 lowered	1

[a] *Penicillium, Mucor, Cladosporium, Botrytis* spp.   [b] *Chrysanthemum leucanthemum*

tion of allergens, the oral symptoms associated with AD have been described in Chap. 2, where mention was made of the frequency with oral itch is encountered; in addition, the relationship between foods and itching of the skin has been noted above. Relevant data, based, mainly on the patient's history, indicate that itch is noted usually some hours after ingestion of food, and this corresponds to the events after exposure by inhalation: similar findings in "alimentary pruritus" were reported by Brenn et al. (1967) (see also Sect 5.3.6). It should also be pointed out that whereas provocation corresponds to a single strong allergen exposure, in real life the exposure is often represented by small, sometimes subclinical stimuli (see also Sect. 5.3.7).

An allergen can lower the itch threshold in AD patients even when skin testing with that substance is negative; but the same can happen even in controls. This leads to the conclusion that these alterations in itch cannot represent only an allergic mechanism but must involve a direct effect of the substance applied. Such a view is in agreement with the concept that nonimmunological mechanisms, including psychic stimuli, may elicit pruritus.

Although it is possible that the first noticeable sign of an incipient AD attack before itch is erythema, as Hanifin (1983) postulates, and edema is also an early sign, the author maintains that the first main, central and for the patient clearly significant manifestation of the consequences of histamine release is pruritus. The arguments for the leading role of itch in AD are listed in Table 3.6.

Table 3.6. *Main arguments for the role of itch in AD*

1. Itch is the primary event in AD, as was expressed by Jacquet as long ago 1904 ("ce n'est pas l'élément éruptif qui est prurigineux, c'est le prurit qui est éruptif").
2. Itch is the main objective or subjective (Schnyder 1961) parameter used to characterize the intensity of AD.
3. The characteristic expressions of AD are consequences of (prurigo/lichenification) or are strictly correlated to (eczematous reaction) itch: "Atopic dermatitis is also largely caused by rubbing and scratching. If the fingers of a patient with AD could be restrained, the skin lesions would virtually disappear, although the itching would doubtless persist" (Ackerman 1978). Protection from scratching via bandage after allergenic exposure may prevent a flare-up of AD in infants and small children (Engman et al. 1936; Rajka, unpublished observations).
4. Immunological (antigen + IgE) as well as nonimmunological (dry skin, sweating) mechanisms can elicit itch in AD.
5. In the field of immunological mechanisms, itch is the first and most persistent symptom of IgE-mediated reactions in the skin following direct skin testing and passive transfer (ad modum Prausnitz-Küstner). Itch is the real indicator of low-level allergenic exposure as occurs in vivo, rather than a positive skin reaction (wheal) following a massive exposure. Itch is the only event, or precedes the inflammatory reaction, e. g., as may be observed in the skin/oral mucosa in food exposure trials.
6. Morphological findings of increased numbers of mast cells and nerve derangement in AD (Mihm et al. 1976; Soter and Mihm 1980) may be related to the intense itch.
7. Itch is the primary event in an experimental model of AD, namely exposure to pollen in dogs (Patterson 1959; Anderson 1975). The characteristic symptom in all dogs with canine AD was facial and pedal itch; not all dogs developed dermatitis (Willemse and van der Brom 1983).
8. Itch is the primary event in nasal/conjunctival atopy and in 40%-70% is a prodromal sign of asthma (Orr 1979; David et al. 1984, Rettig et al. 1984)

References

Aas K (1979) Common immunochemistry in atopic dermatitis and bronchial asthma. Derm Venereol [Suppl] (Stockh) 92: 64

Ackerman B (1978) Histologic diagnosis of inflammatory diseases. Lea & Febiger, Philadelphia p 259

Andersson W (1975) Atopic dermatitis in the dog. Cutis 15: 955

Aoki T, Kushimoto H, Kobayashi E, Ogushi Y (1980) Computer analysis of nocturnal scratch in atopic dermatitis. Acta Dermvenereol [Suppl] (Stockh) 92: 33

Arthur RP, Shelley WB (1955) The role of proteolytic enzymes in the production of pruritus in man. J Invest Dermatol 25: 341

Arthur RP, Shelley WB (1958) The nature of itching in dermatitic skin. Ann Intern Med 49: 900

Arthur RP, Shelley WB (1959) The peripheral mecanism of itch in man. In Wolstenholme GEW, O'Connor (eds) Pain and itch. Nervous mechanism. Ciba Foundation Study Group, No 1, Churchill, London

Bernstein JE, Swift RM, Soltani K, Lorincz AL (1982) Antipruritic effect of an opiate antagonist, naloxone hydrochloride. J Invest Dermatol 78: 82

Bickford RG (1938) Experiments relating to itch sensation, its peripheral mechanisms and central pathways. Clin Sci 3: 377

Bonnevie P (1939) Aetiologie und Pathogenese der Ekzemkrankheit. Barth, Leipzig

Borelli S, Chlabarov S, Flach E (1966) Die atopische Neurodermitis – zur Frage ihres 24-Stunden Rhytmus, ihrer Wetter- und Klimaabhängigkeit. Munch Med Wochenschr 108: 474

Brenn H, Borelli S, Gehrken H (1967) Über den Wert von Kutantestungen bei der konstitutionellen, atopischen Neurodermitis. Z Haut Geschlechtskr 42: 229

Brostoff J, Carini C, Wraith DG, Johns P (1979) Production of IgE complexes by allergen challenge in atopic patients and the effect of sodium cromoglycate. Lancet I: 1268

Cauna N (1976) Morphological basis of sensation in hairy skin. Prog Brain Res 43: 35

Chapman LF, Goodell H, Wolff HG (1960) Structures and processes involved in the sensation of itch. In : Montagna W (ed) Cutaneous innervation. Pergamon, Oxford, p 161 (Advances in biology of skin, vol 1)

Cormia FE (1952) Experimental histamine pruritus. I. Influence of physical and psychological factors on threshold reactivity. J Invest Dermatol 19: 21

Cormia FE, Kuykendall V (1953) Experimental histamine pruritus. II. Nature, physical and environmental factors influencing development and severity. J Invest Dermatol 20: 429

Cormia FE, Doherty JW, Unrau SA (1957) Proteolytic activity in dermatoses : preliminary observations on inflammation and pruritus. J Invest Dermatol 28: 425

Craps L, Inderbitzin T (1957) Anaphylaxie cutanée et proteolyse. Dermatologica 114: 218

Czarnetzki BM, Behrendt H (1981) Urticaria pigmentosa: clinical picture and response to oral disodium cromoglycate. Br J Dermatol 105: 563

David TJ, Wybrew M, Hennessen U (1984) Prodromal itching in childhood asthma. Lancet II: 154

Davies MG, Greaves MW (1981) The current status of histamine receptors in human skin: therapeutic implications. Br J Dermatol 104: 601

Davis MJ, Moursund MP (1955) Electrostatic electricity as a possible factor in pruritus of dry skin dermatoses. Arch Dermatol Syph 71: 224

Denman ST, Wuepper KD (1982) Anatomic and biochemical aspects of *Mucuna pruriens* (abstract) Clin Res 30(2): 581a

Di Prisco Fuenmayor MC, Champion RH (1979) Specific hyposensitization in atopic dermatitis. Br J Dermatol 101: 697

Dolovitch J, Hargreave FE, Chalmers R, Shier KJ, Gauldie Bienenstock J (1973) Late cutaneous allergic responses in isolated IgE dependent reactions. J Allergy Clin Immunol 49: 43

Engman MF, Weiss RF, Engman MFL (1936) Eczema and environment. Med Clin North Am 20: 651

Felix R, Shuster S (1975) A new method for the measurement of itch and the response to treatment. Br J Dermatol 93: 303

Fjellner B (1981) Experimental and clinical pruritus. Thesis, Universtity of Stockholm, Sweden

Fjellner B Arnetz BB (1985) Psychological predictors of pruritus during mental stress. Acta Derm Venereol (Stockh) 65: 504

Fjellner B, Hägermark Ö (1979) Pruritus in polycythemia vera: treatment with aspirin and possibility of platelet involvement. Acta Derm Venereol (Stockh) 59: 505

Fjellner B, Hägermark Ö (1981) Studies on pruritogenic and histamine-releasing effects of some putative neurotransmitters. Acta Derm Venereol (Stockh) 61: 245

Fjellner B, Hägermark Ö (1985) Experimental pruritus evoked by platelet activating factor (PAF-acether) in human skin. Acta Derm Venereol (Stockh) 65: 409

Fjellner B, Arnetz BB, Eneroth P, Kalner A (1985) Pruritus during standardized mental stress. Relationship to psychoneuroendocrine and metabolic parameters. Acta Derm Venereol (Stockh) 65: 199

Gmerek DE, Cowan A (1983) Bombesin – a central mediator of pruritus? Br J Dermatol 109: 239

Graham DT, Goodell H, Wolff HG (1957) Studies on pain: the relation between cutaneous vasodilatation, pain threshold and spontaneous itching and pain. Am J Sci 234: 420

Greaves MW McDonald-Gibson W (1973) Itch: role of prostaglandins. Br Med J 3: 608

Greaves MW, Black AK, Eady RAJ, Coutts A (1981) Aquagenic pruritus. Br Med J 282: 2008

Hägermark Ö (1974) Studies on experimental itch induced by kallikrein and bradykinin. Acta Derm Venereol (Stockh) 54: 397

Hägermark Ö, Strandberg K (1977) Pruritogenic activity of prostaglandin E2. Acta Derm Venereol (Stockh) 57: 37

Hägermark Ö, Rajka G, Bergqvist U (1972) Experimental itch in human skin elicited by rat mast cell chymase. Acta Derm Venereol (Stockh) 52: 125

Hägermark Ö, Strandberg K, Hamberg M (1977) Potentiation of itch and flare responses in human skin by prostaglandins E2 and H2 and a prostaglandin endoperoxide analog. J invest Dermatol 69: 527

Hägermark Ö, Hökfelt T, Pernow B (1978) Flare and itch induced by substance P in human skin. J Invest Dermatol 71: 233

Hanifin JM (1983) Clinical and basic aspects of atopic dermatitis. Semin Dermatol 2: 5

Harnack K (1980) Experimental itch as a diagnostic method. Acta Derm Venereol [Suppl] (Stockh) 92: 87

Haxthausen H (1957) Interpretation and value of skin tests in atopic dermatitis. Acta Derm Venereol (Stockh) Proceedings of 11th International Congress of Dermatology, Vol 3 p 6

Jacquet L (1904) In: Besnier E, Brocq L, Jacquet L (eds) La pratique Dermatologique, Vol 5, Masson, Paris

Jordan JM, Whitlock FA (1972) Emotions and the skin: the conditioning of scratch responses in cases of atopic dermatitis. Br J Dermatol 86: 574

Kaaber K, Veien N (1977) The significance of chromate ingestion in patients allergic to chromate. Acta Derm venereol (Stockh) 57: 321

Keele CA, Armstrong D (1964) Substances producing pain and itch. Arnold, London

Lovell CR, Burton PA, Duncan EHL, Burton JL (1976) Prostaglandins and pruritus. Br J Dermatol 94: 273

Mihm MC, Soter N, Dvorak HF, Austen KF (1976) The structure of normal skin and morphology of atopic eczema. J Invest Dermatol 67: 305

Morsbach P (1962) Über inhalative Provokationsteste bei Atopie. Inaugural dissertation, Juris, Zürich

Nexmand PH (1948) Clinical studies of prurigo Besnier. Rosenkilde and Bagger, Copenhagen

O'Leary PA (1953) Atopic dermatitis. South Med J 64: 67

Orr AW (1979) Prodromal itching in asthma. J R Coll Gen Pract 29: 287

Paganelli R, Levinski RJ, Brostoff J, Wraith DG (1979) Immune complexes containing food proteins in normal and atopic subjects after oral challenge and effect of sodium cromoglycate on antigen absorption. Lancet I: 1270

Patterson R (1959) Ragweed allergy in the dog. JAMA 135: 178

Rajka G (1963) Studies in hypersensitivity to molds and staphylococci in prurigo Besnier (atopic dermatitis) Acta Derm Venereol (Stockh) 13: 54

Rajka G (1967) Itch duration in the involved skin of atopic dermatitis (prurigo Besnier) Acta Derm Venereol (Stockh) 47: 154

Rajka G (1968) Itch duration in the uninvolved skin of atopic dermatitis (prurigo Besnier) Acta Derm Venererol (Stockh) 48: 320

Rajka G (1980a) Itch and IgE in atopic dermatitis. Acta Derm Venereol [Suppl] (Stockh) 92: 38

Rajka G (1980b) Pruritus. In Korting GW (ed) Dermatologie in Praxis und Klinik, vol I. Thieme, Stuttgart, p 239

Rettig A, Rettig PA, Kittredge D (1984) Prodromal itching in asthma. Lancet II: 44

Rocha de Silva M (1940) Beiträge zur Pharmakologie des Trypsins. Arch Exp Pathol Pharmakol 174: 335

Rostenberg A (1955) Atopic dermatitis: a discussion of certain theories concerning its pathogenesis. In: Baer RL (ed) Atopic dermatitis. Lippincott, Philadelphia, p 57

Rothman S (1922) Beiträge zur Physiologie der Juckempfindung. Arch Dermatol Syph 139: 227

Rothman S (1954) Physiology and biochemistry of the skin. University of Chicago Press, Chicago

Rothman S (1960) Pathophysiology of itch sensation. In: Montagna W (ed) Cutaneous innervation. Pergamon, Oxford, p 189 (Advances in biology of skin vol I

Savin JA (1980) Itching. In: Rook A, Savin JA (eds) Recent advances in dermatology, vol V. Churchill Livingstone, Edinburgh, p 221

Savin JA, Paterson WD, Oswald I (1973) Scratching during sleep. Br J Dermatol 93: 296

Savin JA, Paterson WD, Oswald I, Adam K (1975) Further studies in scratching during sleep. Br J Dermatol 93: 297

Schnyder UW (1961) Neurodermitis vom klinisch-dermatologischen Standpunkt. Acta Allergol 16: 463

Serowy C, Klinker L (1971) Über tages- und jahreszeitliche Variationen des Juckreizes bei endogenen Ekzematikern in Ostseebad Heiligendamm. Dermatol Monatsschr 157: 653

Shelley WB, Arthur R (1957) The neurohistology and neurophysiology of the itch sensation in man. Arch Dermatol 76: 296

Solley GO, Gleich GJ, Jordon RE, Schroeter AL (1976) The late phase of the immediate wheal and flare skin reaction. J Clin Invest 58: 408

Soter NA, Mihm MC (1980) Morphology of atopic eczema. Acta Derm Venererol [Suppl] (Stockh) 92: 11

Storck H (1961) Le role de la predispostion, du systeme neurovégétatif et de l'allergie dans le prurigo de Besnier. Arch Belg Dermatol 17: 95

Stüttgen G, Klofat H, Strauch M (1965) Die Reaktion der normalen und krankhaft veränderten menschlichen Haut auf intrakutan und epikutan applizierte Endopeptidasen (Trypsin, Bromelin). Arch Klin Exp Dermatol 222: 580

Summerfield JA, Welch ME (1980) The measurement of itch with sensitive limb movement parameters. Br J Dermatol 102: 275

Swanbeck G, Rajka G (1970) Antipruritic effect of urea solutions. Acta Derm Venereol (Stockh) 50: 225

Tomasch J, Britton WA (1956) On the individual variability of fibre composition in human peripheric nerves J Anat 90: 337

Török L (1907) Über das Wesen der Juckempfindung. Z Psychol 46: 23

Trotter K, Wilkin JK (1986) Cognitive activity povokes changes in cutaneous blood flow (abstract). J Invest Dermatol 86: 512

Tuft L (1949) Importance of inhalant allergens in atopic dermatitis. J Invest Dermatol 12: 211

Ungar G, Hayashi H (1958) Enzymatic mechanisms in allergy. Ann Allergy 16: 542

von Frey M (1910) Physiologie des Sinnesorganes der menschlichen Haut. Ergeb Physiol 9: 351

Wasserman SI (1980) The mast cell: its diversity of chemical mediators. Int J Dermatol 19: 7

Wedell G, Palmer E, Taylor D (1959) The significance of the peripheral arrangements of the nerves which serve pain and itch. In Wolstenhalme GEW, O'Connor M (eds) Pain and itch. Nervous mechanisms. Ciba Foundation Study Grouß No 1. Churchill, London

Whitlock FA (1976) Psychophysiological aspects of skin disease. Saunders, London, p 126

Whitney DK, Bernstein JE (1984) Local action of N-allylnoroxymorphone on histamine induced pruritus. J Invest Dermatol 82: 415

Willemse A, von der Brom (1983) Investigations of the symptomatology and the significance of immediate skin test reactivity in canine atopic dermatitis. Res Vet Sci 34: 261

Zakon SJ, Taub SJ (1938) The inhalation of house and horse danders as an etiologic factor in atopic dermatitis. J Allergy 9: 523

Zotterman Y (1939) Touch, pain and tickling: an electrophysiological investigation on cutaneous sensory nerves. J Physiol (Lond) 95: 1

Zotterman Y (1959) Discussion to Weddel et al. In: Wolstenholme GEW, O'Connor M (eds) Pain and itch. Nervous mechanisms. Ciba Foundation Study Group No 1, Churchill, London p. 13

4 Histopathological and Laboratory Findings

4.1 Histopathological Findings

Considerable difficulties arise in describing the dermatopathological picture in AD because appearances not only differ according to the stage of the disease when the biopsy is taken, but are also modified by such factors as the almost inevitable scratching (Pinkus and Mehregan 1969; Ackerman 1978; see also Chap. 3).

The histological components of the clinical lesions in AD are nonspecific. The major difference between the papules of prurigo (Kocsard 1962) and eczema appears to concern vesicle formation in the epidermis; this, typically, is pronounced in eczema but is less prominent (microvesicles: Greither 1970) or absent in prurigo. Investigation the first visible prurigo reaction, follicular eczematous alterations are seen in the follicular and adjacent epidermis, including multinuclear epidermal cells. The latter have also been found in other eczematous lesions (Uehara 1980).

The following changes were noted in the usual paraffin-embedded biopsy specimens stained with hematoxylin-eosin or toludine blue (Pinkus and Mehregan 1969) but were especially pronounced when a newer technique using thin (1 cm thick) glutaraldehyde-fixed, Epon-embedded sections stained with Giemsa's stain (Dvorak and Mihm 1972) was employed:

Acute vesicular lesions showed epidermal hyperplasia with focal intercellular edema, vesiculation, and an epidermal infiltrate consisting predominantly of lymphocytes and macrophages. In the dermis, the endothelial cells of the superficial venous plexus were enlarged and contained large nuclei with clumped chromatin and prominent nucleoli. A perivenular infiltrate of lymphocytes and macrophages, occasionally neutrophils, basophils, and eosinophils, was noted. Activated histiocytes, often containing melanin, were distributed in the superficial dermis.

In *lichenified* plaques, the additional finding showed psoriasiform hyperplasia and hyper- and dyskeratosis. In the dermis the number of mast cells was significantly increased. The deeper venules were also involved, the basement membrane was thickened, and enlarged pericytes were noted. A conspicuous finding was that the cutaneous nerves showed demyelination and fibrosis at all levels of the dermis.

In *symptom-free* skin all of the described alterations were observed but to a lesser degree, including changes in epidermis, dermal venules, and nerves; the dermal infiltrate was mainly lymphocytic. The significance of these findings is that the symptom-free skin in AD differs from normal skin (cf. Sect. 7.2).

In the *dry, xerotic* skin in AD, moderate but obviously inflammatory changes with discrete mononuclear infiltrate are observed (Van Neste et al. 1985): in other words, similar lesions to those in symptom-free skin.

By applying immunological markers (direct and indirect immunofluorescence with antihuman T-lymphocyte antisera and immune adherence), Braathen et al. (1979) showed T-lymphocytes in the dermal infiltrate. Furthermore, by using monoclonal antibodies and the immuneperoxidase technique, it was found that lymphocytic infiltrate in AD primarily consists of T helper cells, whereas the number of T suppressor cells was low (Leung et al. 1983; Zachary et al. 1985). In addition to reports affirming the T suppressor cell reduction, an opposing view is present by Sarfati et al. 1982. Other important cells of AD skin, like mast cells, Langerhans' cells, and eosinophils will be discussed in Chap. 6.

In the electron microscope, skin from exudative infantile AD was found to show abnormal keratinization: the granular layer keratinocytes were larger and contained aggregates of tonofilaments with a moderate number of lysosomes. In addition, keratinocytes from the upper epidermis contained lysozymes.
In stratum granulosum, as well as in stratum corneum, there were signs of intercellular fluid. In chronic lichenified lesions the changes were less striking (Prose 1965; Prose et al. 1965; Frichot and Zelickson 1972).

Sebaceous glands in the scalp of AD infants were reduced in number and showed retarded development: their basal cells were smaller than normal and lacked evidence of secretory activity in the form of lipids. Furthermore, serial sections revealed no poral occlusion of the sweat gland (Prose 1965).

Although in the above-mentioned papers spongiosis (vesiculation) was reported, the presence of spongiosis is a highly controversial topic. Some authors do not consider it to be a hallmark of the disease (see also Sect. 1.2) and it is probably not related to the mechanism of the lesions, Russell Jones believes that in all "eczemas" the primary event is dermal; it begins with edema of the superficial venular plexus and there is subsequent transepidermal elimination of this papillary edema (Russel Jones and MacDonald 1982).

The microscopic picture of AD shows certain similarities to that of contact dermatitis. The main differences consist of an absence of fibrin deposition, the presence of marked nerve changes, less epidermal involvement, and less dermal infiltration in AD (Soter and Mihm 1980).

4.2 Laboratory Findings

Critical evaluation has made it clear that no significant abnormality occurs, even infrequently, in laboratory investigations of AD patients, despite some reports to the contrary. Although Reinberg and Sidi (1959) and MacCardle et al. (1941) found low levels of calcium and magnesium in the skin, Lipkin et al. (1964) found both their levels to be normal or unspecifically higher. In 65 children with AD, the zinc values in serum were lower compared to controls, independently of the clinical state of the patients (David et al. 1984). Reduced zinc levels were also found by another group (Hinks et al. 1987) but this was connected with unspecific inflammation.

The alkali reserve and the salicylate binding capacity in the blood are normal. Gastric hypoacidity and achlorhydria have reputedly been associated with AD in some cases, but no statistically valid evaluation has yet demonstrated any correlation. However, an association with a flat glucose tolerance curve has been recorded (Rost and Marchionini 1932).

The level of unsaturated fatty acids was found to be lower by Hansen as long ago as 1933. Increased linoleic acid and reduction of its metabolites in serum lecithin were registered by Strannegård et al. (1987). These abnormal fatty acid values were also observed in cord blood (in patients with high IgE) and were interpreted as a basic feature of AD.

In one investigation 23% of AD patients over 18 years of age and 7% of those under that age were found to have an abnormal electroencephalogram (Russel and Last 1955). This unconfirmed finding contrasts with the relationship between age and the intensity of skin lesions in AD. The conclusion is that the mentioned alterations, even if confirmed by further works, can be considered as secondary events in the mechanism of AD.

References

Ackerman B (1978) Histologic diagnosis of inflammatory skin diseases. Lea and Febiger, Philadelphia, p 259, 691

Braathen RL, Forre O, Hovik JB, Eeg Larsen T (1979) Predominance of T-lymphocytes in the dermal infiltrate of atopic dermatitis. Br J Dermatol 100: 511

David TJ, Wells FE, Sharpe TC, Gibbs ACD (1984) Low serum zinc in children with atopic eczema. Br J Dermatol 111: 597

Dvorak HF, Mihm MC (1972) Basophil leukocytes in allergic contact dermatitis. J Exp Med 135: 235

Frichot BC III, Zelickson AS (1972) Steroids, lysosomes and dermatitis. Acta Derm-venereol (Stockh) 52: 311

Greither A (1970) On the different forms of prurigo, pruritus-prurigo. In: Mali JW (ed) Current problems in dermatology, vol 3. Karger, Basel, p 1

Hansen AE (1933) Study of the iodine number of serum fatty acids in infantile eczema. Proc Soc Exp Biol Med 30: 1198

Hinks LJ, Young S, Clayton B (1987) Trace element status in eczema and psoriasis. Clin Exp Dermatol 12: 93

Kocsard E (1962) The problem of prurigo. Aust J Dermatol 6: 156

Leung DYM, Schneeberger E, Geha RS (1983) Characterization of the mononuclear cell infiltrate in atopic dermatitis using mononuclear antibodies. J Allergy Clin Immunol 71: 47

Lipkin G, March C, Gowdey J (1964) Magnesium in epidermis, dermis and whole skin of normal and atopic subjects. J Invest Dermatol 42: 293

MacCardle RC, Engman MF, Engman MF (1941) The spectrograpic analysis of neurodermatitic lesions. Arch Dermatol Syph 44: 429

Pinkus M, Mehregan A (1969) A guide to dermatohistopathology. Appleton, New York

Prose PH (1965) Pathological changes in eczema. J Pediatr 66(2): 178

Prose Ph, Sedlis E, Bigelow M (1965) The demonstration of lysozymes in the diseased skin of infants with infantile eczema. J Invest Dermatol 45: 448

Reinberg A, Sidi E (1959) Tétanie chronique et eczema constitutionnel. Ann Endocrinol (Paris) 20: 186

Rost GA, Marchionini A (1932) Asthma-Eksem, Asthma-Prurigo und Neurodermitis als allergische Hautkrankheiten. Würz Abh Gesamtgeb Prakt Med 27: 10

Russel B, Last SL (1955) Besnier's prurigo: observations on abnormal cutaneous and central nervous relations. Br J Dermatol 67: 65

Russel Jones R, MacDonald DM (1982) Eczema. Immunopathogenesis and histogenesis. Am J Dermatopathol 4: 335

Sarfati M, Rocha C, Delespesse G (1982) Characterization of the cellular infiltrate in the skin lesions of atopic eczema with mononuclear antibodies. J Allergy Clin Immunol 69: 135

Soter NA, Mihm MC (1980) Morphology of atopic eczema. Acta Derm Venereol [Suppl] (Stockh) 92: 11

Strannegård IL, Svennerholm L, Strannegård Ö (1987) Essential fatty acids in serum lecithin of children with atopic dermatitis and in umbilical cord serum of infants with high or low IgE levels. Int Arch Allergy Appl Immunol 82: 422

Uehara M (1980) Prurigo reaction in atopic dermatitis. Acta Derm Venereol [Suppl] (Stockh) 92: 109

Van Neste D, Douka M, Rahier J, Staquet MJ (1985) Epidermal changes in atopic dermatitis. Acta Derm Venereol [Suppl] (Stockh) 114: 67

Zachary CB, Allen MH, MacDonald DM (1985) In situ quantification of T-lymphocyte subsets and Langerhans' cells in the inflammatory infiltrate of atopic eczema. Br J Dermatol 112: 149

5 Pathomechanism:
Genetic and Immunological Factors

5.1 Genetic Factors

Evaluation of much of the early literature on heredity in atopy proves difficult mainly because of the terminology in use at that time. It was imprecise and included atopic manifestations other than the principal ones. A hereditary predisposition to atopy, as postulated by Coca and Cooke (1923), including the transferability of specific antibodies, was subsequently confirmed by several authors. These included Edgren (1943), who demonstrated an increased frequency of respiratory atopic manifestations in patients who had previously suffered from AD. Clinicians investigating atopic subjects found hereditary background of atopy, including asthma, rhinitis, and AD, in 62%–68% in their cases (Rost and Marchionini 1932; Korting 1958; Baer 1955), and, despite possible sources of error, the Scandinavian series of Hellerström and Lidman (1956) and of the author (Rajka 1960) both gave the incidence as 68%. Reports on "allergic" children gave an even higher incidence (Freeman and Johnson 1964; Kaufman and Frick 1976). These and similar findings support the conclusion that the coexistence of AD and atopic respiratory disease is genetically determined (Schwartz 1952; Schnyder 1960; Rajka 1960).

5.1.1 Mode of Inheritance

One fundamental question was the mode of inheritance in atopic disease. Wiener et al. (1936) proposed a genetic model with an allelic pair of genes for the same chromosomal locus. They assumed that the predisposition to an allergic constitution is carried by an abnormal, recessive allele h; the normal allele H of the gene pair is, of course, dominant. Homozygotes with a normal pair of alleles HH are normal, whereas those with an abnormal hh pair always develop allergic manifestations before puberty. Of the heterozygotes, with one normal and one abnormal allele Hh, five-sixths are clinically normal carriers of the trait, the remaining one-sixth developing allergic disease after puberty. In the investigation of heredity in atopic disease this theory has, however, been rejected by most authors, who have assumed that the principal gene predisposing to atopy is dominant with low penetrance: its frequency of expression was given as 38% by Schwartz (1952) and as 50% by Schnyder and Borelli (1965). It has therefore been considered that the mode of transmission is a dominant one, but due to the variability with which the abnormal gene is expressed, it may appear to be "irregularly" dominant. This feature has understandably led other workers to conjecture that the inheritance is polygenic with additional, independently transmitted genes being involved (see below). The author (Rajka 1960) also found the earlier proposed recessive theory improbable, as he had observed nonatopic children both of whose parents had atopic disease. This means that the mode of inheritance is probably not monogenic but is multifactorially determined. Other data support this theory (van Arsdal and Motulsky 1959; Vogel and Motulsky 1979; Marsh et al. 1981).

Progress in studying the mode of inheritance has mostly been achieved by the study of twins. This investigative method has long been used (Spaich and Ostertag 1936, but, not infrequently, small series were considered and the determination of zygosity, mostly according to Siemens polysymptomatic method (1924) and/or based on several blood type systems, was not always mentioned. Thus the results (see Table 5.1) were rather variable: for monozygosity the concordance rate was 40–100% and for dizygosity 0%–67%. Low such rates (15.4% and 4.5% respectively) were given by Edfors-Lubs (1971).

Using the Danish Twin register, which was the first one established in the world (Harvald and Hauge 1956), 1184 mailed questionnaires were sent to like-sexed twins, identified by the central register of personal numbers. Sixty-nine twins from 48 twin pairs were clinically investigated according to the diagnostic criteria of Hanifin and Rajka (1980) (see Chap. 10), including HLA types, IgE titers, and lymphocyte characteristics (Schultz Larsen 1985; Schultz Larsen et al. 1986). His chief conclusion based on this data was that genetic factors play a decisive role in the development of AD (see Table 5.2 and also Chap. 8).

Krain and Terasaki (1973) and Turner et al. (1977) claimed that a relationship might exist between the HLA-ABC system and AD; however, this was disputed by others (Desmons et al. 1976; Scholtz et al. 1977; MacKie and Dick 1979) and recently Schultz Larsen's (1985) studies have confirmed that no such relationship exists.

Table 5.1. Larger series of atopic twins reported in the literature

	Monovular twins		Dizygotic twins	
	Concordance	Discordance	Concordance	Discordance
Atopic manifestations				
Spaich and Ostertag (1936)	6	6	2	19
Haynal and Schnyder (1960)	6	6	1	22[a]
Total	12	12	3	41
AD only				
Spaich and Ostertag (1936)	2	2	2	1
Rajka (1960)	2	3	6	3
Haynal and Schnyder (1960)	2	2	0	1
Niermann (1964)	5	0	3	10
Vogel and Dorn (1964)	1	6		
Lynfield (1974)	1	1	0	2

[a] Rate of concordance for monovular twins, 50%; for dizygotics, about 4%

Table 5.2. Number of condordant and discordant twin pairs with AD and the concordance rates for the two types of zygosity (after Schultz-Larsen 1985)

	Monozygotes	Dizygotes
Concordant twin pairs	17	4
Discordant twin pairs	5	22
Pairwise concordance rate[a]	0.77	0.15
Proband concordance rate[b]	0.86	0.21

[a] Proportion of concordance pairs among affected twin pairs
[b] Proportion of affected co-twins of probands (risk of the disease in background population is 0.03–0.10)

5.1.1.1 Organ Transmission

There can, as yet, be no decision as to whether the atopic gene is pleiotropic, predisposing to both skin and respiratory atopic disease, or whether the various atopic manifestations are expressions of different allelic genes, of genes at different loci, or of both.

According to the studies already discussed, there is a considerable likelihood that AD patients will have an atopic heredity; the probability that they will have a hereditary predisposition specifically to AD is lower (see also Table 5.1 b). In other words, of the two genetic influences – one expressed as the atopic state, the other determining the particular organ affected – the former is the stronger. The results of Schnyder (1972) showed that AD patients more often have a family history of that disease – the incidence being 44.4% – than of atopic respiratory disease; this clearly points to the importance of genetic factors in selecting which organ or organs will manifest atopic disease. Vogel and Dorn (1964) stressed that a separate gene is responsible for transmitting the susceptibility of an organ to atopic disease. Whereas it seems that a "principal" gene is responsible for manifestations of atopy, and a different one for AD, it is possible that the latter and respiratory atopies may be attributable to the same genetic predisposition, a question which can only be answered by further thorough investigation.

5.1.2 Transmission of IgE and Other Features

Before the discovery of IgE, reagin transmission was postulated and studied. A hereditary tendency to produce reagins has been sought in families, but atopic heredity has been shown not to influence the results of skin testes and therefore the production of reagin. Reagin production, however, has been correlated with the presence of respiratory allergic manifestations (Schnyder 1960; Rajka 1960), and generally speaking, positive reactions to skin tests are more frequent in AD patients who have asthma, rhinitis, or both, than in those with the "pure" disease. According to the author's statistics, positive responses to skin tests were found in over 90% of patients with AD and respiratory atopy, but in only 70% of "pure" AD patients. Schnyder (1972) postulated that the genotype plays an important role in determining reagin production in atopic monozygotic twins; the type of reagin produced is, however, environment dependent. The author (Rajka 1960) investigated three monozygotic twin pairs and found that all six twins produced reagins, but that the results of skin tests differed in corresponding twins, and that this applied to all three pairs (see Table 5.3); Schnyder (1972), however, reported that reagin production is identical in 33.3% of AD cases.

All these findings emphasized the possibility of the existence of an independent reaginic gene. Later, the genetic relations to IgE production were studied. Bazarel et al. (1971) found that a separate gene controls IgE, and the same gene may also control the predisposition to atopy (Opreé et al. 1972). Further studies (Billewicz et al. 1974; Gerrard et al. 1974; Blumenthal et al. 1981; Wütrich et al. 1981) showed the complexity of the question. Blumenthal et al. (1981) believed that either multiple alleles at a single locus or more than one major locus are involved. Furthermore, the existence of antigen-specific and -nonspecific immune responses, regulated by different genes, has been postulated (Marsh et al. 1981).

In twin RAST studies it was found that the concordance was greater for monovular than for diovular twins (Wütrich et al. 1981). Possibly, antigen recognition of B- and T-lymphocytes, influencing IgE response, is also under genetic control (Aas 1978). One can thus conclude that IgE production in, for example, AD is partly regulated by genetic factors. Schultz-Larsen (1985) believes that the genetic variance of IgE comprises about 50% of the total phenotypic variance. Other factors may be assumed but not proven. For example, some parameters of AD skin, such as itchy skin (Rosenberg and Solomon 1968, 1971) or sebaceous secretion, may be genetically controlled, whereas, as shown above, the vasomotor function test seems not to be.

AD is more common in females (whereas in childhood AD the reverse may be true). To explain this, Schnyder (1972) proposed that an XX-containing karyotype lowers the threshold of a stimulus eliciting AD.

Table 5.3. Reactivity to allergens injected intracutaneously in three pairs of monovular twins with AD

Positive reactions of extracts of

No. 1. Horse hair, yeast
No. 2. Cat hair, hen's feather, fish
No. 5. Dog hair, yeast
No. 6. Horse hair, dust, mold
No. 9. Horse hair, birch, timothy, *Chrys. leucanthemum,* dust
No. 10. Cow hair, birch, timothy, *Chrys. leucanthemum,* shellfish

Table 5.4. Risk of developing atopy and AD, according to Petersen et al. (1986)

Family history	Risk in percent			
	Atopy	AD	If one sibling already has atopy	
			Atopy	AD
No parent atopic	7	3	15	9
One parent atopic	16	8	34	21
Two parents atopic	Not done	Not done	50	Not done

Material: 188 AD patients; 48% also had respiratory atopies. 2151 family members of AD patients; 72% had additional atopy; 37% had AD

5.1.3 Practical Consequences for the Clinician

Goertler and Schnyder (1975) made calculations on the basis of their patient material and concluded that the possibility of a child's developing AD is 15% if the parents are healthy, 25%–30% if one of them is atopic, and about 66% if both of them are atopic. Studying 188 patients with AD and 2151 family members, the following results shown in Table 5.4 were reported (Petersen et al. 1986).

It is unclear which child of atopic parents will be involved. In a study of AD families with between one and ten children, de Gracianski (1966) found that the youngest child is most prone to have the disease. On the other hand, Harnack and Lenz (1970) stressed that each child has the same possibility of developing atopic symptoms.

A closing remark: many unsolved questions still exist in this field, including the possibility of genetic heterogeneity in AD.

5.2 Atopic Allergens

5.2.1 General Remarks

It follows from the original concept of atopy that an immunological peculiarity, in the form of a demonstrable and special type of antibody, the atopic reagin, is characteristic of AD and of atopic respiratory disease. The relevant immunological traits will be briefly discussed below.

It has long been acknowledged that certain environmental substances, including inhalants, food, and microorganisms, can induce reagin production and are therefore allergenic for atopic subjects although harmless for most persons. Regarding terminology, the broad definition of Strauss (1960) will be used here: "Antigen is any substance capable of producing antibodies. An allergen is thought of as any substance capable of inducing an allergic reaction." In the case of atopic allergens, usually proteins or glycoproteins, the antibody is IgE.

A great deal of detailed knowledge is available about substances allergenic for atopics, including those with AD. In this context a valuable observation was that during hyposensitization for respiratory atopy the first manifestation of an AD not infrequently appeared (Storck 1979). Atopic patients may react to various allergens present in inhaled or ingested substances or in microorganisms reaching the skin. This can be verified by various test methods, primarily skin tests and RAST. Of several hundred different allergens only a few, in Europe probably less than ten, account for more than 96% of all allergies observed (Johansson 1986).

The first person to try to investigate the chemical nature of the atopic allergens was Berrens, who published several reports, dating from 1961, and later combined them in a monograph (Berrens 1971 a). The overall chemical composition of atopic allergens, i. e atopens ranges from almost exclusively protein with small quantities of carbohydrate, to predominantly carbohydrate with a small amount of peptide. Berrens and his co-workers isolated skin-sensitizing allergens from house dust, dandruff, kapok, liquorice, tomato, ipecac, cow's milk and egg-white, and evolved a theory based on a similarity in the chemical structure of these compounds. They proposed that atopens arise from nonphysiological reactions of the Maillard type between glycoprotein and reducing sugar; these create structural sites composed of lysine and ε-amino monosaccharide conjugates in the molecular framework. Berrens (1971 a) considered that, in atopics, the intensity of the reaction with reaginic IgE is determined solely by the number of these reactive, reducing lysine–sugar conjugates present in, and administered with, a carrier macromolecule. Optimal potency as an allergen seems to be possessed by substances having a molecular weight of about 30 000–40 000; this suggests that molecular size plays an important part in the relationship between structure and activity (Stanworth 1963).

Berrens' conclusion was that allergens in atopy differ characteristically from those in the other allergic diseases. Similarly, it has been emphasized that cockfoot pollen contains not only an antigenic factor which elicits IgE production, but also a factor A which evokes IgG precipitins (Augustin and Hayward 1962; Augustin et al. 1971). An opposing view was put forward by King (1980), suggesting that atopic allergens are not different from any other protein antigen. One of his main arguments was that several allergens can elicit both specific IgE and IgG reactions. These include P1 and a rye grass pollen allergen (Chapman et al. 1983) or the peptides from codfish allergen M. (Elsayed et al. 1980). Studies of codfish allergen M (Aas and Elsayed 1969) showed that two tetrapeptides (Asp-Glu-Asp-Lys and Asp-Glu-Leu-Lys) are responsible for the immunoclinical reactivity (Elsayed et al. 1976).

Recent works have verified the earlier assumption that inhalant allergens are complex, consisting of several allergens. These include cow hair (Prahl 1981), cat hair (Löwenstein et al. 1985), horse hair (Wahn et al. 1982) and several molds (see Sect. 5.2.7 and Table 5.5). (H. Löwenstein, personal communication). The purified allergens have in common that their molecular weight is usually 20 000–40 000, that they are the most abundant proteins present in the extract, and that their activity is markedly reduced on denaturation (King 1980). Atopic

Table 5.5. Antigens and specific allergens detected in a selection of allergen extracts (H. Löwenstein, personal communication 1985)

Extract	No. of patients	No. of antigens detected	No. of allergens detected	Patients with positive reactions to the major allergen (%)
Cat	31	15	10	96
Mite (Dp)	27	30	14	89
Timothy	30	36	11	87
Birch	20	40	6	100
Mugwort	29	42	10	100
Ragweed	37	52	22	95
Alternaria	27	44	16	85

allergens used as test substances lack uniformity as a result of differences in (a) sampling of the basic substance; (b) conditions of extraction; (c) methods and conditions of purification; (d) concentration of stock extracts; (e) sterility and toxicity; (f) standardization and quality control; (g) disclosure of composition, and (h) instability of the extract under different conditions, and possibly for other reasons as well. Thus there is an obvious need to standardize and to control the antigenicity of these substances. A great deal of work in this area has already been carried out in Scandinavia (Aas and Belin 1972). It is most essential to check the purity of the allergen, for such tests are known to involve not only important major allergens but also antigens and proteins unrelated to clinical allergy.

5.2.1.1 Improved Allergen Extracts

During the last decade, important progress has been made in the characterization, purification, and standardization of commercial allergen extracts. This was achieved by applying biochemical, chromatographic, electrophoretic, and immunological methods. Regarding the latter, particular attention has been focused on crossed immuno- and radioimmunoelectrophoresis (CIE and CRIE), which can indentify and compare allergens and control the composition and stability of the extracts. Furthermore, these methods may be used for measuring allergenic potency; in vitro the latter can be assessed by means of the RAST inhibition method (for further information, see, e. g., Einarsson 1985).

5.2.2 Skin Testing

The various commercial or laboratory allergenic extracts have previously been generally applied as intracutaneous tests, injecting no more than 0.02 ml extract and taking into consideration several factors. These include; the site of injection (on lower or upper arm or even on the back, which is more sensitive), the ambient temperature and season, and drugs (particularly antihistamines, to some extent corticosteroids, and also immunotherapy) being administered to the patient (Van der Bijl 1960). In addition, testing in severe systemic or generalized skin diseases is contraindicated, and the testing should not, of course, be performed during a very active or secondarily infected phase of AD (see below).

Besides allergenic extracts it is always necessary to apply negative (physiological saline) and positive (histamine) controls for biological comparison.

The ensuing reaction, a wheal, is read on average after 15 min and the size calculated in mm^2 (area) or in mm (diameter). The reading and evaluation of skin test responses is subject to considerable variation. Reactions seen include the "pseudopositive", which is nonspecific and polyvalent; such a reaction is usually due to mechanical trauma (tests may be too close to each other), to a very active phase of the skin disease, or to the presence of mechanical urticaria. The "pseudonegative" response is due, for example, to unstable extracts or a local tissue unresponsiveness, and here evaluation is complicated by the frequent absence of a flare or halo around the wheal in AD (see Sect. 7.4.4). It is further advisable to read the test after 6–8 h for a possible late cutaneous reaction.

Criteria for grading the reactions are unfortunately far from uniform. This lack of comparability is particularly evident in studies from countries where standardization has not been attempted, but may also be seen even in reports from Scandinavia, despite the official recommendations of the Northern Allergy Society.

Weakly reacting skin tests show the most marked differences in interpretation and grading, and have the least agreement with results of the RAST (Öhman 1971). Furthermore, on being repeated 6 months later, 27% have a grading different to that of the first testing, compared with only 5% in the case of stronger reactions (Gottlieb et al. 1960). These facts highlight the discrepancies in skin test statistics. Since the 1920s (Engman and Wander 1921; Haxthausen 1925), a large number of researchers have carried out skin test series on AD patients, and the relevant data, presented below, are derived from several series, each with upwards of 100 patients. Some of these series included cases of AD coupled with respiratory atopy (Table 5.6). The author's statistics for over 1200 patients tested with 48 extracts are given in Fig. 5.1 and Table 5.7, the high proportion of positive reactions probably being due to the application of so much allergen (Rajka 1961).

The intracutaneous type of testing was later considered to use a greater amount of allergens and thus to be less safe for testing purposes. It has generally been replaced by prick or scratch methods, which are simple to perform. According to most authors, the skin prick test methods give an adequate degree of specificity – provided that satisfactory allergens are used – in addition to being safe in that only minimal amounts of allergen are introduced into the skin (about 100 times less than in intracutaneous tests). Safety is particularly important when testing AD infants and children. To improve the skin test results, a new prick test method has recently been introduced, namely the Phazet (i. e., allergen-coated sterile lancets ready to use for skin prick testing). The lancets are individually wrapped in an envelope of aluminum/paper laminate (Österballe and Weeke 1979; Dreborg 1985).

Table 5.6. References on frequency of immediate-type reactions in AD

	No. of patients with AD	Positive immediate skin reactions (%)
Adults:		
Alexander (1931)	11 443	52.7 (compilation of 44 U.S. authors)
Brunsting (1936)	100	70
Norrlind (1946)	100	78
Hellerström and Lidman (1956)	311	90 (including patch tests)
Schnyder (1957)	136	57
Oddoze (1959)	117	69.2 (excluding molds, bacteria)
Children (infantile eczema):		
O'Keefe and Rackemann (1929)	239	52
Epstein and Palacek (1951)	231	75
Kesten (1954)	2 000	75 (about ¼ of the patients were over 6 years)
Meara (1955)	112	65
Ratner and Collins-Williams (1958)	114	97

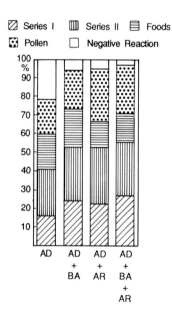

Fig. 5.1. Positive intracutaneous reactions according to atopic symptoms. *AD*, atopic dermatitis; *BA*, bronchial asthma; *AR*, atopic rhinitis. *Series I:* inhalants (especially animal hair); *series II:* inhalants (especially dust and molds)

5.2.2.1 The Value of Skin Testing

There are considerable differences of opinion about the value of skin testing and especially about the data provided by skin test results from different sources. The differences in allergen extracts have already been mentioned. Among other relevant variables are the conditions of exposure and those allergens, such as fungi, which may be peculiar to different geographical areas. Of even greater importance are the patients under study, for whether or not AD is

Table 5.7. Results of immediate skin tests in 643 patients with AD and in matched controls

	Series I		Series II		Foods[a]		Egg		Pollen		Negative	
	Number of positive reactions	%	Number of positive reactions	%	Number of positive reactions	%	Number of positive reactions	%	Number of positive reactions	%	Number of positive reactions	%
Group I[b]: 123 patients[c]	17	11.5	12	8.1	43	29.1	18	12.2	15	10.1	43	29.1
Group II: 131 patients	32	15.9	46	22.9	29	14.4	4	2.0	41	20.4	49	24.4
Group III: 174 patients	47	15.9	74	25.1	38	12.9	4	1.4	66	22.4	66	22.4
Group IV: 207 patients	65	18.4	119	33.7	45	12.7	–	–	64	18.1	60	17.0
Group V: 8 patients	1	7.7	5	38.5	4	30.8	–	–	2	15.4	1	7.7
Total 643	162	16.0	256	25.3	159	15.7	26	2.6	188	18.6	219	21.7
50 patients without allergic symptoms or known history	1	2.0	1	2.0	3	6.0			1	2.0	44	88.0
50 patients with a skin disease other than AD	15	19.5	19	24.7	13	16.9			4	5.2	26	33.8

Series I: inhalants (especially animal hair)
Series II: inhalants (especially dust and molds)
[a] Food allergens excluding egg
[b] Group I: 0–6 years; group II: 7–12 years; group III: 13–18 years; group IV: 19–45 years; group V: 46 years and over
[c] One patient had several reactions
χ^2 test between A and B:
Series I: $P < 0.1\%$
Series II: $P < 0.1\%$
Foods: $0.1\% < P < 1\%$
Pollen: $P < 0.1\%$

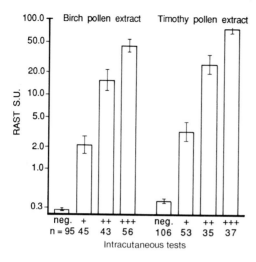

Fig. 5.2. Correlation between results of 470 RAST and skin tests. The *bars* represent mean strength of the RAST reaction with ±SE indicated at the top. (Wide et al. 1972)

"pure" or is combined with respiratory atopy determines a difference in skin reactivity; thus the sum of a patient's atopic manifestations is essential information. Finally, it is most important to know the age group of the patients studied (Hill and Sulzberger 1935), as dietary allergens predominate in the younger, and inhalant allergens in the older age groups. In order to illustrate the reliability of the skin tests, comparison with other methods is necessary.

In the past, passive transfer, as used by Prausnitz and Küstner (1921) and de Besche (1923), or its modifications, was used to supplement and to check skin reactions to certain allergens. Later, a reliable in vitro method, the radioallergo-sorbent test (RAST), was designed, and this can be used instead of passive transfer as both methods measure circulating reaginic antibody and seem to have a similar degree of sensitivity (Wide and Wiholm, quoted by Wide et al. 1972). Very good agreement between skin tests and the RAST was demonstrated by Wide et al. (1972) (see Fig. 5.2), who subsequently compared, in 220 cases, the RAST with nasal and inhalation provocation tests and found a 95% correlation between the two. Other in vitro biological tests demonstrate reagins by releasing histamine from sensitized leukocytes (Lichtenstein and Osler 1964) or from passively sensitized human and monkey lung (Parish 1967; Ishizaka et al. 1970).

5.2.2.2 Comparison of Skin Tests with Clinical Findings

Adequately performed skin tests alone have no great significance in AD, and, although provocation tests and the RAST are helpful in their evaluation, to be meaningful their results have to be assessed in the light of, and be consistent with, the patient's history and clinical course. This point of view is considered in the following discussion on allergic groups. The available information on this subject is valid only for "pure" AD cases, in which several of the positive skin test reactions may represent latent sensitization or an immunological warning that respiratory atopic symptoms may appear in the future.

Principally skin tests could be compared with provocation tests. Provocation tests are considered to be reliable clinical methods for demonstrating the presence of antibodies, provided certain precautions are taken, particularly in inhalation and nasal tests. These precautions are:

1. Patients should not be taking drugs that could influence the tests.
2. The concentration and the method of administration of the allergens should be capable of eliciting an allergic but not a nonspecific reaction in the target organ.
3. Control tests should be performed by the simple blind method; suitable control substances are allergen extracts to which the patient is known to be nonallergic.
4. The test site should be examined before and after testing, and the reaction should be recorded.

The test is positive if the local changes in appearance or in function are characteristic of allergy and are beyond the bounds of normal variation, but it is of diagnostic value only when the corresponding control test is negative (Aas 1970). Unfortunately the easy and reliable nasal or conjunctival provocation test in respiratory atopics has no strict counterpart in AD. Intracutaneous and subcutaneous provocation tests are easily carried out, but it is doubtful whether they adequately reproduce the mode of entry of allergens in AD, and, while inhalation tests would seem to be more appropriate from an immunological point of view, they seldom produce objective skin changes. Furthermore, the most appropriate timing of their reading is uncertain, suggestions ranging from a few minutes to several hours. In fact, it is the author's experience that pruritus is the cardinal and often the only sign observed (see also Chap. 3). The significance of immediate reactions in AD is still controversial. Thus, the old discussion as to whether or not skin testing in AD has any value, has not yet been settled. In the opinion of the author, it is of value for the following reasons:

1. It provides evidence for or against an atopic background in the patient.
2. It provides information on some allergens; if the significance of this information is confirmed by the history, it may enable advice to be given on elimination of the allergen concerned (e. g., certain food allergens in infants).
3. It may reveal inhalant allergens significant for respiratory atopy coexisting with AD, with obvious therapeutic consequences.
4. It provides information which can be scientifically evaluated (e. g., disappearance rate of some allergic responses, one of the methods for standardization of new allergens).

5.2.3 Inhalants: Pollen

There is no doubt that, in a minority of AD patients, pollen sensitivity may play a not insignificant role in the pathogenesis of their disease, as a seasonal aggravating factor for example. In this respect ragweed pollen has been incriminated by several authors (Feinberg 1939; Rowe 1946; Tuft and Heck 1952). However, it has already been noted that, in the author's series, grass pollen could be credited with only a trivial, and tree pollen with a minor role in influencing the seasonal course of AD. In similar investigations, Eichenberger (1963) noted only slight seasonal differences, and Schnyder (1957) found none. Nevertheless, a positive reaction to allergen, inhaled as a provocation test in "pure" AD patients, strengthens the hypothesis that pollen may play an etiological role.

Indeed, Storck et al. (1960) noted both clinical exacerbation and the development of new lesions in AD patients after pollen inhalation, and Nilzén (1958) recorded positive reactions in inhalation tests in four of eight AD patients. An interesting property of pollens is their possible content of a component that is not allergenic either for animals or for man, but which nonspecifically enhances vascular permeability; this ingredient possibly resembles bradykinin in character (Eriksson 1965; Kind et al. 1967). Thus, while pollens are significant allergens in atopic rhinitis and asthma, and may play an important pathogenetic role in a minority of AD cases, in the majority they play no great part. The finding that serum IgE levels in these patients show no tendency to increase during the pollen season supports this view (Öhman et al. 1972).

Positive skin tests to pollens occurred in 18% of the author's AD cases, but in only 2%–5% of the controls (Rajka 1961). Such reactivity in "pure" AD patients may indicate that hay fever will later develop. For example, of nine children with a high serum IgE level, two had developed symptoms of allergic rhinitis when reinvestigated just 1 year subsequently (Öhman et al. 1972).

Reports in the literature given a similar incidence of pollen sensitivity in AD; however, in many instances no distinction is made between those cases with, and those without, respiratory atopic disease.

There are several indications that the month of birth has a relation to the development of atopy to pollen (see, e. g., Björksten and Suoniemi 1981).

5.2.4 Inhalants: Animal Hair

Domestic animal hair is a well-known allergen. Feathers are included under this heading and, although they may provoke skin reactions in AD, it is suspected that their house dust content is responsible for their allergenicity (Voorhorst 1962). Haxthausen (1925) was one of the first investigators to skin test AD patients with animal hair extract; many other researchers, including Brunsting (1936), Hill (1937), Zakon and Taub (1938), and Bonnevie (1939), followed suit. The author found that 10%–15% of his AD cases were sensitive to hair (Rajka 1961), and, although analysis of the data showed that only one-third of these had a history of direct contact with domestic animals, there are everyday sources of possible contact with animal products such as hair-containing mattresses and upholstered furniture, meat products, and sometimes horse serum (Hård 1950; Stanworth 1957). Furthermore, only 18% of those with positive skin tests had a history of sensitivity to animals, which was usually provoked by horse-riding, grooming, or involuntary contact with horse hair; in exceptional cases, contact with guinea pigs or rabbits was incriminated.

Most contact with animals took place in summer, yet, when the patients's history could be checked, it was found that the dermatitis improved in that season. In this respect, therefore, skin test results correlated poorly with clinical data. The keeping of pets is common among children; over 50% had furred pets at home (Kjellman and Petterson 1983). Cats are more frequent elicitors of respiratory atopy in children, presumably due to a more intimate contact than is usual with dogs (Murray 1983). It is unclear whether this also is relevant for AD. It should be mentioned in this context that eight of ten AD patients who gave positive reactions to skin tests with animal hair displayed clinical deterioration when given provocation tests (Nilzén 1958). Zakon and Taub (1938) described the production of pruritus by nasal challenge tests, whereas in the AD patients studied by Bonnevie (1939), a positive response to provocation tests was the exception.

Characterization of the allergenic components after gel filtration in RAST investigations showed that, as might be predicted, horse epithelial extracts vary greatly in their composition. However, an additional, unpredicted finding was that atopic individuals react to different components of the extract (Wide et al. 1972).

5.2.5 Inhalants: Human Dandruff

The possibility that human epidermis might be allergenic was suspected by early investigators (Keller 1924; Hampton and Cooke 1941) and was investigated by Simon (1944, 1949). Despite criticism being leveled against the results, on the grounds that different extracts and concentrations had been used, their clinical significance has been confirmed (Magnusson 1954). The contribution made by Berrens (1971 a) gave new relevance to this question, for his chemical analyses led him to the view that allergenic activity may be imparted to glycoprotein carrier molecules by the formation of monosaccharide-conjugated lysine residues.

Although human and horse dandruff have no proven allergenic determinant in common, their allergens share functional properties. Human dandruff allergens are absent from sweat as secreted, but are present in sweat collected from the skin surface (Berrens 1971 a). Furthermore, Hénocq et al. (1966) found cross-reactivity between house dust and human dandruff in some cases of AD. Positive RAST reactions have also been demonstrated (Berrens and Guikers 1980). Therefore, the existence of an allergen in human dandruff is not in dispute, but its significance in AD needs further evaluation.

The discovery that human dandruff is allergenic raises the question as to whether this chemically modified, and therefore not entirely native, skin component might be a potential autoallergen. In this respect, the investigations of Hashem et al. (1963) are particularly pertinent. They demonstrated that lymphocyte transformation was induced by autologous and homologous skin extracts from normal subjects tested with lymphocytes from children with AD. These findings were not confirmed in adult AD cases by some later investigators, including Borelli (1970), and the author's results (Rajka, unpublished observations) were inconclusive, but the role of autosensitization in AD remains relevant.

A new perspective was given by reports that human dander may elicit positive patch test reactions in 66% of AD patients (Uehara and Ofuji 1976). Human dander fractions gave positive patch reactions after stripping the stratum corneum in AD patients but not in controls. The same patients also showed delayed reactions to mite extracts (cross-reactivity?), which argues against a specific role of dander reaction in AD. However, human dander preparations have the capacity to elicit not only immediate but also delayed reactions in AD patients (Young et al. 1985).

5.2.6 Inhalants: House Dust and House Dust Mites

This conglomerate of assorted allergens, derived from such sources as epidermis, fungi, seeds, food particles, pollen, and acari, has, since the initial studies of Rost (1929), been widely investigated in connection not only with atopy but also with "pure" AD. The importance of dust as an allergen in AD was further stressed by Brunsting (1936), Hill (1937), and Zakon and Taub (1938), although it was pointed out a long time ago by Sulzberger (1940) that it might be nonallergic in character; indeed, in the opinion of later researchers, skin testing with the usual commercial extracts is of very limited value. Although positive responses in AD patients on challenge with house dust have frequently been reported (e. g., Tuft 1949; Storck 1955), provocation test results cannot be considered as valid evidence for an allergic mechanism. Such caution seems justified by the normal or only slightly elevated serum IgE levels in house dust sensitive atopic subjects (Johansson et al. 1970), and by the fact, pointed out by Schnyder (1957), that dust sensitivity cannot explain clinical deterioration in winter. On the other hand, after taking up residence in a dust-free highland environment, or after removing dust-producing items such as carpets or bedclothes from the house, clinical improvement has frequently been noted. Moreover, Lobitz and Jilson (1958) reported that an eczematous lesion subsequently developed on the site of a positive wheal reaction to house dust, and that there was an associated exacerbation of the AD.

The purification of house dust allergens has been approached from several angles with different interpretations of the results by the various researchers, including Berrens (1971 a). A polysaccharide fraction was used by Musso et al. (1959) to skin test AD patients, and as they found that a positive reaction was very common (in fact it was found in 91%), they suggested it to be indicative of atopy. However, Eichenberger (1963) as well as other authors were less successful in eliciting this reaction.

A new and fruitful field was opened by the demonstration that house dust mites are the main allergen and the cardinal factor in eliciting atopic respiratory symptoms. The prime offenders are *Dermatophagoides pteronyssinus* in Europe and Japan, and *D. farinae* in other parts of the world (Voorhorst et al. 1967; Maunsell et al. 1968; Pepys et al. 1968). The complexicity of *Dermatophagoides* allergens was shown, for example, in respect of *D. pteronyssinus*, which contains 49 antigens (Lind et al. 1984). Its main allergen, isolated from feces, was called P1 extract (Chapman et al. 1980). This glycoprotein with a molecular weight of 24 000 is found in high levels in dust from carpets, furniture, and clothing (Tovey et al. 1981). The most important habitat of mites is the mattress and there are optimal conditions, including temperature and human scales, for mites in beds. Mite body antigens were also isolated (Lind and Löwenstein 1983). Immediate skin test positivity and specific IgE antibodies were not only observed in asthma and rhinitis but also in AD (Alani and Harlov 1972; Chapman et al. 1983). A correlation with the clinical state of AD was also reported (Barnetson et al. 1987). The possible role of mites in AD was further supported by observed improvement of the disease after reduction of their number (August 1984; Zimmermann 1987). AD children born during the months of maximal mite exposure, i. e., the summer months, showed a higher prick test reactivity (Beck and Hagdrup 1987).

5.2.7 Inhalants: Molds

Sensitivity to molds is a very complex subject due to the large number of different species, geographical variations, and the presence of cross-reacting or specific allergens. Molds are present in house dust, but commercial extracts give more reliable results in mold than in house dust allergy and in skin testing. MMP extracts (Prince 1961) from molds grown on modified synthetic media were especially useful in the past.

As mentioned above, isolation of major allergenic fractions was performed for several mold species. RAST, RAST inhibition, and other techniques, were used to investigate the allergenic composition of *Alternaria,* (Yunginger et al. 1976), *Cladosporium* (Aas et al. 1980), and *Aspergillus* (Kerr et al. 1981).

The cross-reactivity of mold antigens, is a complex topic, both shared and unique antigens having been reported. In a thorough study of different strains from several species, primarily *Cladosporium herbarum,* minimal cross-reactivity was demonstrated despite multiple clinical sensitivities. These multiple sensitivities thus seem to be parallel to, but independent of, allergies.

Feinberg (1939) pointed out the significance of positive skin tests and of local reactions to molds, and noted a correlation between atmospheric mold counts and seasonal deterioration of AD in 14 patients. In subsequent larger series of Kesten (1954), Oddoze (1959), Hellerström and Lidman (1956), Norrlind (1946), and Jillson (1957), the frequency of positive skin test reactions to molds was found to lie between 10% and 29%. Jillson (1957) stressed the importance of the observation that delayed skin test reactions to molds may persist for 1–2 weeks, and be subsequently associated with a flare-up of the dermatitis. As almost 25% of the author's 643 patients with "pure" AD gave positive

Table 5.8. History of 30 AD patients with skin reactivity to molds

Patients	Question groups					Summary of "mold history"	Remarks	Role of other noxae[a] in the history
	I-II	IIb	III	IV	V			
AI	−	+	−	+	+	+++		Animals
AB	−	−	−	+	−	+		Foods
AH	(+)	−	−	+	+	++	(+)=living in wooden house	Foods
BP	−	−	−	?	(+)	(+)	(+)=uncertain	Perfumes, rubber
BSG	++	+	−	+	+	+++++		Foods
BSO	+	−	−	+	−	++		−
BI	+	+	−	+	+	++++		Foods
DB	(+)	−	−	+	−	+	(+)=living in wooden house	Foods, animals
EC	−	−	−	+	−	+		Foods
EK	(+)	−	−	+	+	++	(+)=wood fuel	Foods
EL	−	+	−	+	+	+++		−
GA	−	−	−	+	+	++		Foods
HB	−	−	−	+	+	++	Earlier bad housing conditions	−
HC	−	−	−	+	+	++		Foods, animals
HM	−	−	(+)	?	+	+	(+)=contact with old books	−
IL	−	−	−	(+)	−	(+)	(+)=uncertain	−
JE	(+)	+	+	+	+	++++	(+)=living in wooden house and uses wood fuel	Foods, animals(?)
JK	−	−	−	+	+	++		Foods, animals
KR	−	−	−	+	+	++		−
MG	(+)	−	−	−	+	+	(+)=living in wooden house	Foods
MO	−	−	(+)	+	−	+	(+)=works in confectionery	Foods
MB	(+)	−	−	+	+	++	(+)=living in wooden house	Foods
NR	++	−	−	+	−	+++		Foods
NT	−	+	−	−	−	+		Foods, animals, pollen
NC	−	+	−	+	+	+++		Foods
PP	−	−	−	+	−	+		−
RU	−	+	−	+	+	+++		Foods
SK	−	−	−	+	+	++		Foods
SB	++	+	−	+	+	+++++		Foods
UM	−	−	−	+	−	+		−

[a] They may act as allergens and/or irritants

Question groups:

I-II: housing conditions

IIb: staying in wooden summer residences } and influence on skin disease

III: working conditions

IV: course of the disease: improvement in summer and deterioration in autumn

V: influence on skin disease of different exposure factors related to molds (for example when cleaning, eating Roquefort cheese, drinking beer)

skin test reactions to molds (see Table 5.7), the significance of mold allergy was analyzed in 30 patients. This was achieved by scrutinizing their domestic and working environments, by skin testing with extracts of molds collected from their homes and with commercial nongeneric mold extracts, and by carrying out several other investigations, including passive transfer, in vitro neutralization and thrombocytopenic tests, patch tests, inhalant provocation tests, and gel identification tests. The findings are summarized in Tables 5.8–5.10 and Fig. 5.3. In addition, passive transfer was positive in 76% of 55 cases, neutralization tests were inconclusive, patch tests were invariably negative, and serum precipitins could not be demonstrated in those patients on whom tests were performed. Evaluation of all these results showed that in about 50% of the AD cases tested, and in 10%–15% of all the "pure" cases, there was in fact a clinically significant mold sensitivity (Rajka 1963).

Mold reactivity has important correlations with sensitivity to trichophytin. In an earlier work the author (Rajka 1963) showed that a cross-reactivity exists between airborne molds and trichophytin in AD, since 15 of 19 patients with *Cladosporium–Alternaria–Botrytis–Rhizopus* reactivity were positive to trichophytin. By comparing immediate skin tests and RAST in AD patients with and

Table 5.9. Intracutaneous reactions to molds in 30 AD patients

Concen-trations	Allergens	Immediate reactions		Delayed reactions	
		+ + or +	(+)	+	(+)
0.1%	1 *Alternaria tenuis*	11	3	1	2
0.1%	2 *Hormodendrum cladosporoides*[a]	12	3	2	–
0.1%	3 *Helminthosporium interseminatum*	5	2	1	2
0.1%	4 *Curvularia specifera*	10	6	2	4
0.1%	5 *Stemphylium botryosum*	8	6	2	3
0.1%	6 *Spondylocladium sp.*	10	4	1	1
1.0%	7 *Penicillium notatum*	15	7	1	2
1.0%	8 *Penicillium expans*	14	9	–	–
1.0%	9 *Penicillium brevicompactum*	12	6	1	1
1.0%	10 *Phoma betae*	12	7	–	1
1.0%	11 *Pullularia sp.*	12	4	–	1
1.0%	12 *Rhizopus nigricans*	13	5	1	1
1.0%	13 *N. sitophila*	8	7	–	1
1.0%	14 *Mucor racemosus*	14	4	–	2
1.0%	15 *Mucor mucedo*	7	6	–	4
1.0%	16 *Fusarium sp.*	10	4	–	2
1.0%	17 *Botrytis cinerea*	11	6	–	2
1.0%	18 *Aspergillus niger*	5	6	2	1
1.0%	19 *Aspergillus fumigatus*	2	3	–	–
1.0%	20 *Cladosporium*	14	3	–	1
		205	101	14	31

[a] *Hormodendrum* and *Cladosporium* are synonyms
Extracts 1–6 are MMP extracts; 7–20 are species extracts from a laboratory

Table 5.10. Evaluation of mold allergy in 30 AD patients

Patients	Immediate test category (Concentration 0.1% or 1.0%[a])	Delayed reaction (Concentration 0.1% or 1.0%[a])	Focal reaction after i.c. test	Subcutaneous injection				Inhalant exposure				Evaluation[b]
				Concentration 0.5% or 1% (dose in ml)	Local reaction	Focal reaction	Thrombocytopenic test	0.1% concentration (dose in ml)	Focal reaction	10% concentration (dose in ml)	Focal reaction	
AI	(+)	−	+	0.5	−	+	−					++
AB	++	−	−	2	−	−	−			2	−	++
AH	++	−	−	2	−	−	−					+?
BP	++	−	−	2	−	−	+	1	−			+?
BSG	+	−	−	0.5	−	−	−					−
BSO	++	(+)	−	0.5	−	−	−	1.5	−			++
BI	++	+	+	0.5	+	+	−					++
DB	(+)	−	−	0.5	−	−	+					+?
EC	−	−	−	0.5	−	−	−					−
EK	(+)	(+)	−	0.5	−	−	−					(+)+[c]
EL	(+)	−	−	2	−	+	−	3	−			−
GA	−	+	−	2	−	+	−					+
HB	(+)	+	−	2	−	+	+					++
HC	++	−	−	0.5	−	−	−					++
HM	++	(+)	+	0.5	−	−	+					+?
IL	+	−	−	0.5	−	+	+	1.5	−	2	−	(+)+[c]
JE	++	(+)	−	0.5	−	+	−					+?
JK	+	−	−	2	−	−	+	1	−			−
KR	+	−	−	2	−	−	−	1	−			+?
MG	(+)	+	−	2	−	+	+	1.5	−	2	−	++
MO	(+)	−	−	2	−	−	+					++
MB	++	(+)	+	2	−	−	+					−
NR	−	−	−	0.5	−	−	−					−
NT	+	−	−	2	+	−	−					++
NC	++	−	−	0.5	+	−	−	1.5		2	+	+

PP	(+)	−	−	0.5	+	−	+			+	++
RU	++	−	+	2	+	+	+		2		++
SK	+	−	−	2	−	+	−	1			(+)+ᶜ
SB	++	+	+	0.5	−	−	+	−			++
UM	++	+	+	0.5	+	−	−				++
30	11: ++ 8: + 8: (+) 3: −	5: + 4: (+) 21: −	7: + 23: −	16: 0.5 14: 2	5: + 25: −	9: + 21: −	11: + 19: −	8: −	2: + 3: −		15: ++ (+)+ 8: +, +? 7: −

ᵃ MMP extracts 0.1%, others 1%

ᵇ Criteria:
If local and/or focal reactions present: ++, (+)+
If only immediate test ++ positive: +
If (+) or + immediate and/or delayed reaction as well as positive thrombocytopenic test: (+)
If only positive thrombocytopenic test: (+)
If (+) or + immediate and/or (+) delayed reaction: (−)
If no reaction at all: (−)

ᶜ One plus to two plus

According to the results given in this table

Correlations existed:

Between: Focal reactions after i. c. tests and immediate tests: out of 7 patients with focal reactions, 6 had ++ and 1 (+) immediate test

Correlations were not observed:

Between: Thr. test and local/focal reactions

Between: Focal reactions after i. c. test and focal reaction after exposure test

Between: Delayed reactions and immediate test category

Between: Delayed reactions and thrombocyte tests

Between: Exposure doses and focal/local reactions, thrombocytopenic test

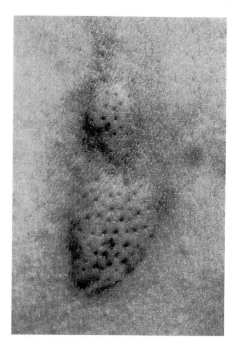

Fig. 5.3. Immediate reaction to 1% mucor racemosus *(top)* and to 1% mucor mucedo *(bottom).* (Rajka 1975)

Table 5.11. Intracutaneous reactions and RAST positivity in AD patients with tinea infections and controls (given as percentages)

	Intracutaneous reactivity								RAST		
	Trichophytin		*Penicillium*		*Cladosporium*			*Alternaria*		*Penicillium*	*Cladosporium*
	Immed	Del.	Immed.	Del.				Immed.	Del.		
					Immed.	Del.					
10 patients with AD + tinea	50	0	50	0	40	0		30	0	50	40
35 patients with AD	40	0	50	0	40	9		40	3	50	50
15 patients with LL tinea	66	33	0	0	6	0		0	0	0	6
15 controls	0	0	0	0	6	0		0	0	0	6

Abbreviations: AD, pure atopic dermatitis; LL, long-lasting; Immed., immediate; Del., delayed

without tinea infection, a later investigation (Rajka and Barlinn 1979) demonstrated parallel reactions between mold species and trichophytin (Table 5.11). Similar cross-reactivity was observed in asthmatic children (Jones et al. 1973 b). Since no evidence of dermatophyte infection could be found in these children, and in the author's material the signs of tinea infections in children with AD were very slight, tinea reactivity may be considered as secondary. In other words, a positive trichophytin reaction in AD does not necessarily mean sensitization to dermatophytes, but is primarily an indication of cross-sensitivity to molds to which AD patients have been exposed at an early age. It is tempting to speculate that impaired immunological reactivity in AD is followed by decreased resistance and is associated with high immediate reactivity to molds and, by cross-reactivity, to dermatophytes. In a proportion of AD patients this may be followed by clinical dermatophyte infection with a chronic course, especially if elicited by *Trichophyton rubrum* (see also Sect. 2.9).

5.2.8 Other Inhalants

Allergens in seeds, cotton seed, castor oil, coffee beans, and similar substances are significant in atopic respiratory disease, but not, so far as is known, in AD. *Lycopodium* extract was used by the author to test AD patients, but the results produced no conclusive evidence to show that this allergen plays any role in the disease. Plant-powder allergens, such as pyrethrum and liquorice, seem to be similarly irrelevant. Of the plant fibers, cotton may be present in house dust, and kapok allergen has been thought possibly to elicit inhalative allergy in some AD cases, but its significance has been very restricted since the introduction of synthetic fibers such as polyesters. In one report (Osborne and Murray 1953), wool was considered to be an inhalant allergen, but this was disproved. Finally, Champion (1971) reported five patients with both AD and mild respiratory allergies in whom skin exacerbations were provoked both by inhalation and by direct contact with algae. The algal content of house dust may be important in dust sensitivity (Bernstein and Safferman 1970). A stinging insect may elicit skin lesions by allergic or by pharmacological mechanisms (see Sect. 5.4.3), but airborne scales or dust shed by insects may also induce sensitization in atopic subjects (Perlman 1958). However, investigations of this occurrence in patients with AD are lacking. It is well-known to clinicians that food allergens like egg (MacKie et al. 1979) and fish (Aas 1967) can also act as inhalant allergens.

5.2.9 Inhalants Eliciting Contact Reaction

Using P1 mite antigen in a larger quantity for patch testing on the mildly abraded skin of AD patients, a delayed response was produced (Mitchell et al. 1982), which corresponded to a cutaneous basophil hypersensitivity. This is considered to be a form of delayed skin hypersensitivity (Dvorak et al. 1976). Repeated application gave rise to a mast cell hyperplasia replacing the earlier basophil infiltration (Mitchell et al. 1986), a phenomenon suggested to occur in AD (Mihm et al. 1976).

Eczematous lesions were produced on AD skin by scratching and continuous application of a mite antigen, and its entry into the skin was visualized by ferritin labeling (Gondo et al. 1986). Furthermore, specific IgE antibodies were shown in AD as having the highest level against mite body antigens (Carswell and Thompson 1986). House dust mite solution, applied under a crepe bandage, led to the exacerbation of AD when applied on mildly eczematous or to symptom-free skin (Norris et al. 1988). Tanaka et al. (1989) observed in such experiments presence of Langerhans' cells in the skin. These observations raised the possibility that mite body antigens directly penetrate the skin. Such direct penetration was proven for concentrated birch extracts in AD patients with hypersensitivity to this pollen, as positive patch thest reactions with typical histology were registered on the normal (nonabraded) skin (Reitamo et al. 1986). These results were confirmed in some cases by Bruynzeel-Koomen et al. (1988) and by our group (Langeland and Braathen, unpublished observations), and were in agreement with the history of the patients, (Adinoff et al. 1988).

Using the indirect immunoperoxidase technique, Bruynzeel-Koomen et al. (1986) observed positive anti-IgE staining of dendritic cells in the epidermis and dermis, which, through labeling experiments and immunogold electron microscopy, proved to be Langerhans' cells. Based on the presence of IgE molecules on Langerhans' cells, Bruynzeel-Koomen (1986) suggested a new concept. According to her hypothesis, inhalant allergens penetrate the epidermis of AD patients and bind to IgE molecules on Langerhans' cells, which migrate to the dermis, where allergen presentation occurs to sensitized T-lymphocytes. The latter cells give rise to a delayed-type hypersensitivity reaction, via the lymphokines, which results in skin alterations with subsequent increased permeability of the epidermis. As a consequence, inhalant allergens may penetrate the dermis directly and bind to IgE molecules present on mast cells. This binding is followed by an immediate-type skin reaction which may also occur after contact with inhalants. In recent patch test experiments with inhalant allergens the participation of eosinophils was revealed; this occurred first in the dermis and then in the epidermis, and electron microscopy showed the eosinophils to lie in close contact with Langerhans' cells. Thus, eosinophils are assumed to participate in these patch reactions to inhalants (Bruynzeel-Koomen et al. 1988) (see Sect. 6.2). Applying birch, timothy or egg white allergens Langeland et al. (1989) observed patch reaction with 30–50% T helper/inducer and 25–40% T cytotoxic/suppressor cells as well as 10% CDl positive cells, which points to the possibility that these allergens may penetrate normal skin. Successfull passive transfer test indicated that IgE-antibodies are involved in this type of reaction.

5.3 Foods

Only some aspects of the vast amount of information in this field can be mentioned here.

5.3.1 General Remarks

Several foods, including cow's milk, egg, fish, shellfish, nuts, and cereals, are known to elicit clinical symptoms in the skin and the gastrointestinal (see Chap. 2), bronchial, and nasal mucosa in varying frequency. Milk and egg often give parallel reactions in the skin and in the gastrointestinal tract. Reactions in the skin are itch/AD and urticaria. These reactions mostly depend on the immunological state of the subject and are strongly influenced by regional dietary habits. Foods can elicit specific antibody response in low frequency and transiently even in healthy persons (Rothberg et al. 1965; Kletter et al. 1971) who can also sometimes experience clinical reactions, but they primarily cause serological and clinical responses in atopics (Hattevig et al. 1984). The mechanism is either immunological (allergic) or nonimmune; the former group predominantly includes IgE-mediated reactions, but non-IgE-mediated reactions may also occur. IgE-mediated reactions can be demonstrated by skin and challenge tests and by RAST, which replaced the previously usual passive transfer. In atopics IgE-mediated cross-reactions may occur, the best studied being group reactions between milk or egg originating from different animal sources. Furthermore, cross-reactions involving two toods in the same biological group (Hansel 1953), such as eggs and chicken or two or more cereals, have often been reported (Borelli and Berova 1965; and others) but were seldom found in the author's series.

Cross-reactivity of birch pollen with apples, nuts, carrots, and potatoes may be a source of food reactions Andersen and Löwenstein 1978; Lahti et al. 1980; Alberse et al. 1981; Eriksen et al. 1982).

5.3.1.1 Food Allergens

Commercial food extracts are unreliable test substances, as they do not represent the allergen actually responsible for the skin reaction; the "true" allergen is probably an end product of food degradation in the gastrointestinal tract. As Ruiz-Moreno (1959) wrote: "an unknown world of germs, ferments, putrifications and complex processes of a physicochemical nature which take place in the intestines, must be a source of an immense quantity of allergenic substance of which we know very little, originating from foodstuffs, but chemically and biochemically different from the foods we eat". Consequently, while some investigators have preferred to test using the raw materials (Freedman and Sellars 1959), others have used enzyme-digested preparations.

Immediate reactions to fruits and vegetables are more adequately studied by the scratch-chamber method (Hannuksela and Lahti 1977).

Food allergy reactions generally appear early in life, a fact tentatively explained by immaturity and increased vulnerability of the gastrointestinal tract and the immune system to foodstuffs introduced in different frequencies and quantities (Mathew et al. 1977; Hansen et al. 1977). Food antigens penetrate the normal gastrointestinal tract even in adults as demonstrated by applying serum from a fish-sensitized individual to recipients who developed at this site an urticarial reaction after ingesting fish (Brunner and Walzer 1928).

There is an interesting suggestion that initial exposure of the neonate to small quantities of food allergens, such as cow's milk, could elicit higher levels of specific (IgE) antibodies (Jarrett 1977; Björksten and Saarinen 1978). During breast feeding, babies who are developing AD may be sensitized by foods eaten by their mothers and develop AD (Cant et al. 1985). On the effect of breast feeding, see Chap. 11.

Late reactions appearing some hours after contact with dietary allergens have been reported (Dannaeus et al. 1977; Firer et al. 1982). An initial IgE-mediated mechanism is assumed, with subsequent participation of several mediators, but there are as yet no definite data in this field.

Antibody responses to food allergens include antibodies other than IgE, i. e., IgA and IgG. (Secretory) IgA is present in the gastrointestinal mucosa and probably participates in the immune defense of the gut, primarily against microorganisms. Similarly, IgG and its subclasses are produced against food antigens even in healthy subjects. Their role in the atopic process is, however, unclear, and it is possible that they only indicate food absorption from the gut. It has also been stated that foods may elicit other types of allergic reaction, such as anaphylactic, delayed (Livingood and Pillsbury 1949; Minor et al. 1980), or even type III reactions (Werner 1972). On food-evoked immune complexes, see Sect. 5.5.2.

5.3.2 Food Reactivity

The evidence for food reactivity in AD (Table 5.12) is conflicting and has long been debated. Because of the many contradictions in assessing the role of foods in AD and in evaluating the vast and increasing literature, both enthusiastic support for and total rejection of food reactivity may be found. The early authors' postulates on and overemphasis of this subject were replaced in the middle of the century by strong criticism and serious doubts. Recently, a new wave of reports has again emphasized a correlation between foods and AD (Atherton et al. 1978; Bonifazi et al. 1978; Barnetson 1980; Hannuksela 1980). These

Table 5.12. Food intolerance in AD

I. Food allergy	*Some examples:*
Immune mechanisms are elicited by food allergens penetrating the intestinal mucosa and involving gut-associated lymphoid tissue. There the interaction with immunoglobins in the gut wall results in liberation of mediators which (by enhancing penetration of allergens through mucosa and thus reaching the circulation or by immune complexes?) elicit itch and IgE-associated inflammation in the involved (or sometimes symptom-free) skin.	Milk, egg, fish, nuts
II. Food idiosyncrasy	
Elicited on basis of enzymatic/metabolic changes by food penetrating the intestinal mucosa and liberating mediators (due to weakness of individual regulatory mechanisms?). Food metabolites reaching the circulation elicit itch in the involved skin as well as inflammation.	Citrus fruits, some spices, smoked/roasted food, foods liberating histamine locally (e. g., strawberries, tomatoes, chocolate), histidine- or histamine-rich food (?) (e. g., cheese, sausages, tuna)
Subgroup: Lectins binding unspecifically to IgE molecules.	Wheat, soya, tomato

have been paralleled by a demand for stronger criteria and, in general, the best-controlled studies have failed to show that early allergen avoidance is of any benefit in preventing AD (Halpern et al. 1973; Kjellman and Johansson 1979; Kramer und Moroz 1981).

Note that the patient material of dermatologists, pediatricians, and allergists may differ somewhat. It is important to stress that only pure AD cases (without respiratory allergies) can give direct evidence for the etiological role of foods in AD.

A given food may aggravate AD by either sensitization, resultting in specific IgE antibodies, or intolerance including idiosyncrasy (a revived, unfortunate but accepted term), with nonimmunological, enzymatic, or metabolic liberation of mediators, such as histamine, causing vasodilatation and itching. This distinction is necessary, although allergy predominates, but is frequently ignored in evaluating patients. Idiosyncrasy is typically provoked by tart or sour items, such as citrus fruits (but oranges are also known allergens), spices, vinegar, and smoked or roasted foods, or by foods liberating or containing histamine (and possibly also by histidine-rich food). It is assumed that in such cases gastrointestinal symptoms are infrequent; however, congenital lactase deficiency or gluten enteropathy can mimic the symptoms. Regardless of the mechanism, the resulting symptoms are itching, aggravation of AD, and sometimes new lesions. The urticarial reaction is not a characteristic of AD, but contact urticaria does often occur and points to the tendency of atopic persons to react to ingested allergens with type I reactions. A relationship may also exist between atopy and lectin-containing foods which cause symptoms simulating immune reactions (Andersen and Löwenstein 1978; Eriksson et al. 1982).

Strong food reactions have been described in infants immediately upon commencement of breast feeding (Kaufman 1971). This gives rise to suspicion of sensitization in utero, even if this possibility has been questioned by several authors. IgE can be demonstrated by RAST in the cord blood. This IgE originates from the infant since IgE cannot pass the placental barrier, and production of IgE is assumed to start when the fetus is only 3 months old.

Infantile AD constitutes a special problem in relation to food sensitivity. The greater permeability of the gut (see Chap. 2) and immaturity of the immune state are mostly quoted in this context.

Food allergy, or at leat food intolerance, is most noticeable in the first years after birth, and the types of food incriminated differ in younger and older chil-

Table 5.13. Fluctuation of food and inhalant allergens on the basis of repeated intracutaneous tests in 75 AD patients

Age groups	Food reactivity		Inhalant reactivity	
	Acquired	Lost	Acquired	Lost
0– 6	2	3	5	1
7–12	3	0	5	0
13–18	0	8	19	12
19–45	4	7	18	10

dren. As the child grows older, food reactivity diminishes and the importance of inhalant allergens becomes increasingly evident; this was seen in a study of 75 patients who were skin tested at intervals of at least 1 year to demonstrate which sensitivities had been lost and which acquired (see Table 5.13). There is therefore, a tendency for food reactivity to regress gradually and for inhalant reactivity to increase. The decrease in clinical food sensitivity relates to a general tendency for type I food allergies, such as egg or milk allergy, to disappear; however, not all such reactions display such a tendency, and fish or nut sensitivity, for example, may remain for longer periods. Furthermore, idiosyncrasy does not show any tendency to disappear with aging (see Table 5.14).

5.3.3 Frequent Food Allergens

Allergy to *cow's milk* may play a not insignificant role in the infantile phase of AD (Hill and Sulzberger 1935), the disease being more common in babies fed on cow's milk than in those exclusively breast fed (Grulee and Sandford 1936). β-Lactoglobulin and lactalbumin are held to be the principal allergenic components, but it is suspected that other allergens as well as nonimmunological factors may also be relevant (Collins-Williams 1956; Fries 1959), and, in consequence, the results of skin tests with milk extracts show considerable variation.

Recently the roles of α-lactalbumin and of the heat-stable casein have been emphasized; furthermore, cross-sensitivity between β-lactoglobulin and calf meat is possible (Wütrich 1987).

Firer et al. (1982) found that atopic patients allergic to cow's milk had significantly higher specific IgE and lower IgG antibody levels than controls, whereas in AD patients all Ig catagories were elevated. Thus they postulated that non-IgE milk antibodies have a regulatory effect on clinical manifestations of IgE-associated hypersensitivity disorders. Wütrich (1987) points out that milk sensitivity, which frequently involves the gastrointestinal and respiratory mucosa in addition to the skin, mostly disappears after 3–5 years if milk is eliminated from the diet.

Reactivity to *egg* albumin is very frequent in early life, its incidence in AD cases having been reported as 100% during the 1st year and as 49% during the 2nd year (Epstein and Palacek 1951), although other authors (Ratner and Untracht 1952; Sedlis et al. 1966) have reported a lower incidence, such as 35%–38%. It has been postulated that this reactivity is based on sensitivity (Hill 1955; Jadassohn 1958), but, because of its peculiar age incidence, it is regarded as only indicative of AD. Theories proposed by several authors, and which can-

Table 5.14. Incidence of mechanisms of reactivity to foods in AD

	Food allergy	Food idiosyncrasy
Infants	+ +	+ +
Children	+ − + +	+ +
Adults	(+)	+ +

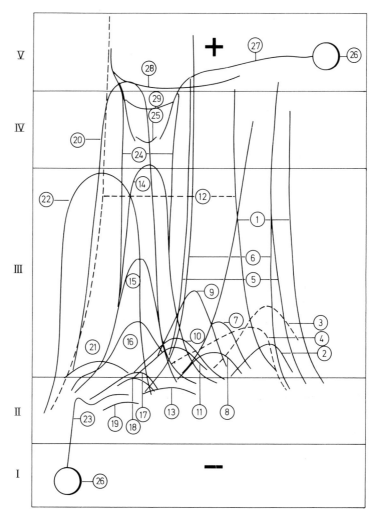

Fig. 5.4. Drawing of the CIE reference precipitation pattern of hen's egg white. Precipitates drawn with *dotted lines* are detectable in CRIE only, using selected patient sera. Gels I and V: first dimensional gels; gels II and IV: intermediate gels; gel III: antibody-containing gel. (Langeland 1982b)

not be discounted, suggest (a) that egg albumin may, if fact, be absorbed more readily by a young infant's intestine, (b) that positive skin test reactions and passive transfer may be elicited by nonspecific histamine liberation, or even (c) that the lack of immunological tolerance in younger infants is relevant (Glaser 1965). In any event, certain authors do not include sensitivity to egg albumin in their statistics.

In the studies of Schur et al. (1974), clinical egg sensitivity showed a significant correlation with egg-white RAST, but not with total IgE levels. Low levels of IgE antibodies to egg proteins compared to house dust mite antigen were seen in 60 AD patients, who on the other hand had high IgG levels (Rowntree et al. 1987).

In work on our department on the significance of egg allergy in AD, crossed immunoelectrophoresis demonstrated three major allergens (ovalbumin, ovomucoid, and ovoferrin) and several intermediate and minor allergens in the egg-white (Langeland 1982 a, b) (see Fig. 5.4). Analyzing the data of 84 AD Infants with egg allergy, Langeland found that egg allergy usually developed before the introduction of egg into the diet (exposure during pregnancy and through breast milk?). The clinical manifestations were in general itching or exacerbation of the skin condition. Comparing this group with 72 AD children without egg allergy, it was found that egg allergy is associated with high IgE levels and with a clinically more active and severe form of AD (Langeland 1983).

Fish allergy also merits mention for, although the relevant allergen commonly elicits manifestations and primarily causes asthma or urticaria in young children, several authors have suspected that it may be related to AD. This sensitivity has a long history which dates back to Küstner's own fish allergy and to the subsequent discovery of the Prausnitz-Küstner transfer test (1921). Aas (1967) succeeded in isolating a very potent allergen from white muscle of the cod (*Gadus callarias* 1) and partially purified the principal component allergens. Major antigens from fish have proved valuable research tools in allergology and immunology (see Sect. 5.2); however, the fish allergen extracts also contain components of minor importance to many fish-hypersensitive patients. Steam from cooking fish contains allergens in trace amounts, which are, nevertheless, sufficient to elicit reactions in susceptible individuals; these allergens are identical to one or more of the major antigens mentioned above, demonstrating that fish can also be classed as a source of inhalant allergens.

Many other foods are incriminated as frequent allergens in AD. If we consider only reliable food challenge results, then the following may be added to the above-mentioned dietary antigens: wheat, peanuts, soy and chicken (Sampson and Albergo 1984). This list, with the exception of wheat, is primarily of importance for United States' dietary conditions. Soy proteins are however, being used increasingly in a number of foods and food products in different parts of the world and both specific IgE and IgG antibodies to crude soy were elevated in AD patients with positive challenge (Burks et al. 1988).

5.3.4 Skin Reactivity

Statistical surveys of large series of AD patients tested for foodstuff sensitivity have shown positive results in 29%-75% (Nexmand 1948; Kesten 1954; Rowe and Rowe 1951; Brunsting 1936; Hill 1934; Balyeat 1930; Hopkins and Kesten 1935). The author, however, found an incidence of 15.7%; an additional 2.6% of his cases had egg reactivity. Characteristically, there was no difference in food reactivity between AD patients and controls with other skin diseases; in fact, in 50 controls with neither a history nor symptoms of allergy, positive responses occurred in 6%, an incidence which differs statistically very slightly

Table 5.15. History of food sensitivity and immediate skin reactions in patients with AD

History of food sensitivity	Results of skin tests			No history of food sensitivity	Results of skin tests	
	Positive and fits with history	Positive to other food allergens	Ne-ga-tive		Positive to foods	Negative to foods
25 patients, group I[a]	5	6	14	25 patients, group I	7	18
25 patients, group II	7	4	14	25 patients, group II	1	24
25 patients, group III	5	5	16	25 patients, group III	9	16
25 patients, group IV	4	5	16	25 patients, group IV	7	18
100	21	20	60	100	24	76

[a] Group I: 0-6 years; group II: 7-12 years; group III: 13-18 years; group IV: 19-45 years

from that in AD patients ($P > 0.05$) (Rajka 1961). Even normal infants may, for a short period, produce anibodies to newly introduced foods.

Furthermore, in this study by the author there was only a weak correlation between a history of sensitivity to food and the results of skin tests (see Table 5.15), although there was a valid agreement in some cases for cocoa, eggs, and oranges. In this series, positive skin tests were in fact elicited most commonly by fish, oranges, tomatoes, and apples, whereas the history usually incriminated those common food allergens mentioned by many other authors, namely eggs, shellfish, nuts, and, in infants, milk.

Skin reactivity is generally thought to be of little significance and that is why, at an earlier symposium on infantile AD, there was a consensus against the use of food extract skin tests either as a diagnostic procedure or as a guide in formulating elimination diets for management of the disease: a view strongly supported by, among others, Sedlis (1965). This was in marked contrast to the previous overestimation of the value of skin testing with foods in AD, although some authorities (Sulzberger 1940; Cooke 1947) had long advised against attaching too much importance to them. Recently, it was pointed out that skin testing should be considered a good test for excluding immediate food hypersensitivity but only a suggestive positive indicator of hypersensitivity due to the high rate of clinically insignificant positive skin tests (Sampson and Albergo 1984).

The author believes that skin tests are of very limited value, but that exposure to some foods undeniably may aggravate existing lesions and perhaps elicit new lesions in AD. In fact, foods have been seen to play a role in some cases of the disease and, provided patients are thoroughly interrogated, a positive history is found more often in AD than in respiratory atopy. These positive histories may appear to be surprisingly frequent; furthermore, a tendency for manifestations to occur in a particular organ could be determined (see Table 5.16).

There are several possible sources of error in any history of food reactivity, e. g., parental overestimation of the significance of foods in the child's skin dis-

Table 5.16. History of food-induced symptoms in atopic patients

	Symptoms				
	Skin	Lung	Nasal	Oral	Intestinal
50 patients with bronchial asthma	3	11	5	6	5
50 patients with allergic rhinitis	6	0	4	10	0
50 patients with AD	34	0	1	6	0
50 patients with infantile AD	34	0	0	4	0

ease, attribution by parents of excessive relevance to food items, such as food color and other additives [which for the dermatologist seem to be of less importance (Young et al. 1986)], and the frequent confusion of allergic and idiosyncratic mechanisms. Such sources of error often make the history unreliable. Correlation of skin tests with RAST is often emphasized. They are closely related procedures, deviations of findings depending on the fact that the former are influenced by IgE level and the age of the patient. The RAST, which can be used in infants or when there are difficulties with skin test evaluation, is also often inadequate due to a lack of reliable food allergens. There may be certain discrepancies between RAST and skin tests (Öhman and Johansson 1974), but clearly positive skin tests and higher classes of RAST show parallelism. Thus, combining the results of skin tests and RAST is of no advantage compared with the use of prick tests alone. (Sampson and Albergo 1984); the most appropriate means of evaluating skin test results, in addition to history and clinical symptoms, are challenge tests.

5.3.5 Challenge Tests

Oral provocation tests with foods in AD, and particularly in infantile AD, have been abundantly reported in the literature. Most studies have been on egg and milk sensitivity, with the selection of cases for study being based on positivity of skin tests and a convincing history.

Concerning milk, the rate of sensitivity has usually been found to be high (Goldman et al. 1963; Hammar 1977; Juto et al. 1978; exception: Bonifazi et al. 1978). In the case of egg, a lower incidence of positivity was found (Meara 1955; Bonifazi et al. 1978). In addition to itch and flare-up of the AD, urticaria was also provoked by egg in some instances, in addition to other allergic symptoms, listed in Table 5.17 (Sedlis 1965).

One must, however, be cautious when evaluating the provocation data as several sources of error may be present: patients may not have strictly avoided the substance before the test, tests may have been repeated too soon (as nonreactive latent periods after exposure may occur), or itch may have been overlooked at evaluation. One positive challenge is insufficient, as multiple factors may contribute to a possible pseudopositivity of provocation. The performance of double-blind tests, using appropriate placebo tablets, is recommended al-

Table 5.17. Results of challenges to egg[a] in 27 patients with infantile eczema who were skin sensitive to egg (Sedlis 1965)

Negative	6
Urticaria and/or angioneurotic edema	16
With vomiting	8
With inconstant exacerbation of eczema	4
Inconstant exacerbation of eczema only	1
Immediate erythema	2
Vomiting, scratching, sneezing	2

[a] Whole egg given dally, usually as eggnog

though such tests have been carried out only infrequently in the past (Bock et al. 1978).

A thorough study with placebo challenge was performed by Sampson (1983) in 26 children with AD. He found 23 positive challenges in 15 patients, and of them 21 were a manifestation of itch and erythema leading to scratching and subsequent eczematoid lesions. There was only limited agreement between positive skin tests and food challenge tests, and the extent of this agreement varied from food to food; moreover, a high rate of skin reactions were without clinical significance. On the other hand, some challenges were positive where the skin test had been negative but the patients had been selected due to their convincing history, i. e., a certain pseudonegativity also occurred. Despite some agreements, the history in general proved quite unreliable for predicting clinical food sensitivity.

Recently Sampson and Jolie (1984) broadened the evaluation of double-blind placebo-controlled multiple food challenges in 33 children with AD via determination of their plasma histamine levels. Only patients with positive oral challenge showed a significant rise in plasma histamine, which was interpreted as involving mast cell or basophil mediators, including histamine, with subsequent itch and eczematoid skin changes. Thus the rise in histamine level after challenge can be considered as a significant parameter for such studies, as was confirmed in some patients by Boner et al. (1985) and in severe, but not mild, food-allergic adult subjects by Atkins et al. (1985).

The counterpart of challenge, the elimination trial, may also give false results, mostly due to inadequate completeness or duration of the withdrawal. Food elimination is most reliably performed under hospital conditions, even if not every author (e. g., Atherton 1981) shares this opinion.

5.3.6 Late and Non-IgE-Mediated Food Reactions

Late reactions, i. e., reactions appearing between 12 and 24 h after food exposure, were described by Hammar in 1977, and have also frequently been demonstrated by RAST (Wraith et al. 1979). In 37 AD patients, Benton and Barnetson (1985) reported late reactions – including urticaria, itch, and exacerbation of AD – in addition to immediate and to dual reactions. According to these authors, late reactions were elicited either by alcoholic beverages and colorings (based on nonimmunological histamine release), or by allergens such as milk and wheat, acting by an unknown mechanism. Sampson (1988) reports in AD patients immediate skin reactions (within 3 hours) after food challenge. In addition, many patients developed long-lasting itch and less frequently a macular pruritic rash 6–8 hours after the initial response. These interesting studies concur with observations (a) that late reactions are elicited by an initial IgE-mediated reaction (see Sect. 5.3.1) and (b) that there is a correlation between late reactions and itch (see Chap. 3). Furthermore, it is of considerable interest that it was possible to elicit an eczematous reaction after applying egg-white for 72 h in a patch test on an egg-sensitive girl with AD (Langeland and Braathen, unpublished studies); this finding is similar to the results of experiments with contact inhalants (see Sect. 5.2.9).

In the past interest was focused on IgA, which is a protective factor of mucosal surfaces, including the gut. It has previously been speculated whether or not IgA deficiency, which occurs at a frequency of 1:500 (Hobbs 1968), could result in increased antigen absorption and therefore overstimulation of IgE-producing cells (Soothill 1974). A transient IgA deficiency was postulated in early infancy in AD (Taylor et al. 1973) but no later reports have confirmed this. IgA often occurs complexed to dietary allergens (Brostoff et al. 1979), which are considered to be harmless and biologically inert (Atherton 1982). In one report increased prevalence of IgA antibodies to food antigens was demonstrated in AD children (Dannæus et al. 1977).

IgG antibodies also seem to be increased to dietary allergens in children (Dannæus et al. 1977) as well as to milk and gliadin (Finn et al. 1985). Precipitins to food antigens have been reported in 15% of adult AD patients without, and in 45% with food allergy (Barnetson et al. 1983). Of IgG subclasses, IgG4 has not infrequently been reported as elevated in AD against food antigens, but such elevation is without apparent clinical significance (Shakib et al. 1985). The same conclusion was reached by Rowntree et al. (1987), although they found a certain relationship between egg-specific IgG4 levels and both IgE levels and skin test results. Barnetson et al. (1981) also reported raised IgG4 levels to egg but these authors added to their conclusion that the significance of the findings remained to be elucidated. Similarly, Husby et al. (1986) reported β-lactoglobulin-elicited specific IgG4 levels to be higher in AD, but without relevance to the clinical state or IgE levels. All these findings possibly only indicate increased gut permeability to food antigens in AD. On the other hand Gondo et al. (1987), on the basis of high IgG4 but low IgE levels to ovalbumin in children with AD, believe that IgG4 is a blocking antibody. Higher IgG-3 antibody levels to codfish were found in children with AD by Lea et al. (1980).

5.3.7 Concluding Remarks

In the author's personal view, propositions that food reactions have only an allergic mechanism rest on a rather insecure basis. Many foods can influence only skin that is already inflamed; thus when the skin disease is quiescent in the summer, the AD patients often tolerates foods of which he/she is intolerant in the winter. This fact clearly points to an idiosyncratic mechanism. The primary connecting link between foods acting by immunological and nonimmunological mechanisms and the symptoms of AD is presumably itch (foods can also elicit vasodilatation).

The demonstration of food hypersensitivity is often difficult, mostly due to variable reliability of allergens and because the idiosyncratic mechanism is not always clear to doctors (and still less so to the public). Therefore, dermatologists and pediatricians who frequently observe negative food provocation tests and achieve poor therapeutic results through diets (which include food allergens to which the patients have positive tests) are of the opinion that foods have little importance in AD. Many data and personal experiences indicate, however, that foods play a contributory role in the mechanism of AD, particularly in the early phases of the disease.

From the clinical point of view, it is essential to realize that positive skin tests and/or RAST demonstrating an IgE-mediated reaction do *not* automatically indicate clinical sensitivity. Therefore, the tests should be evaluated in conjunction with history, clinical symptoms, and, if possible, challenge tests. Of these, the (repeated double-blind) challenge test, usually leading first to itch (and erythema) and subsequently to flare-up of the AD process, is considered to indicate an immunological mechanism if it agrees with the result of immediate tests, while if it does not, a nonimmunological mechanism seems probable.

The situation is more difficult where there are positive food tests but no clinical reactivity after exposure. A certain significance of the foods in question cannot totally be excluded, as it may be assumed that by repetition or in conjunction with other reactions at a subclinical level they can contribute to the mechanism of AD, e. g., by lowering the itch threshold (Rajka 1963; MacKie et al. 1979).

In short:

1. Positive challenge and immediate tests = clinical significance.
2. Positive challenge and negative immediate tests = probably nonimmunological mechanism (idiosyncrasy).
3. Positive immediate tests but negative challenge tests = uncertain significance.

In addition, the result of elimination and/or treatment may confirm or weaken these postulates (see Chaps. 11, 12).

5.4 Other Allergens from Living Agents

5.4.1 Staphylococci and Other Bacteria

Several techniques and various extracts differing in antigenic quality have been used to study allergy to staphylococci. However, despite intensive work on the subject, many problems remain unsolved, particularly with regard to identification of the "appropriate" allergen. The role of bacterial allergens in AD was first demonstrated by Norrlind (1946), who found that 37 of 39 patients with the disease and with a history of infections produced positive immediate skin reactions when tested with composite bacterial products from organisms such as staphylococci, *Klebsiella pneumoniae* (Friedländer's bacillus), and *Hemophilus influenzae* (Pfeiffer's bacillus). Furthermore, 6 of the 78 patients tested reacted only to bacterial products. The present author used laboratory-prepared staphylotoxoid and staphylovaccine to skin test AD patients; the results are summarized in Table 5.18. In further studies, using repeated local injections of staphylotoxoid, neutralization techniques, and biopsies, it was shown that altered immunity, and not a hypothical skin-bound antitoxin, is the cause of the diminished delayed reactivity. The frequency of immediate reactions is in keeping both with the tendency of AD patients' skin, in general, to react to allergens, and with the results of studies on other dermatological patients using staphylotoxoid or staphylococcal polysaccharides (Swineford and Holman 1949; Rudzki et al. 1965).

Hénocq et al. (1982) found antistaphylococcal IgE levels to be elevated in superinfected AD, but only slightly or not at all elevated in other atopic patients. On the other hand, Bergquist and Nilzén (1959) reported that skin reactions to staphylococci were not significant in AD.

The staphylococcal cell wall antigen protein A binds to the Fc portion of IgG and to the Fab portion of IgE (Inganäs and Johansson 1981). Thus it not only has a specific but also a nonspecific binding activity and therefore, compared with other cell wall constituents, it is seldom used in experiments. After intradermal injection of protein A in AD patients, White and Noble (1985) registered a reduced immediate reaction.

In most studies of staphylococcal antigens the Wood 46 *Staphylococcus aureus* strain was used, since its nonspecific binding is minimal and the specific antistaphylococcal IgE antibodies can be shown by radioimmunoassay. In such studies, antistaphylococcal IgE antibodies were reported by Hénocq et al. (1982) in superinfected but not in other atopic AD cases, by Abramson et al. (1982) in most of their AD patients, and by Motala et al. (1986) in 29% of their child and 23% of their adult AD patients. In half of their AD patients, Hauser et al. (1985) noted IgE to purified cell wall antigens which did not correlate with whole body or unpurified extracts but did show a parallelism to total IgE values and to the presence of regional lymphadenopathy. The delayed reactivity was decreased; however, the immediate skin tests were normal. Gabrielsen and Brandtzæg (1985) demonstrated via ELISA in 45 AD patients increased IgE antibodies and at the same time also elevated IgG antibodies

Table 5.18. Changes in immediate/delayed reactions to staphylococcal substances[a] and Asta

	Controls	AD patients	Infection-sensitive AD patients
In childhood:			
Immediate reactions		Mostly negative	Mostly negative
Delayed reactions		In ½: (+)	Others: 0
In adult age:			
Immediate reactions	In ⅔: (+)	In ⅔: (+)	In all: (+)
Delayed reactions	In ⅔: +[b]	In ½: 0. In ½: +	In ½: 0. In ½: +
Asta titers	Various[b]	Relatively high	Relatively high
After a cure with CSV[d]:			
Immediate reactions	In ⅓ increased	In ½ increased	In ⅓ decreased
Delayed reactions	Unchanged	Unchanged	Unchanged
Asta titers	Increased	Relatively small increase[c]	Relatively small increase[c]

[a] Staphyloalphatoxoid 0.02 E and 600000 organisms of staphylovaccine
[b] Showed spontaneous variations
[c] Only if high dosage was given
[d] CSV: Combined staphylovaccine 0.03 E alphatoxoid + 1.2 million organisms

Evaluation:
+ reaction = over 20 mm (sum of two largest perpendicular diameters)
(+) reaction = 12–20 mm[b]
0 = without macroscopic reaction

whose level corresponded with the severity of the disease. By contrast Friedman et al. (1985) observed increased IgE antibodies in only 3 of their 25 AD cases, and in a similar series of 13 patients, only one had raised antistaphylococcal levels (Christophersen et al. 1986).

Although these studies mostly showed antistaphylococcal IgE responses in a proportion of AD patients, these responses did not correspond with the clinical state. Furthermore, atopic (Hénocq et al. 1982) or hyper-IgE cases (Schopfer et al. 1979) without AD may also show elevation of antistaphylococcal IgE values. On this basis Hanifin (1986) suggests that one can speak only of an association between staphylococcal infections and AD, and not of an etiological relationship (see also Chap. 2).

Finding antistaphylotoxin (Asta) titer to be a rather insensitive indicator of staphylococcal disease, Mustakallio (1966) tried to ascertain the cause of the high titers usually found in AD (Sonck and Widholm 1954; Eberhartinger and Landes 1960; Bergquist and Nilzén 1960). It was shown, from statistical analysis of 593 cases, that the severely affected patients with extensive lesions had the highest titers. The explanation offered was that, when staphylococci abundantly colonize the diseased skin (Cooke and Buck 1963), they penetrate the skin barrier which has been damaged by scratching, chapping, and allergic inflammation. Thus the Asta titer reflects the skin barrier defect rather than the presence of pyogenic foci in the skin.

5.4.1.1 A Short Comment on Streptococci

Conflicting reports on the antistreptolysin O (ASO) titer in AD have appeared in literature. Some authors (Sonck and Widholm 1954; Zezschwitz 1957) have reported higher levels in most patients as compared with controls. Other authors, however (Craps et al. 1959; Huriez 1966), have reported higher levels in only a minority of patients, for example, 20%–33%. In the author's series, raised ASO titers, of the order of 200–500 Todd units, were found in 34% of the AD patients and in 19% of the controls. This was of marginal statistical significance.

5.4.2 Dermatophytes and Candida

As mentioned in Sect. 2.9.4, chronic dermatophytosis is not infrequent in AD and in these cases a positive immediate skin reaction to trichophytin and a positive RAST test are usually found. This indicates a greater susceptibility to dermatophyte infections in AD patients, primarily due to a deficient delayed reactivity.

In the context of food intolerance, the possible role of *Candida albicans,* or of intestinal parasites, should be considered. *Candida* has been reported to be a frequent cause of urticaria, a conclusion based on the results of intradermal (Holti 1966), prick (James and Warin 1971), and challenge tests. AD patients have also been shown to give positive reactions to skin tests or challenge tests or both using *Candida* antigen, but these results are probably of very doubtful value. Positive challenge tests with yeasts and a yeast-free diet are more likely to have some clinical relevance in this disease.

5.4.3 Scabies Mite, Insects, and Helminths

An immediate reactivity resulting in positive immediate skin tests, higher IgE, and positive transfer tests was detected in AD patients having scabies, as was cross-reactivity to house dust mites (Falk and Bolle 1983 a, b), (see Sect. 2.9.5).

Stinging insects (arthropods) can cause local or systemic, toxic or allergic symptoms in both atopic and nonatopic subjects, the allergic reactions being immediate anaphylactic, serum sickness, or delayed in type.

Immediate-type responses, being considered analogous to drug reactions (see p. 41 Sect. 2.14.1), are assumed to occur more frequently in atopics (Miyachi et al. 1979), but there is as yet insufficient documented evidence supporting the hypothesis. On the contrary, Frankland (1968), who examined more than 100 cases of bee and wasp sting sensitization, reported that more than 70% had "no other stigma of atopy". There has been no report of an association between insect sting sensitivity and AD.

There is no evidence that atopics with or without AD differ in any way from the normal population in their pattern of reaction to helminths, and there have been no reports providing conclusive evidence for an association between type I or type IV reactivity and AD. Theoretically, one might expect to find that the high serum IgE levels in atopic subjects are associated with enhancement of some of the defense mechanisms against helminths.

5.5 The Atopic Antibody

5.5.1 General Remarks

The serum factor responsible for the allergic reactivity, which Prausnitz and Küstner transferred from allergic to nonallergic individuals, was later investigated by Coca and Grove (1925). They demonstrated that a response was no longer elicited by intracutaneous administration of the relevant allergen if it had previously been mixed with serum of the type transferred; they referred to antibodies contained in the serum as reagins. Subsequent discovery of their physiochemical properties, such as heat lability and low molecular weight, and of their biological attributes, including skin sensitization, failure to fix complement, and failure to cross the placenta, left their immunoglobulin class to be determined; they were, however, generally assumed to belong to the IgA class.

A decisive development was the discovery, in 1967, independently, by Johansson and Bennich (1967 a, b) and by Ishizaka et al. (1967), of a special class of immunoglobulins, present in the serum in nanogram quantities; this was IgE, corresponding to the atopic reagin. A most important feature of these immunoglobulins is their avidity for skin and certain other tissues. Further discoveries followed the introduction of new, sensitive, radioimmunological techniques for detecting IgE; examples of such procedures include the radioimmunosorbent technique (RIST) of Wide and Porath (1966), as applied to IgE determinations by Johansson et al. (1968). Immunofluorescence and autoradiographic techniques have demonstrated the formation of IgE in plasma cells and in the germinal centers of lymphoid tissues; they have also shown IgE bound to the surface of mast cells and of basophil leukocytes (Ishizaka et al. 1970; Hubscher et al. 1970; Tada and Ishizaka 1970), and to lymphocytes in the peripheral blood (Lobitz et al. 1972).

Later it was shown that mast cells and basophils have a high number of surface receptors which bind IgE with high affinity whereas lymphocytes, eosinophils and platelets, and, most importantly, Langerhans' cells (see Sect 5.2.9) and

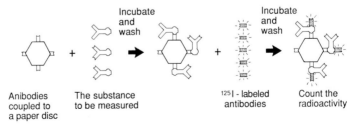

| Anibodies coupled to a paper disc | The substance to be measured | 125I - labeled antibodies | Count the radioactivity |

Fig. 5.5. Phadebas IgE PRIST test principle (Yman 1985)

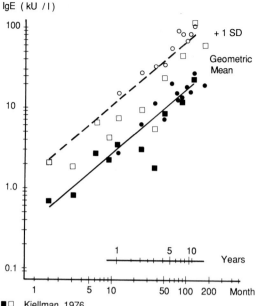

Fig. 5.6. IgE values in children (Yman 1985)

macrophages (Dessaint et al. 1979) have low affinity binding receptors. The lymphocytes correspond to T-lymphocytes. In the original radioimmunoassay, ^{125}I-labeled anti-IgE was covalently coupled to Sephadex particles. This was later modified by applying a paper disc as the solid phase (Phadebas PRIST), or in a variant by enzyme-labeling (Phadezym IgE PRIST), and further by a double antibody radioimmunoassay (RIA), by which methods very low values can also be demonstrated. Recently, microtiter modifications or use of monoclonal antibodies have been developed (Yman 1985; Schröder et al. 1985; Berglund et al. 1985).

The relatively simple PRIST test (see Fig. 5.5) has been used worldwide for routine purposes and the consequence has been a variation of reported IgE levels (the newer values are lower than the original ones) due, among other things, to improvement in selection criteria (e. g., exclusion of smokers), in test methods, and in statistics. The upper limit of the normal range, i. e., the value above which pathology can be suspected and investigations are usually started, is 100 kU for adults (1 kU = 2.4 ng). Unfortunately some authors work with higher values. For children, the values are shown in Fig. 5.6 (Kjellman et al. 1976; Bhalla et al. 1982). IgE in cord blood is of fetal (and possibly also of maternal) origin. When higher values (e. g., over 1 U/ml) are present, this has a predictive value for atopy (Kjellman 1976; Michel et al. 1980; Croner et al. 1982). The month of birth also has some influence on a high genetic risk population, since there was a higher risk for atopy when the child was born in May (Croner and Kjellman 1986).

Free IgE in the serum has a short half-life, only 2 days, but when fixed to the skin it is presumed to disappear more slowly. It has been demonstrated that IgE is present in normal serum in a mean concentration of 250 ng/ml, the levels found showing a certain scatter. In addition, the RAST has "verified" that IgE comprises two elements, a nonreaginic and a reaginic part; therefore allergen-specific reagins may be present in low concentrations in serum which has no elevation of the total IgE level as determined by the RIST. In addition, circulating reagins, demonstrated by the RAST, can be found in children with either high or normal serum IgE levels (Wide et al. 1967). IgE binds to IgE receptors (Fc) on mast cells, present in large numbers, and on basophils, and the reaction with allergens causes cross-linking of the receptors with a subsequent release of histamine and other mediators. The number of IgE receptors on lymphocytes and monocytes is high in severe AD and in hyperimmunoglobulinemia E syndrome (Spiegelberg 1986).

IgE titers are influenced by several factors, including viral infections (Johansson 1981), cigarette smoke (Zetterström et al. 1981; Bahna et al. 1983), and graft versus host reaction (Geha et al. 1980; Ringden et al. 1983), but not by short corticosteroid or azathioprine courses (Johansson and Juhlin (1970). Long-term therapy with these drugs may reduce IgE levels (Ring 1985).

In addition to atopy and parasitic infestations, higher serum IgE levels were found in several conditions, such as hyperimmunoglobulinemia E, Wiskott-Aldrich syndrome, and certain skin diseases (O'Loughlin et al. 1977); however, they were usually lower than in AD. The in vivo regulation of IgE production investigated in rodents and in atopic sera showed a complex interaction of T-cell-produced suppressive (which may be relevant to high IgE response in T cell immunodeficiency states) and potentiating factors, influenced by glycolization. These binding factors are supposedly part of IgE receptors (Ishizaka 1984; de Weck et al. 1986).

The clinical significance of the recently discovered anti-idiotypic (IgE) antibodies is still unclear (therapeutic possibility?).

A rapidly increasing number of reports provide details on the presence of IgE in different conditions and on its relation to various clinical and immunological problems, but the present discussion will be restricted to the relation between IgE and AD, and to some relevant points already mentioned in discussing allergens in AD.

5.5.2 IgE in AD

The first large relevant study to be undertaken (Juhlin et al. 1969) revealed that the majority of in-patients with severe AD had high serum levels of IgE. In subsequent studies, elevated IgE values were found to varying degrees in AD patients: from 43% (Johnson et al. 1974) to 80% (Juhlin et al. 1969). The variations could be explained by differences in the patient material, but on the other hand it is probable that there exists an AD subgroup with normal IgE values (Stone et al. 1976), i. e., high and low responders may be genetically coded at

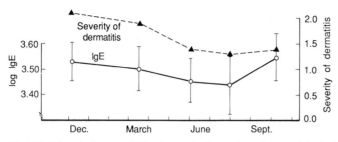

Fig. 5.7. Means of serum IgE value and of severity of dermatitis during 1 year in adult patients with AD and high serum IgE values. The *vertical lines* indicate mean ± SE. The severity has been graded as: mild = 1; moderate = 2; severe = 3. (Öhman et al. 1972)

birth (Croner et al. 1982). Regarding the details, it was shown that IgE values in the serum:

1. Are increased in the presence of atopic respiratory disease, or if there is a positive history of such disease (Ogawa et al. 1971; Öhman et al. 1972; Johnson et al. 1974; Jones et al. 1975; Wittig et al. 1980; Uehara 1986).
2. Are related to the severity of AD (Johansson and Juhlin 1970; Ogawa et al. 1971; Wütrich et al. 1973; Jones et al. 1975) [although this has not always been reported (Stone et al. 1976; MacKie et al. 1979)]. Consequently the IgE decreases if AD is healed (Johansson and Juhlin 1970).
3. Are related to the extent of AD (Ogawa et al. 1971; Öhman et al. 1972; Gurevitch et al. 1973; Clendenning et al. 1973), contrary to Jones et al.'s (1975) report.
4. Are correlated to duration of itch in the AD patient (Rajka 1980).
5. Are uninfluenced in AD by the pollen season (Öhman et al. 1972, see Fig. 5.7).
6. Are unrelated to skin test results (Jones et al. 1975). Rajka (1960) claimed they are also unrelated to vasomotor test results, but evidence is equivocal since Stone et al. (1976) did observe correlations with the results of such tests.
7. If massively increased, indicate an unfavorable prognosis in that individual (Wütrich et al. 1973).

5.5.2.1 IgE in Skin

The connection between T cells and IgE will be discussed below. In secretions, the concentration of IgE has been found to be higher than that of other immunoglobulins. Tada and Ishizaka (1970) verified, by the immunofluorescence technique, that IgE-forming cells are to be found primarily in respiratory and gastro-intestinal mucosae and in regional lymph nodes. Analogous to local immunity due to IgA, production locally, of IgE may be responsible for sensitization phenomena which are restricted to that area and which may well be independent of serum levels; in fact, local IgE formation can be assumed to play a significant role in the skin. It may be relevant in this context that IgE levels have been shown, using the RIST, to be raised twofold in uninvolved, and threefold in involved, skin of AD patients (Jansén et al. 1973).

A higher incidence of IgE-staining (mast) cells in AD patients than in controls was also seen by Anan (1976), and the occurrence of IgE-positive cells even in symptom-free skin in AD was confirmed by Hodgkinson et al. (1977), whereas Secher et al. (1978) could not find any IgE deposits in ten investigated AD patients. Small proportions of $Fc_\varepsilon +$ cells were found in the eczematous skin in AD, whereas their number in the serum was correlated with severity (Takigawa et al. 1989). IgE-positive Langerhans' cells have also been detected in the skin (see Sect. 5.2.9). Anti-IgE antibody, when injected into the skin, reacts with cell-bound IgE, which is normally present there, to elicit an urticarial response (Ishizaka and Ishizaka 1968); in AD this reaction is not correlated with the serum IgE level (Ogawa et al. 1971; Öhman 1971). It should also be mentioned that IgE can be demonstrated in sweat, the highest levels being in the presence of AD (Föström et al. 1975).

It was found that atopic patients have an abnormally high level of naturally occurring IgG antibodies against the Fab portion of IgE (Williams et al. 1972). Similar circulating antibodies to the Fc portion of IgE were later found, which has great importance as they also react with undegraded IgE in atopics, including those with AD (Inganäs et al. 1981). Such complement-fixing immune complexes were previously demonstrated in AD in connection with food allergens (Brostoff et al. 1977; Paganelli et al. 1981) and were confirmed by radioimmunological assay (Kazmierowski et al. 1981; Ferguson and Salinas 1984). Quinti et al. (1984) reported, in an important work, a correlation between serum IgE and IgE-containing immune complexes of larger molecular weight (over 19 S: over 90000 daltons). This was present only in AD (and hyperimmunoglobulinemia E), not in respiratory atopy. On this basis Johansson (1984) and Geha and Leung (1986) suggest that these circulating anti-IgE antibodies might play a putative role in the mechanism of AD, by affecting (T) lymphocytes or mast cells. High molecular weight immune complexes have also been demonstrated in AD by special techniques, such as liquid chromatography (Swainson et al. 1985) and a polyethylene glycol precipitating method (Kapp et al. 1986). According to Kapp et al. (1986), C3 is also elevated in these immune complexes (in addition to significant amount of IgE), but is unrelated to skin involvement. These findings point to the possibility of type III mechanisms in AD.

5.5.2.2 In Vitro IgE Synthesis

In AD peripheral blood mononuclear (lymphocytic) cells might produce IgE, which can be demonstrated in the supernatants of cell culture, optimally after 1 week. This was shown in a few AD patients by Buckley and Becker (1978) and was found more frequently in severe AD cases by Hovmark (1979) and Hemady et al. (1983). Of the factors studied for their influence on IgE secretion, radiation and mitogens, particularly pokeweed mitogen (PWM), gave no uniform results, mostly no effect at all or merely a slight effect being reported (Cook et al. 1985; Ring et al. 1987), by contrast a correlation was observed with serum

IgE levels (Ring et al. 1987). Although these studies constitute an important argument for the role of IgE in AD, it is debatable whether the IgE produced by mononuclear cells is preformed and only released during the culture period, or whether it is a de novo B cell synthesis (Massicot and Ishizaka 1986). Regarding the latter, alternative T cell released helper factors (Geha et al. 1981) may be necessary, as mentioned above in connection with the regulation of IgE synthesis.

5.5.3 RAST

In 1967 Wide et al. developed a radioimmunological allergen-specific IgE in vitro assay technique, the RAST (see Fig. 5.8). The original RAST was later modified for various reasons, including interference with IgE blocking antibody and in order to increase sensitivity. The resulting refinements include the mini-RAST (Gleich et al. 1980) and the Phadezym RAST microtiter test, a procedure giving fluorimetric or colorimetric readings within a day (Schröder et al. 1985). Recently a multidisc method, i.e., several allergens of the same group coupled to the same disc, has been used for screening purposes (Kalveram 1985), or 12 different allergens have been used (Phadiatop, Gustafsson and Danielsson 1988). In addition, the enzyme-linked immunosorbent assay (ELISA) can also demonstrate allergen-specific IgE (and IgG) antibodies. The role of RAST in AD was thoroughly investigated in a monograph by Wütrich (1975). RAST studies have increased to such a degree that Steigleder organized three symposia in Cologne (1978, 1979 and in 1981), which included several important lectures on problems related to AD. [The second and third have been published (Steigleder 1979, 1981)]. The author considers skin tests and RAST to be closely related procedures, deviations in their findings depending on the fact that the former are influenced by IgE level and age of the patient. The correlation is best when higher (3–4) RAST classes are compared with skin or chal-

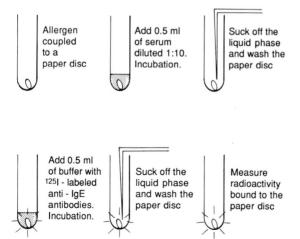

Fig. 5.8. The principle of the RAST with the use of allergens coupled in paper discs (Wide et al. 1972)

Table 5.19. The correlation of RAST to skin test in AD

Results of skin tests		Results of RAST	Interpretation of RAST
Varying according to allergens: 55%–89%	+	+	Equivalent with skin test
Certain foods	+	+ +	False-positive
Some cases	+ +	−	False-negative (no circulating reagin)
In 11%	−	+ +	Highly diagnostic
Respiratory atopies, pollen	+	+	Equivalent with skin test
Some ragweed allergics	+ +	+	Less diagnostic than skin test

Table 5.20. Main indications for RAST in AD

1. If skin tests should be avoided; dependent upon:
The person (infants, neurotics, etc.)
The state of skin inflammation (acute or generalized AD)
Difficulties in evaluation due to paradoxical skin reactivity
Medication (antihistaminics, steroids)
2. If equivocal history and/or skin tests are found concerning an important allergen
3. If total IgE level is high but the history of reaction to allergens is negative
4. For prospective studies of immunological development of AD in a high-risk pediatric population

lenge tests; otherwise RAST is, in general, less reliable in food sensitivity. Quantitative sequential variations may depend upon allergen exposure and possibly on the activity of the disease (Wütrich 1975). An interpretation of RAST results in AD compared to skin tests is given in Table 5.19, on the basis of data from several reports (Öhman and Johansson 1974; Wütrich 1974, 1975; Hoffman et al. 1975; Takahashi et al. 1977; MacKie et al. 1979; Berrens and Guikers 1980). The main indications for the performance of RAST are listed in Table 5.20.

5.5.4 Non-IgE Antibodies

It is possible that immunoglobulins other than IgE, subclasses of IgG for example, may have some reaginic activity (Parish 1970; Hubscher et al. 1970), and whether other immunoglobulin classes are related more closely to atopy or to AD is of considerable interest. The available information is conflicting, for several authors have been unable to find abnormal immunoglobin levels in sera from atopics (Huntley et al. 1963; Momma 1965; Buckley et al. 1968) whereas others have reported raised levels of individual immunoglobulins, including higher IgG levels in atopic children (Varelzidis et al. 1966; Berg and Johansson 1969) and higher IgA (Ortiz 1968) and IgD (Kohler and Farr 1967) levels in atopic sera. The findings of higher IgD, however, were not verified in atopic children by an electroimmunodiffusion technique by Brasher et al. (1973) or by Öhman and Johansson (1974).

IgG S-TS (short-term sensitizing anaphylactic IgG antibodies) seem to be absent in AD, but there are similarities in biological activity to IgG subclasses IgG4 and IgG2 (Parish 1981). IgG4 has already been discussed in connection with food allergens (see Sect. 5.3.6) but inhalants too can (although less markedly than food allergens) elicit antigen-specific reactions of the IgG4 type in AD patients, as demonstrated by RAST (Bruynzeel and Berrens 1979; Barnetson et al. 1981; Wütrich et al. 1983) or by an RIA technique (Rowntree et al. 1987). Gondo et al. (1987) found that patients with severe AD have a small amount of mite-specific IgG4, whereas those with mild AD have a high amount. In children with "pure" AD, Wütrich et al. (1983) reported normal IgG4 levels; only in cases in which respiratory allergy was also present were IgG levels elevated. For clinical significance, see Sect. 5.3.6.

The role of IgA has already been mentioned in Sect. 5.3.6. It was reported that while atopic children have normal levels of IgA in their saliva, patients with AD who suffer repeated upper respiratory tract infections have reduced salivary IgA levels (Brasher and Deiterman 1972).

Mediators of immediate-type skin reactions are mentioned in Chap. 6.

5.5.5 Evaluation of Immediate Type Skin Reactions

The following are objections customarily raised against attributing clinical significance to positive immediate-type skin reactions in AD:

1. Skin tests or passive transfer can produce only urticaria, a reaction which does not adequately reflect the skin lesions of AD.
2. Exposure to inhalation or food allergens by different techniques induces no typical lesions.
3. The use of positive skin tests to select those allergens for elimination or for use in specific hyposensitization is followed usually by neither a rapid nor even a consistent or convincing clinical improvement.

These objections have been voiced for a long time and have had strong supporters, including Sulzberger (1936), Cooke (1944), Nexmand (1948), Haxthausen (1957), and Jadassohn (1958), all of whom claimed that positive skin reactions are without clinical significance in AD and merely reflect the atopic state. Other authors, however, have considered that inhalants may be of some etiological significance (see Sects. 5.2.3–5.2.9) (Feinberg 1939; Rowe 1946; Tuft 1949; Storck 1954, 1955).

In the author's opinion, the primary and adequate symptom in AD is pruritus produced by allergic or nonimmunological mechanisms (see Sect. 3.2). Therefore the itch itself should be evaluated, not the concomitant wheals, for they are just a consequence of the introduction of an allergen or of a histamine-liberating substance into a shock tissue, namely the superficial capillary area of the corium. In the majority of cases the wheal may be etiologically nonspecific and should then be correlated with the atopic disposition. In fact, the occurrence of multiple positive skin reactions in AD ought to be regarded as evidence of nothing more than the primary atopic state, the reactions themselves being interpreted as "immunological markers"; nevertheless, type I reactivity may be of etiological importance in some cases. Likewise, the transformation of a wheal to lichenification has never been witnessed and was supposed to require and additional "X" factor (Hill 1952). Thus a single application of an allergen in a skin or a provocation test cannot elicit the essential prurigo or lichenification of AD, which are induced by repeated stimuli and are closely correlated with itch. This view, that repeated stimuli are necessary, is supported by the reported development of a plaque of eczema on a site where dust allergen had been repeatedly applied in the process of hyposensitizing an asthmatic patient (Derbes and Caro 1957). Sometimes, a positive skin reaction, which can be checked by RAST, is in accordance with the history and clinical facts; it is then possible to challenge with the relevant allergen, which may exacerbate the AD and occasionally, especially after challenge by inhalation, even induce new lesions, as has been observed by many workers, including Zakon and Taub (1938), Nexmand (1948), Tuft (1949), Hellerström and Lidman (1956), Nilzén (1958), Storck (1961), and Glaser (1965). It is generally assumed that a positive challenge involves an allergic mechanism, but it should be noted that nonimmunological pathways may be implicted instead. Clearly, elimination of or immunological measures (hyposensitization) against a reputed allergen will be effective only if that substance is in fact allergenic. This can be evidenced clinically by clinical improvement in a minority of AD patients when they take up residence in an environment lacking the allergen or are specifically hyposensitized to it.

5.5.5.1 Immediate-Type Reactions in AD and Respiratory Atopy

It has been assumed that different genes determine reagin production and select which organ manifests AD disease. Although it has been established that reaginic IgE production is higher in respiratory atopics than in AD patients, the major discrepancy between these two disease categories seems to lie in the *clinical* significance of the reagins (see Sect. 5.5.5), for, generally speaking, IgE (reagin) is of major significance in respiratory atopy whereas in AD it either plays only a minor etiological role or is of importance in only a small group of patients. This may be related to the fact that AD develops in only a small percentage of patients [10%–15% according to Engel et al. (1934)] with respiratory atopy and a good reagin-forming capacity.

As a concluding remark, confirmation that reagin may be of clinical importance in AD is provided by the presence of high levels of IgE and of specific IgE in the serum of the most severe cases and by the predominance of IgE in the peripheral lymphocytes and Langerhans' cells in the disease (see Sect. 5.5.2.1).

5.5.5.2 Immediate-Type Reactivity in Nonatopics

It is well-known that reagin is not confined to atopics but also occurs in nonatopics (Lindblad and Farr 1961; Curran and Goldman 1961), as can be seen from Table 5.7. Type I skin reactivity, after the injection of protein or of the poly-saccharide dextran as allergens, did not differ quantitatively in atopic an non-atopic subjects (Simon and Rackemann 1934a, b, Leskowitz and Lowell 1961); however, it should be noted that "induced" allergens were used in these experi-ments. Immediate-type skin reactivity in nonatopic subjects could be due to reaginic IgE, which is sometimes produced in normal persons, particularly those exposed to parasite antigens. Berrens (1971b) calculated from reports in the literature that the frequency distribution curve for type I responses to com-mon allergens is similar in shape in nonatopic and in AD subjects, even when the allergen dose administered is increased 100- to 1000-fold.

The essential difference in immediate-type reactivity between atopic and nonatopic subjects seems to be that atopics react to spontaneous exposure to natural allergens having a certain chemical structure and generally poor anti-genicity, whereas nonatopics do not. The route of exposure to the allergen seems to be of considerable significance, as intranasal administration results in greater skin test reactivity in atopics (Salvaggio et al. 1964). Several workers have emphasized the role not only of the allergen's penetration of the mucosae, including those of the respiratory and gastrointestinal tracts, but also of the dif-ferent allergens such as pollens; probably these phenomena are related to a finding by Tada and Ishizaka (1970) that IgE-producing cells are localized mainly in these mucosal areas.

5.6 Contact Reactivity

Immediate-type skin reactions were the first to be considered in this book be-cause they occur so commonly in AD. However, as this disease is usually classi-fied as an "eczema" or is described as having eczematous lesions, it can be as-sumed that delayed-type reactivity is also significant. The following is an attempt to analyze this complex problem.

5.6.1 Allergic Contact Dermatitis

Sensitivity in AD to contact allergens has frequently been recognized, and the responsible allergens may be any of the commonly incriminated substances present in the environment or belong to a large group of medicaments (some of which are potent sensitizers) used in topical application. The relevance of these sensitizing agents may be dependent, in part, on their increased percutaneous absorption consequent on the pathophysiological changes characteristic of AD skin, e. g. inflammation and damage by scratching.

Sulzberger et al. (1932) and Hill and Sulzberger (1935) were the first to state that epicutaneous reactivity is less pronounced in AD. This was confirmed by several other authors (Blumenthal and Jaffe 1933; Bonnevie 1939; Norrlind 1946), and data from larger series supported these findings. Rostenberg and Sulzberger (1937) investigated a large series and compared the frequency of

Table 5.21. Reactions to epicutaneous routine series in patients with AD

Patch test done in 535 patients	
Positive in 126 patients $= 23.5\%$	
Analysis of the 126 positive cases:	
$K_2Cr_2O_7$	49 reactions $= 9.2\%$[a]
Formaldehyde	45 reactions $= 8.4\%$
p-Phenylenediamine	44 reactions $= 8.2\%$
Nickel	39 reactions $= 7.3\%$
Oil of turpentine	8 reactions $= 1.5\%$
$HgCl_2$	5 reactions $= 0.9\%$

[a] Percentages relate to the total number of patients (535) tested

positive patch test reactions by using a sensitivity index: they found this index to be lower in AD patients (2.1) than in patients with other varieties of eczema (3.2) and distinctly lower than in patients with allergic contact dermatitits (5.2). The incidence of positive patch test reactions in the series of Skog and Thyresson (1953) was similar, the figures being 19.1% for AD patients, 31% for nondescript eczema patients, and 43% for allergic contact dermatitis patients. Fuchs (1960) obtained positive patch test responses in 14.3% of patients with seborrheic dermatitis, and in as many as 17.6% of 1704 persons free of skin disease. Investigating adults with earlier AD, the rate of positive patch tests was somewhat less in those with severe disease (Rystedt 1985). The lower response in AD to contact allergens is also valid for children (Angelini and Meneghini 1977).

The incidence of positive contact reactions to epicutaneous allergens in AD was 23.5% in the author's series (Rajka 1961, 1967) (see Table 5.21). Similarly, Cronin et al. (1970) found a frequency of 26% in their extensive material. This average, with a range of 15%–39%, was later also shown in other statistics (Bandman et al. 1972; Marghescu 1985). The concept of reduced contact reactivity in AD was also investigated by sensitization studies. The capacity in AD to be sensitized was found to be reduced in respect of DNCB (Palacios et al. 1966; Forsbeck et al. 1976), *Rhus* (Jones et al. 1973 a), and nitrosodimethylaniline (Forsbeck et al. 1976), but in respect of 3-pentadecylcatechol it was identical to that in a contact dermatitis patient group (Skog 1960).

However, not all authors share the above opinion, and some have demonstrated normal (Lammintausta et al. 1982; Huber et al. 1987) or even high reactivity in AD to contact allergens, particularly to topical medicaments (Epstein and Moharejin 1964). Of these drugs neomycin played a leading role and, in a later study, Epstein (1965) found that between 55% and 75% of 120 neomycin-sensitive patients were atopic. Epstein, however, used the latter term in its widest sense and included persons who produced wheals on skin testing with protein antigens, and Fisher (quoted by Epstein 1965), using the usual criteria, could not confirm his findings.

Although a high exposure exists in AD patients to topical medicaments which might also easily penetrate the damaged epidermal barrier, obviously the proven immunological alterations in AD (see Sect. 5.7.1) are a more potent factor in the incidence of contact reacitvity. On the other hand, special situations may emerge concerning some contact allergens such as balsam of Peru, fragrance substances, nickel (see below), and neomycin. On the basis of positive intracutaneous and epicutaneous tests to neomycin in AD, Epstein (1956, 1965) tried to explain the frequent sensitization in this disease through the concept of dermal contact dermatitis (Jillson et al. 1959). In short, a substance as a hapten combines with a component of the dermis rather than of the epidermis, as usually occurs in ordinary contact dermatitis. The resulting inflammation mostly affects the dermis and for diagnosis, intracutaneous tests are more adequate than patch tests.

5.6.1.1 Hybrids (Atopic Contact Dermatitis)

The combination of allergic contact dermatitis and AD has long been acknowledged and the term "hybrid" was introduced for this group by Malten (1968); others speak of atopic contact dermatitis. Combination with contact dermatitis involves only a proportion of AD patients. One of the known examples is baker's eczema, which in some cases corresponds to AD (Järvinen et al. 1979). In such patients, who have inhalatory as well as skin contact with wheat flour, a positive patch reaction was induced to flour (Pigatto et al. 1987). In this context it is of interest to read the remark of Meneghini and Bonifazi (1985) that special clinical characteristics are to be found among these patients, such as later onset, a predominance of females, more frequent hand and foot localization, and a lower incidence of asthma and food allergy, probably due to their lower IgE levels. In these hybrid cases both IgE-bearing lymphocytes, typical of AD, and IgD-bearing lymphocytes are present, which would be characteristic of contact dermatitis (Cormane et al. 1974). One can speculate that some immunological traits are important in the acquisition of contact allergy in these AD subjects; in particular the rate and function of T cells and their relation to B cells, as well as Langerhans' cells, may play a part here.

There are also examples of immediate reactions influencing allergic contact dermatitis. In five patients with AD plus respiratory symptoms responding to protein allergens with an immediate reaction, Strauss and Kligman (1957) observed that the administration of such allergens per- or subcutaneously or intranasally evoked a flare-up of a contact dermatitis due to a completely different allergen, i.e., Rhus toxicodendron. Food handlers' eczema may be considered a subgroup of such reactions: its occurrence indicates that contact with (food) proteins to which the subject shows an immediate-type reaction may elicit hand dermatitis in, among others atopics (see Sect. 2.15.5). Further complexity is added to this problem by the demonstration that inhalants (Reitamo et al. 1986; Bruynzeel-Koomen et al. 1986) or food allergens (Langeland and Braathen unpublished observations) may also cause positive eczematous patch reactions in AD (see Sects. 5.2.9 and 5.3.2).

5.6.1.2 Nickel Sensitization and AD

In contrast to the above-mentioned hybrids, the occurrence of nickel allergy in atopy and/or AD is frequent (Epstein 1956; Dobson 1963; Watt and Baumann 1968; Huber et al. 1987), being putatively correlated to familial or personal atopy (Wahlberg and Skog 1972; Christensen 1982) or to pompholyx (Christensen 1982). Others (Calnan 1956; Wilson 1956; Marcussen 1959; Caron 1964) could not, on clinical grounds, find such a connection between nickel allergy and atopy. However, several biases hinder the solution of this problem, such as:

1. The criteria for atopy are interpreted differently in various studies (Malten 1972; Christensen 1982).
2. The high incidence acknowledged in "healthy" women (Menné 1978; Prystowski et al. 1979; and others) is not always considered, and values reported are thus in the normal range (Rystedt 1985; Marghescu 1985; Schubert et al. 1987).
3. Pustular reactions related to sweat ducts (Wells 1956) or to irritation (Uehara et al. 1975) may occur in both atopic and nonatopic subjects (Epstein 1956; Caron 1964).

Additional data, such as normal IgE (Wahlberg and Skog 1971; Christensen 1982) or a lowered (Kim and Schöpf 1976) or normal (Silvennoinen-Kassinen 1981) lymphocyte transformation test, have failed to resolve the question of nickel allergy in AD. In a thought-provoking study, Möller and Svensson (1986) found that patients with a positive history of metal sensitivity but a negative patch or even intracutaneous test were mostly atopics, and similar findings were reported by Fischer and Rystedt (1985). Möller and Svensson (1986) consistently maintain that a positive metal history but a negative test indicates atopy. According to the author (Rajka unpublished observations), the incidenc of nickel allergy in diagnostically proven AD cases is so frequent that it could be discussed as a minor diagnostic criterion, a view shared by Huber et al. (1987) (see Chap. 10). However, for the moment the real cause of this correlation remains a mystery.

5.6.2 Irritative Contact Dermatitis

According to common clinical experience, the AD skin, probably due to its impaired lipid and water content and barrier damage, has a lower resistance to irritants, including lipid solvents and substances like SLS or cantharidin. Concerning cantharidin, results of earlier experiments by the author (Rajka 1975) are shown in Table 5.22. Allison and Bettley (1958) reported larger and more protein-rich blisters in AD, putatively due to inhibition of magnesium utilization in atopics (Allison and Williamson 1960). Contradictory results have been reported in respect of other chemical irritants. The nature of the agent probably plays a role: ditranol (Heite and Kleinhans 1961) and chrysarobin (Rajka 1962) evoked milder responses in AD patients than in controls, while pentadecylcate-

Table 5.22. Epicutaneous reaction to cantharidin of different concentrations in patients with AD

Concentration of cantharidin	AD group: 18 women + 7 men Number of reactions						Control group: 17 women + 8 men Number of reactions					
	−	(+)	+	2+	3+	4+	−	(+)	+	2+	3+	4+
100%	–	2	9	12	–	2	–	6	16	3	–	–
50%	1	1	15	6	1	1	3	7	13	2	–	–
25%	5	6	11	2	1	–	6	10	8	1	–	–
12%	8	9	6	2	–	–	5	13	6	1	–	–
6%	11	8	4	2	–	–	11	13	1	–	–	–
Total	25	26	45	24	2	3	25	49	44	7	–	–

Evaluation:	<2+	≥2+	
AD group	96	29	125
Control group	118	7	125
	214	36	250

χ^2 test between AD and control groups: $P < 0.001$

chol, in the irritant concentration of 1%, caused similar reactions in AD patients and controls (Skog 1960). These data correspond with the concept that susceptibility to irritants varies greatly among individuals (Kligman and Wooding 1967) and that it is impossible to predict the strength of a reaction to one irritant by knowing the strength of the reaction to another (Björnberg 1968). Further examples of an impaired tolerance of AD patients to irritants are their reactivity to soaps/detergents and wool.

5.7 Delayed (Tuberculin-Type) Reactivity

5.7.1 In Vivo Reactivity

During an investigation of skin reactivity to staphylococcal allergens the author noted that delayed reactions were much less frequent in AD patients than in controls, and consequently a more extensive investigation was designed to test these patients with common microbial antigens such as tuberculin and streptococcal and staphylococcal extracts, and in further studies also with diphtheria toxin, mumps antigen, and trichophytin. The results clearly revealed a significantly reduced incidence of delayed reactivity to these agents (Rajka 1963, 1967; 1968) (see Table 5.23).

This first demonstration of reduced delayed reactivity contrasted with observations that AD patients may produce delayed reactions on exposure to, for example, bacterial or environmental allergens and to such experimentally applied antigens as ascaris extract (Good et al. 1962). It also contrasted with reports of normal delayed (tuberculin-type) reactivity in AD "to intradermal injection of bacterial and mycelial antigens" (Palacios et al. 1966) and with works on der-

Table 5.23. Positive delayed reactions in AD and control groups

Allergens	I. AD	II. Controls with skin diseases	III. Respiratory atopics
Streptococcal extract	3/50	27/50	15/25
Staphylococcal extract	5/50	29/50	14/25
Tuberculin 0.1 mg	0/50	13/50	5/25
PPD 0.002 mg/ml	11/16	16/16	
Mumps vaccine 1:10	8/16	15/16	
Schick test	6/16	10/16	
Trichophytin 1:50	1/30	7/20	

mal reactivity to contact allergens (see Sect. 5.6.1). On the other hand, it indicated a decreased delayed reactivity to living agents in AD which corresponded to the known experience of clinicians about the frequent occurrence of such diseases in AD.

The reduced delayed reactivity to living agents was confirmed by Rudzki et al. (1965) concerning staphylococcal and streptococcal antigens and by Lobitz et al. (1972), who demonstrated a hyporeactivity against a series of these – in modern terminology – recall antigens. This was followed by reports by Hovmark (1975), Grove et al. (1975), Rogge and Hanifin (1976), Buckley (1976), Young et al. (1985), and many others, so that the reduced delayed reactivity is now accepted as a basic characteristic of AD.

The reduced cell-mediated immunity (CMI) is often parallel to the severity of AD (e. g., Buckley 1976), but may also be present in remission (Leung and Geha 1986). Furthermore, it should be stressed that as an argument for impaired CMI, it is, as an vivo test, more convincing and may show greater impairment (Buckley 1976) than in vitro methods. The latter, even though of great help in experimental work on CMI in AD, in principle throw light only on some parts of the complex mechanism of delayed reactivity in comparison to the intracutaneous test, which imitates the events occurring in clinical situations. This was demonstrated by negative skin tests but normal lymphocyte tests to *Candida* and streptokinase/-dornase (Elliot and Hanifin 1979).

Investigating the reactivity to tuberculin in AD, Uehara (1980 b) concluded that its strength was inversely related to the severity of the disease. Similar results were achieved by the same author in contact dermatitis, i. e., the suppression of the CMI might be subsequent to the inflammatory process (Uehara 1980).

5.7.2 In Vitro Reactivity

Lobitz et al. (1972), investigating two adults with AD, proved that they had depressed lymphocyte transformation. This study gave rise to a large number of in vitro studies – already started by his group (Pass et al. 1966) and by Fjelde and Kopeczka (1967) – which were also facilitated by a new simple method for separating mononuclear cells from peripheral blood (Bøyum 1969).

5.7.2.1 Lymphocytes

The effect of mitogens such as phytohemagglutinin (PHA) and concanavalin A (Con A) was first investigated, and a hyporeactivity to PHA was found in AD (Lobitz et al. 1972; Strannegård et al. 1976; Rachelefsky et al. 1976; Thestrup-Pedersen et al. 1977; Birkeland et al. 1981). On the other hand, only slightly reduced (Schöpf and Boehringer 1974; Andersen and Hjorth 1975; Hovmark 1975; Saraclar et al. 1977) or normal (Gottlieb and Hanifin 1974; Grove et al. 1975) reactivity was reported by several other authors. Reduced Con A stimulation in AD was also reported (Thestrup-Pedersen et al. 1977; Strannegård et al. 1976; Guilhou et al. 1978; Rola-Pleszcynski and Blanchard 1981). It should, however, be mentioned that differences in culture conditions and mitogen concentrations (e. g., Con A is mostly used suboptimally) could explain these divergent results. The next phase included the E rosette technique, i. e., binding to sheep erythrocytes. Reduced values for AD were reported (Luckasen et al. 1974; Gottlieb and Hanifin 1974; McGeady and Buckley 1975; Carapeto et al. 1976; Blaylock 1976; Strannegård et al. 1976; and others), whereas normal conditions were noted by Bjerring et al. (1982). A further step consisted of a method using the affinity of lymphocytes to IgG receptor, characteristic for T suppressor cells, or to IgM receptor, indicating T helper cells (Moretta et al. 1976; Canonica et al. 1979). T suppressor cells, also mediating cytotoxicity, were shown be susceptible to Con A, and particularly on this basis, T suppressor cell hyporeactivity was confirmed in most reports (Strannegård et al. 1978; Schöpf et al. 1978; Stingl et al. 1981; Jensen et al. 1981; Rola-Pleszcynski and Blanchard 1981; and others).

Constrasting results, i. e., normal function, were described by Schuster et al. (1980). Evidence was also found to show that the ability to generate Con A induced T suppressor cells was dependent on disease activity (Stingl et al. 1981). The T suppressor cell is more suspectible to cAMP and apparently to the inhibitory effect of histamine (Strannegård 1977; Ogden et al. 1979), though the latter finding was not confirmed by Martinez et al. (1979). Beer et al. (1982) found that a deficiency in H_2 receptor-bearing T cells correlated with a reduced production of histamine-induced suppressor activity in AD. Furthermore, the presence of thymosine (a bovine thymic hormone extract) inducible T cells, viewed as immature or blocked T suppressor cells, was reported by Byrom et al. (1979).

The recent trend in identification of T cell subgroups started with the development of monoclonal antibody techniques (Reinherz and Schlossman 1980). The OKT 8 (Leu 2) subgroup was identified as roughly corresponding to suppressor/cytotoxic T cells and OKT 4 (Leu 3) cells as helper/inducer cells, whereas a common T cell antigen (OKT 3) defined all peripheral T cells.

In AD decreased numbers of T3 and particularly T8 suppressor cells were found (Leung et al. 1981; Fulton et al. 1981; Willemze et al. 1983; Faure et al. 1982; Braathen 1985).

Consequently, there is a selective increase in the ratio of T4 to T8 cells. This ratio was increased even if the number of T4 cells was low (Miadonna et al.

1985; Klene et al. 1986). Furthermore, other reactions based on T cell function also showed impairment in AD, such as the local xenogeneic graft versus host reaction, i. e., the reaction obtained by, injecting patient lymphocytes into rat skin (Shohat et al. 1980). The autologous mixed lymphocyte reaction, indicating a proliferative T(8) cell response in cultures with autologous non-T cells, was reported to be reduced in AD by Leung et al. (1983) although this was disputed by Hwang et al. (1983).

Based on all these observations, the major hypothesis was that T suppressor cell deficiency is responsible for the elevated IgE levels in AD. Arguments for this theory include:

1. The results of animal experiments (Tada 1975)
2. Clinical observations in hypergammaglobulinemia E (Geha et al. 1981) and other immunodeficiency diseases
3. The fact that elevated in vitro IgE production may be suppressed by T8 cells from nonatopic donors (Geha et al. 1981; Saryan et al. 1983)
4. The secretion by atopic T cells of IgE binding factors (which together with suppressing factors isolated from nonatopic sera regulate IgE synthesis), see Sect. 5.5.2.2
5. The existence of an inverse relation between T suppressor cells and IgE levels (Cooper et al. 1980; Schuster et al. 1980; Stingl et al. 1981)

One consequence of the impaired T suppressor cell function may be production of naturally occurring autocytotoxic cells with a potential skin damaging effect (Leung and Geha 1986), although this was not confirmed due to the insignificant presence of NK cells (Zachary et al. 1985a). The decreased T cell function is already present in early life (Juto and Strannegård 1979), and in patients without overt disease it seems to be a primary event in AD.

There are also indications for other impaired cell immune functions, since Leung et al. (1983) found that T4 cells were deficient in AD. Furthermore, a defect was demonstrated in the generation of pokeweed mitogen-recruitable B cells (Cooper et al. 1983). Thus multiple immunoregulatory deficiencies may exist in AD (Leung and Geha 1986).

The mentioned immunological impairment has important clinical consequences, and is primarily significant in severe cases, mild cases showing, for example, a normal T4/T8 ratio (Braathen 1985). There is also a normalization in healed AD cases (Geha and Leung 1986; Rajka, unpublished observations). However, not all patients with severe AD show this immunological defect, and it may therefore be speculated that there are some subgroups without these features.

Notwithstanding the lack of agreement on every detail, the present general view concerning the T suppressor cell deficit represents a fruitful hypothesis which may be linked to other findings in AD (see below).

5.7.2.2 Recent Knowledge

The latest development of our knowledge on T cell receptors is still partly hypothetical. T cell receptors consist of a polymorph part which varies from T cell to T cell, i. e., a T idiopathic (Ti) molecule which is responsible for the binding of antigen and the major histocompatibility complex (with its class I and II antigens), and a monomorph part, i. e., CD (clusters of differentiation) 3, which has an effector function but which also strengthens the binding. T cytotoxic cells, CD8, recognize antigen together with class I (HLA A, B, C) molecules, whereas helper T4 cells recognize antigen together with class II (HLA DR, DP, DQ) molecules (Haskins et al. 1983; Goverman et al. 1986; and others). The practical consequence of the theory is that one now speaks of, for example, CD4 or CD8 cells instead of T4 or T8 cells.

5.7.2.3 Natural Killer (NK) Cells

A role of cytotoxic cells in AD was postulated by Parish and Champion in 1973. The "third" lymphocyte population, in addition to T and B cells, is the population of natural killer (NK) cells with cytotoxic activity. It can be identified by Leu 11 or Leu 7 (which also identifies K cells, which are probably similar to, or identical with, the former). It is assumed to play a role against tumor cells and viral infections, among other means by producing interferon (see below), and is demonstrated experimentally against target cells such as P3HR1 or 51 Cr-labeled K 562 cells, i. e., a human myeloid cell line.

Strannegård and Strannegård (1980) found increased activity of NK cells in children with AD, which was explained by faulty regulation by impaired suppressor cells; furthermore they produced less interferon. Viander et al. (1982), however, reported normal NK activity in AD.

Further studies showed a significant reduction of the cytotoxic capacity of NK cells in AD. Jensen et al. (1984) demonstrated that the reduction was related to the severity of AD, but it can be considered as secondary to the skin disease. The reduction in NK effect may be due to loss or moderation of activity of the NK cell (Jensen 1985). Decreased NK activity was also reported by other authors (Leung et al. 1982; Kusaimi and Trentin 1982; Lever et al. 1985; Schultz Larsen et al. 1985; Reinhold et al. 1986).

In addition to AD, reduced NK activity was reported in respiratory atopy (Frajman et al. 1987), and higher cytotoxicity was described in AD cases combined with respiratory atopy than in "pure" AD (Chiarelli et al. 1987).

5.7.3 Leukocytes and Monocytes

Several leukocyte functions were reported to be impaired in AD, such as chemotaxis, e. g., studied by the Boyden chamber method (Hill and Quie 1974; Uehara and Ofuji 1974; Snyderman et al. 1977; Furukawa and Altman 1978; Dahl et al. 1978; Rademecker and Maldogue 1981; Chiarelli et al. 1987), and phagocytosis (Michaelsson 1973; Rogge and Hanifin 1976). The putative cause of the chemotactic defect might lie in inhibitory plasma factors (Hanifin et al. 1980). Leukocyte migration was observed to be diminished in AD by a new technique based on production of leukocyte migration inhibiting factor (Horsmanheimo and Horsmanheimo 1979). Furthermore, diminished leukocyte adherence was found in response to histamine and isoproterenol (Thulin et al. 1980).

A reduced liberation of lysosomal enzymes, represented by 13 β-glucuronidase from leukocytes to different stimuli, was shown in AD by Ring and Lutz (1983).

The chemiluminescence response of neutrophils was reduced after stimulation with zymosan-activated serum and explained by specific in vivo leukocyte desensitization by C5a (Schöpf and Kapp 1987). Defective monocyte chemotaxis related to the active phase was first demonstrated by Rogge and Hanifin (1976) and confirmed by later investigations (Snyderman et al. 1977; Furukawa and Altman 1978). Normal chemotaxis, but inhibition after histamine, was seen in 11 AD patients by de Shazo et al. (1982). Monocytes were the effector cells in antibody-dependent cellular cytotoxicity (ADCC), which was found to be diminished in AD independent of clinical state of IgE levels. On the other hand, extrinsic asthma and rhinitis showed normal values (Kragballe et al. 1980; Herlin and Kragballe 1980).

The mechanism of ADCC in AD seems to be diminished respiratory burst, i. e., the signals created by the binding process are defective in activating monocytes (and neutrophils) (Kragballe and Borregaard 1981). The important monocyte (macrophage) function of production of interleukin-1 is reduced in AD (Mizoguchi et al. 1985; Räsänen et al. 1987).

5.7.4 Antigen-Presenting Cells

Due to epidermodermal changes and defective skin responses in AD, the role of antigen-presenting cells was investigated. The Langerhans' cell, which has structural and immunological similarities to monocytes and macrophages, is primarily involved. It is assumed that its main function is the uptake, processing, and presentation of various types of antigens of T (helper) lymphocytes and that its relevant efficacy is greater than that of monocytes (Braathen and Thorsby 1983). The antigens concerned include bacterial antigens (like PPD), herpes simplex virus, candida antigen, and trichophytin (Braathen and Thorsby 1980; Braathen et al. 1980; Braathen and Kaaman 1983). Langerhans' cells are involved in contact allergy (Silberberg 1973; Shelley and Juhlin 1977; Braathen 1980) and they are the only cells in the epidermis that express class II HLA/ DR antigens (Klareskog et al. 1977), furthermore, Langerhans' cell produce interleukin-1 (Sauder et al. 1984).

Uno and Hanifin (1980) were the first to, via the L-dopa histofluorescence method, report an increased number of Langerhans' cells in chronic (lichenified) skin lesions with occasional focal accumulation. Via monoclonal antibody techniques (i.e., OHT-6 positivity), an increased number of Langerhans cells' was seen in the skin by Rocha et al. (1984) and Sillevis Smith et al. (1986). In addition, other dendritic interdigitating reticulum cells (IRCS) (which can have a role in the presentation of gut-derived antigens) were found – as in other in- flammatory conditions (Janossy et al. 1981) – and were located adjacent to T helper cells (Zachary et al. 1985b). Similarly, anti-IgE staining was noted around T-lymphocyte clusters in the dermis by Lever et al. (1987). Via double labeling experiments interleukin-2 receptor positive T helper cells, indicating functional activation in association with antigen-presenting cells, were demon- strated (Dupuy et al. 1985). In connection with the presentation of epicutane- ously administered inhalant allergens (see Sect. 5.2.9), Bruynzel-Koomen (1986) and Bruynzel-Koomen et al. (1986) found positive IgE staining on Langerhans' cells, including symptom-free skin, only in AD. It was also hypotesized that Langerhans' cells, after having bound the antigen in the epidermis, migrate to the dermis in order to present the antigen to sensitized T cells.

The presence of IgE receptors on epidermal Langerhans' cells was a strong argument for the participation of these cells in the mechanism of AD, similar to in contact hypersensitivity, and also for a possible link between immediate and delayed sensitivity. This has, however, been disputed, as the expected class II HLA antigens were not found in AD in contrast to the observations in contact hypersensitivity (Barker and MacDonald 1987).

5.7.5 Skin Infiltrate

The cellular composition of the skin infiltrate in AD has also been investigated using an enzyme (acid α-naphtylacetate esterase) staining technique (Hovmark 1977a), rabbit anti-T cell serum (Braathen et al. 1979), or a monoclonal anti- body technique (Leung et al. 1983, and others). The infiltrate mostly consisted of T4 cells (Willemze et al. 1983, Leung et al. 1983) with a smaller number of T8 cells, i.e., there were changes similar to those in peripheral blood in AD, partic- ularly in the acute phase (Rocha et al. 1984). Furthermore, an increased num- ber of Langerhans' and IRCs was seen (see above).

These data are in accordance with the concept that there is a type IV hyper- sensitivity in AD which is clinically expressed as an eczematous inflammation (Zachary et al. 1985b, and others).

5.7.6 Anti-Infectious Resistance

The above-mentioned impaired delayed reactivity, as well as the defective leu- kocyte and monocyte functions, has obvious clinical consequences such as re- duced resistance against living agents (see Sects. 2.9.1–2.9.3), and there are simi- larities to certain immunodeficiency diseases (Saurat et al. 1985). Turk stated in 1970 that "raised immunoglobulin levels in AD are associated with some de- gree of lowered cell-mediated immunity in that the patients may have a lower

resistance to the viruses of herpes simplex and vaccinia and are readily susceptible to secondary infections." Using the Sendai virus model technique, α-inter-
feron production was found to be reduced in AD (Strannegård and Strannegård 1980). On the other hand, α or γ-interferon production was reported to be
normal in AD subjects with reduced T cell mitogen responses (Kapp et al.
1987). In AD patients with a history of severe cutaneous viral infections, the
ADCC (see Sect. 5.7.2) was depressed under certain experimental conditions
(Fritz et al. 1980). Raised Epstein-Barr virus titers were shown in AD, and in
one case AD was precipitated by infectious mononucleosis that had been
caused by this virus (Strannegård et al 1985; Barnetson et al. 1981).

Furthermore, herpesvirus hominis-induced T cell proliferation was normal
but in autologous mixed cell reactions a defect was reported (Räsänen et al.
1987). David et al. (1987) found no differences between AD patients and controls in neutral herpes simplex antibodies, whereas in one AD child with recurrent severe herpes simplex infections IgG2 deficit was detected (David and
Longson 1985). In eczema herpeticum patients impaired suppressor cell function seems to be of importance (Vestey et al. 1988).

Molluscum contagiosum in its widespread form was reported in AD by Solomon and Telner (1966) and Ganpule and Garretts (1971), while in its chronic
form it was observed in an AD patient with high IgE and depressed cell-mediated immunity (Pauly et al. 1978). It has been postulated by Currie et al. (1971)
that there is an increased incidence of viral warts in patients with three or more
atopic stigmata.

In summary, the majority of investigators found decreased resistance against
cutaneous viral infections. The contorversies can, in the opinion of the author,
be explained by the fact that several factors are operative in virus-host interactions (see e. g., Giannetti 1987) and all of these have to be considered when investigating the host reactions. The relation to staphylococcal infections has already been discussed (see Sect. 5.4.1).

5.7.7 Cell-Mediated Immunity in Respiratory Atopies

There exists a strong parallelism between AD and bronchial asthma from the
point of view of immunochemistry (Aas 1979); however, some divergencies
may be found.

5.7.7.1 Induced Reactivity

Several reports have dealt with the capacity of respiratory atopic patients to respond with delayed reactivity (Vaughan 1929, and others). Findings relevant to
this topic include: the report by Simon and Rackemann (1934 a, b) that delayed
reactivity occurs in atopic after intradermal or intranasal administration of guinea pig serum; the demonstration by Feinberg et al. (1962) that atopic subjects
are not "constitutionally incapable" of producing delayed reactions to pollen
emulsions; and the observation by Salvaggio et al. (1964) that delayed reactivity

was seen in nonatopic subjects only when they used ribonuclease. It is noteworthy, however, that all these reports dealt with induced and not with spontaneous sensitization.

5.7.7.2 Reactivity to Allergens

There are problems in evaluating delayed reactivity in hay fever and asthma, as demonstrated in the studies of Brostoff and Roitt (1969), in which they had to block with antihistamines the predominant immediate-type reactivity of their hay fever patients in order to demonstrate the presence of delayed reactivity. It is not possible to determine from the available literature the frequency or the importance of this delayed reactivity. From the author's investigations of AD and of respiratory atopic patients, it was found that delayed reactivity was as low in respiratory atopics as in nonatopic controls but much higher than in AD.

5.7.7.3 Cell-Mediated Immunity in General

There are a number of data on depressed CMI in respiratory atopics, primarily asthmatics, particularly in respect of parameters indicating T cell decrease. In children, normal values have usually been detected (Hsieh 1976; McGeady et al. 1976), but slight (Saraclar et al. 1977) or even considerable reductions have also been reported (Grove et al. 1975; Strannegård et al. 1976; Khan et al. 1976; Byrom 1980).

In adult asthmatics T cell lymphopenia was reported by Gupta et al. (1975), but in the majority normal or only slightly subnormal levels of T cells were registered (Blaylock 1976). Martinez et al. (1979) and Leung et al (1981) also found normal levels in patients with asthma and rhinitis, and Yocum et al. (1976) reported normal levels in 17 subjects with atopic rhinitis.

5.8 Other Reaction Types

The *late cutaneous reaction* has already been mentioned in connection with itch (see Sect. 3.1) and food reactivity (see Sect. 5.3.6). In short, it is assumed that an IgE-based immediate reaction releases different mediators, including histamine, kallikrein, leukotrienes, thromboxane, and PAF (Dorsch 1988) and that these, by a complex interaction (including chemotaxis of inflammatory cells) are responsible for a reaction appearing 4-24 h later (Dolovitch et al. 1973; Dorsch and Ring 1981; Gleich 1982; Kaliner 1984). The inflammatory cells appearing in the experimental clinical reaction are at first neutrophils and eosinophils (Ting et al. 1980; Gleich 1982), but later mononuclears predominate (Lemanske et al. 1983). Leiferman et al. (1989) mean, however, that due to the difference in elastase deposition, AD can not be explained simply as an ongoing late phase reaction.

Type II and type III reactivity: Type II sensitivity, often involved in autosensitization, is an interesting possibility even in AD, but it is too early to draw conclusions on this point. If it is accepted that dandruff is an important or even the principal allergen in AD, then an autosensitization process is feasible. Although AD patients may develop type III reactions, they have a greater tendency to respond with type I reactivity (Pepys 1969).

Here it should be mentioned that the *occurrence of malignant neoplams,* despite depressed CMI, does not differ from that in a normal population (Kaaber 1976). Blaylock (1976) mentions briefly that there is clinical evidence that atopic patients have a lowered incidence of leukemia.

5.9 Concluding Remarks

It is well documented that inhalants (which, like mites, may obviously reach the skin by contact) and food allergens frequently elicit a specific IgE response; however, they have an etiological role in AD in only a minority of cases. Usually their role in producing itch and subsequent flare-up is probably of more relevance for the mechanism of AD. It is thus appropriate to speak of AD as a disease in which allergic (IgE mediated) factors are more or less represented, rather than as an allergic disease per se.

The impaired CMI, as earlier reported by the author (Rajka 1963, 1967), by Lobitz et al. (1972), and by several others, can be confirmed as characteristic of AD even if not present in all patients. The possibly only secondary impairment

Table 5.24. Some important typical immunological responses in AD

Immediate reactivity to inhalants	Increased
Immediate reactivity to food	Increased
Immediate reactivity to mites (inhalant/contact)	Increased
Skin test positivity in general	Increased
IgE/Serum	Increased
Spontaneous in vitro IgE synthesis	Increased
Contact urticaria, frequency	Increased
Late cutaneous reactivity, frequency	Normal (increased?)
Contact allergy in general	Reduced
Contact allergy to nickel	Increased
Sensitization to DNCB	Reduced
Cell-mediated immunity in general	Reduced
Delayed reactivity to microbial agents	Reduced
In vitro lymphocyte response to mitogens	Reduced
T suppressor cell quantity/function	Reduced
T helper cell quantity/function	Normal (increased?)
NK/monocyte/leukocyte functions	Reduced
Resistance to viral infections	Reduced
Resistance to staphylococci/dermatophytes	Reduced
Langerhans' cell function	Normal (increased?)
Allograft rejection/GVH reactivity	Normal[a]
Occurrence of malignant neoplasms	Normal

[a] Local xenogeneic GVH was reduced (Shohat et al. 1980)

of NK, monocyte, and leukocyte functions has important clinical consequences as regards certain living agents. Some data on immediate and delayed reactivity are shown in Table 5.24.

The bridge between immediate and delayed reactivity in AD may be exemplified by the evident interplay between T and B cells and by IgE-bearing Langerhans' cells; the late cutaneous reactivity may also have some relevance here. Further relations are connected with the immunochemistry and the role of mediators in AD (see Chap. 6).

References

Aas K (1967) Studies in hypersensitivity to fish. Int Arch Allergy Appl Immunol 29: 346
Aas K (1970) Bronchial provocation test in asthma. Arch Dis Child 45: 221
Aas K (1978) What makes an allergen an allergen. Allergy 33: 3
Aas K (1979) Common immunochemistry in atopic dermatitis and bronchial asthma. Acta Derm Venereol [Suppl] (Stockh) 92: 64
Aas K, Belin L (1972) Standardization of diagnostic work in allergy. Acta Allergol 27: 439
Aas K, Elsayed S (1969) Characterization of a major allergen (cod.) Effect of enzymic hydrolysis on the allergenic activity. J Allergy 44: 333
Aas K, Leegaard J, Auktrust L, Grimmer O (1980) Immediate hypersensitivity to common moulds. Allergy 35: 443
Abramson JS, Dahl MV, Walsh G, Blumenthal MN, Douglas SD, Quie PG (1982) Antistaphylococcal IgE in patients with atopic dermatitis. J Am Acad Dermatol 7: 105
Adinoff AD, Tellez P, Clark RAF (1988) Atopic dermatitis and aeroallergen contact sensitivity. J Allergy Clin Immunol 81: 736
Alani MD, Harlov N (1972) The house dust mite: a possible source of allergen in the environment of patients with atopic dermatitis. J Natl Med Assoc 64: 302
Alberse RC, Koshte V, Clemens JGJ (1981) Immunoglobulin E antibodies that cross-react with vegetable foods, pollen and Hymenoptera venom. J Allergy Clin Immunol 68: 356
Alexander HL (1931) An evaluation of the skin test in allergy. Ann Intern Med 5: 52
Allison JH, Bettley FR (1958) Investigations into cantharidin blisters raised on apparently normal skin in normal and abnormal subjects. Br J Dermatol 70: 331
Allison JH, Williamson DH (1960) The abnormal cantharidin blister in atopy: an explanation on its production. Br J Dermatol 72: 383
Anan S (1976) Cellules porteuses d'immunoglobulines au niveau de la peau. Études en immunofluorescence dans les lésions d'eczéma atopique. Rev Fr Allergol 16: 65
Andersen E, Hjorth N (1975) B lymphocytes, T lymphocytes and phytohaemagglutinin responsiveness in atopic dermatitis. Acta Derm Venereol (Stockh) 55: 345
Anderson KE, Löwenstein H (1978) An investigation of the possible relationship between allergen extracts from birch pollen, hazelnut, potato and apple. Contact Dermatitis 4: 73
Angelini G, Meneghini CL (1977) Contact and bacterial allergy in children with atopic dermatitis. Contact Dermatitis 3: 163
Atherton DJ (1981) Allergy and atopic eczema. II. Clin Exp Dermatol 6: 317
Atherton DJ (1982) Atopic eczema. In: Brostoff I, Challacombe SJ (eds) Food Allergy, vol 12. Saunders, London, p 77
Atherton DJ, Sewell M, Soothill JR, Wells RS, Chivers CED (1978) A double blind controlled crossover trial of antigen avoidance diet in eczema. Lancet I: 401
Atkins FM, Steinberg SS, Metcalfe DD (1985) Evaluation of immediate adverse reactions to food in adult patients. II. A detailed analysis of reaction patterns during oral food challenge. J Allergy Clin Immunol 75: 356
August PJ (1984) House dust mite cause atopic eczema: a preliminary study (abstract). Br J Dermatol (Suppl 26): 10

Augustin R, Hayward BJ (1962) Grass pollen allergens. Immunology 5: 124

Augustin R, O'Sullivan S, Davies I (1971) Isolation of grass pollen allergens failing to induce IgE reagin formation although capable of inducing IgG antibody formation. Int Arch Allergy Appl Immunol 41: 144

Baer RL (1955) Atopic dermatitis. Lippincott, Philadelphia

Bahna SL, Hiener DC, Myhre BA (1983) Immunoglobulin E pattern in cigarette smokers. Allergy 38: 57

Balyeat RM (1930) Allergic eczema. J Allergy 1: 516

Bandmann HJ, Breit R, Leutgeb C (1972) Kontaktallergie und Dermatitis atopica. Arch Dermatol Res 244: 332

Barker JNWN, Alegre VA, MacDonald DM (1988) Surface-bound immunoglobulin E on antigen-presenting cells in cutaneous tissue of atopic dermatitis. J Invest Dermatol 90: 117

Barnetson RSC (1980) Hyperimmunoglobulinæmia E in atopic eczema (atopic dermatitis) is associated with "food allergy". Acta Derm Venereol [Suppl] (Stockh) 92: 94

Barnetson RSC, Drummond H, Ferguson A (1983) Precipitins to dietary proteins in atopic eczema. Br J Dermatol 109: 653

Barnetson R, Hardie RA, Merrett TG (1981) Late onset atopic eczema and multiple food allergies after infectious mononucleosis. Br Med J 283: 1086

Barnetson RSC, Macfarlane HAF, Benton EC (1987) House-dust mite allergy and atopic eczema. Br J Dermatol 116: 857

Barnetson RSC, Merrett TG, Merrett J, Burr M (1981) IgG 4 in atopic eczema (abstract). Br J Dermatol 108: 220

Bazaral M, Orgel HA, Hamburger RN (1971) IgE levels in normal infants and mothers and an inheritance hypothesis. J Immunol 107: 794

Beck HI, Hagdrup HK (1987) Atopic dermatitis, house dust mite allergy and month of birth. Acta Derm Venereol (Stockh) 67: 448

Beer DJ, Osband ME, McCaffrey RP, Soter NA, Rocklin RE (1982) Abnormal histamine-induced suppressor cell function in atopic subjects. N Engl J Med 306: 454

Benton EC, Barnetson RSC (1985) Skin reactions to foods in patients with atopic dermatitis. Acta Derm Venereol [Suppl] (Stockh) 92: 129

Berg T, Johansson SGO (1969) Immunoglobulin levels during childhood with special regard to IgE Acta Pædiatr Scand 58: 513

Berglund A, Kober A, Ahlberg M, Persson E (1985) Monoclonal antibodies in IgE assays. Allergy 40 (Suppl 4): 14

Bergquist G, Nilzén Å (1959) Gesichtspunkte zur Hauttestung mit Bakterienvakzinen bei Asthma und Ekzem (Prurigo Besnier). In: Findeisen DGR, Hansen K (eds) Aktuelle Allergiefragen vol 4. Barth, Leipzig

Bergquist G, Nilzén Å (1960) The thrombocyte index after injection of staphylococcus vaccine in man. Acta Derm Venereol (Stockh) 40: 58

Bernstein L, Safferman RS (1970) Viable algae in house dust. Nature 227: 851

Berrens L (1971a) The chemistry of atopic allergens. Monogr Allergy 7

Berrens L (1971b) An analytic approach to the frequency distribution of positive skin reactions to atopic allergens. Ann Allergy 29: 118

Berrens L, Guikers CLH (1980) RAST with human dander allergen in atopic dermatitis. Acta Derm Venereol [Suppl] (Stockh) 92: 116

Bhalla RB et al. (1982) Serum IgE levels in a Northeast Unites States Caucasian population. In: Bensen AA (ed) Advanced interpretation of clinical laboratory data. Decker, New York, p 295

Billewicz WZ, McGreger IA, Roberts DF, Rowe DS, Wilson RJM (1974) Family studies in immunoglobulin levels. Clin Exp Dermatol 16: 13

Birkeland SA, Ølholm Larsen P, Schultz Larsen F (1981) Subpopulations of lymphocytes and lymphocyte transformation tests in atopic dermatitis: an evaluation of a systemic treatment with a new chromone compound and comparison with a normal group. J Invest Dermatol 76: 367

Bjerring T, Thestrup Pedersen K (1982) E-rosette formation of lymphocytes from patients with atopic dermatitis. Acta Derm Venereol (Stockh) 62: 31

Björksten F, Saarinen UM (1978) IgE antibodies to cow's milk in infants fed by breast milk and milk formulæ. Lancet II.: 624

Björksten F, Suoniemi I (1981) Dependence of immediate hypersensitivity on the month of birth. Allergy 36: 263

Björnberg A (1968) Skin reactions to primary irritants in patients with hand eczema. Isacson Tryckeri AB, Gothenburg

Blaylock WK (1976) Atopic dermatitis: diagnosis and pathobiology. J Allergy Clin Immunol 57: 62

Blumenthal F, Jaffe K (1933) Ekzem und Idiosynkrasie. Karger, Berlin

Blumenthal MN, Namboodiri K, Mendell N, Gleich G, Elston RC, Yunis E (1981) Genetic transmission of serum IgE levels. Am J Med Genet 10: 219

Bock SA, Lee WY, Remigio LK, May CD (1978) Studies of hypersensitivity reactions to foods in infants and children. J Allergy Clin Immunol 62: 327

Boner AL, Antolini I, Zambelli M et al. (1985) Preliminary report on histamine release, circulating immune complexes and complement activation in children with atopic dermatitis after oral challenge with milk and egg antigens. Ann Allergy 54: 442

Bonifazi E, Garofalo L, Monterisi A, Meneghini CL (1978) Food allergy in atopic dermatitis: experimental observations. Acta Derm Venereol (Stockh) 58: 349

Bonnevie P (1939) Aetiologie and Pathogenese der Ekzemkrankheit. Barth, Leipzig

Borelli S (1970) Untersuchungen am Kranken mit atopischer Neurodermitis. Hautarzt 21: 335

Borelli S, Berowa N (1965) Vergleichende allergologische Untersuchungen bei Neurodermitis constitutionalis atopica. Hautarzt 16: 269

Böyum A (1969) Separation of leucocytes from blood and bone marrow. Scand J Clin Lab Invest 21 (Suppl 97): 1

Braathen LR (1980) Studies on human epidermal Langerhans' cells. III. Induction of T lymphocyte response to nickel sulphate in sensitized individuals. Br J Dermatol 103: 517

Braathen LR (1985) T-cell subsets in patients with mild and severe atopic dermatitis. Acta Derm Venereol [Suppl] (Stockh) 114: 133

Braathen LR, Kaaman T (1983) Human epidermal Langerhans' cells induce cellular immune response to trichophytin in dermatophytosis. Br J Dermatol 109: 295

Braathen LR, Thorsby E (1980) Studies on human epidermal Langerhans' cells. I. Alloactivating and antigen-presenting capacity. Scand J Immunol 11: 401

Braathen LR, Thorsby E (1983) Human epidermal Langerhans' cells are more potent than blood monocytes in inducing some antigen-specific T-cell response. Br J Dermatol 108: 139

Braathen LR, Förre O, Natvig JB, Eeg-Larsen T (1979) Predominance of T lymphocytes in the dermal infiltrate of atopic dermatitis. Br J Dermatol 112: 149

Braathen LR, Berle E, Mobeck-Hansen U, Thorsby E (1980) Studies on human epidermal Langerhans' cells. II. Activation of human T lymphocytes to herpes simplex virus. Acta Derm Venereol (Stockh) 60: 381

Brasher GW, Deiterman LH (1972) Salivary IgA and infection in children with atopy. Ann Allergy 30: 241

Brasher GW, Hall FF, Bourland PD (1973) Serum IgD concentrations in children with atopic diseases. J Allergy Clin Immunol 52: 167

Brostoff I, Carini C, Wraith DG, Paganelli R, Levinsky R (1979) Immune complexes in atopy. In: Pepys J, Edwards AM (eds) The mast cell: its role in health and disease. Pitman, London, p 380

Brostoff J, Roitt I (1969) Cell-mediated (delayed) hypersensitivity in patients with summer hay fever. Lancet II: 1296

Brunner M, Walzer M (1928) Absorption of undigested proteins in human beings: the absorption of unaltered fish protein in adults. Arch Intern Med 42: 173

Brunsting LA (1936) Atopic dermatitis (disseminated neurodermitis) of young adults. Arch Dermatol Syph 34: 935

Bruynzeel PLB, Berrens L (1979) IgE and IgG4 antibodies in specific human allergies. Int Arch Allergy Appl Immunol 58: 344

Bruynzeel-Koomen C (1986) IgE on Langerhans' cells: new insight into the pathogenesis of atopic dermatitis. Dermatologica 172: 181

Bruynzeel-Koomen C, van Wichen DF, Toonstra J, Berrens L, Bruynzeel PLB (1986) The presence of IgE molecules on epidermal Langerhans' cells in patients with atopic dermatitis. Arch Dermatol Res 278: 199

Bruynzeel-Koomen CAFM, van Wichen DF, Spry C, Venge P, Bruynzeel P (1988) Active participation of eosinophils in patch test reactions to inhalant allergens in patients with atopic dermatitis. Br J Dermatol 118: 229

Buckley RH (1976) The functions and measurement of human B- and T-lymphocytes. J Invest Dermatol 67: 381

Buckley RH, Becker WG (1978) Abnormalities in the regulation of human IgE synthesis. Immunol Rev 41: 288

Buckley RH, Dees SC, O'Fallon WM (1968) Serum immunoglobulins. I. Levels in normal children and in uncomplicated childhood allergy. Pediatrics 41: 600

Burks AW jr, Brooks JR, Sampson HA (1988) Allergeni city of major component proteins of soybean determined by enzyme-linked immunosorbent assay (ELISA) and immunoblotting in children with atopic dermatitis and positive soy challenges. J Allergy Clin Immunol 81: 1135

Byrom NA (1980) Thymosin-inducible "null" cells in atopic children. Acta Derm Venereol [Suppl] (Stockh) 92: 63

Byrom NA, Staughton RCD, Campbell MA, Timlin DM, Chooi M, Lane AM, Copeman CWM, Hobbs JR (1979) Thymosin-inducible "null" cells in atopic eczema. Br J Dermatol 100: 499

Calnan CD (1956) Nickel dermatitis. Practitioner 177: 303

Canonica GS, Mingari MC, Mellioli G, Colombatti M, Moretta L (1979) Imbalances of T-cell subpopulations in patients with atopic diseases and effect of specific immunotherapy. J Immunol 123: 2669

Cant A, Marsden RA, Kishaw PJ (1985) Egg and cow's milk hypersensitivity in breast fed infants with eczema. Br Med J 291: 932

Carapeto FJ, Winkelmann RK, Jordon RE (1976) T and B lymphocytes in contact and atopic dermatitis. Arch Dermatol 112: 1095

Caron GA (1964) Nickel sensitivity and atopy. Br J Dermatol 76: 384

Carswell F, Thompson S (1986) Does natural sensitisation in eczema occur through the skin? Lancet II: 13

Champion RH (1971) Atopic sensitivity to algæ and lichens. Br J Dermatol 85: 551

Chapman MD, Platt-Mills TAE (1980) Purification and characterization of the major allergen from *Dermatophagoides pteronyssinus* antigen P1. J Immunol 125: 587

Chapman MD, Rowntree S, Mitchell EB, Di Prisco Fuenmayor MC, Platt-Mills TAE (1983) Quantitative assessment of IgG and IgE antibodies to inhalant allergens in patients with atopic dermatitis. J Allergy Clin Immunol 72: 27

Chiarelli F, Canfora G, Verrotti A, Amerio P, Morgese G (1987) Humoral and cellular immunity in children with active and quiescent atopic dermatitis. Br J Dermatol 116: 651

Christensen OB (1982) Prognosis in nickel allergy and hand eczema. Contact Dermatitis 8: 71

Christophersen J, Badsgaard O, Christiansen J (1986) IgE antibodies to *Staphylococcus aureus*. Arch Dermatol 122: 971

Clendenning WE, Clark WE, Ogawa M, Ishizaka K (1973) Serum IgE studies in atopic dermatitis. J Invest Dermatol 61: 233

Coca AF, Cooke RA (1923) On the classification of the phenomena of hypersensitiveness. J Immunol 8: 163

Coca FA, Grove EF (1925) Studies in hypersensitiveness. J Immunol 10: 445

Collins-Williams C (1956) The incidence of milk allergy in pediatric patients. Pediatrics 48: 39

Cook RM, Deards MJ, Rhodes EL, Moran DM (1985) In vitro production of IgE and IgG protein by blood mononuclear cells from non-atopic and atopic donors. Allergy 40: 115

Cooke RA (1944) A consideration of some allergic problems. J Allergy 15: 203

Cooke RA (1947) Allergy in theory and praxis. Saunders, Philadelphia

Cooke EM, Buck HW (1963) Self-contamination of dermatological patients with *Staphylococcus aureus*. Br J Dermatol 75: 21

Cooper KD, Hanifin JM, Wuepper KD (1980) Tγ and Tμ cell subsets in atopic dermatitis (abstract). Clin Res 28: 20A

Cooper KD, Kazmierowski JA, Wuepper KD, Hanifin JM (1983) Immunoregulation in atopic dermatitis: functional analysis of T-B cell interactions and the enumeration of Fc receptor-bearing T cells. J Invest Dermatol 80: 139

Cormane RH, Husz S, Hamerlinck F (1974) Immunoglobulin and complement-bearing lymphocytes in allergic contact dermatitis and atopic dermatitis (eczema). Br J Dermatol 90: 597

Craps L, Meets P, Boncoin-Beckman S (1959) Les antistreptolysines en dermatologie. Analyse de cinq cent observations. Arch Belg Dermatol 15: 153

Croner S, Kjellman NIM (1986) Predictors of atopic disease: cord blood IgE and month of birth. Allergy 41: 68

Croner S, Kjellman NIM, Eriksson B, Roth A (1982) IgE screening in 1701 newborn infants and the development of atopic disease during infancy. Arch Dis Child 57: 364

Cronin E, Bandmann HJ, Calnan CD, Fregert S, Hjorth N, Magnusson B, Maibach HI, Malten K, Meneghini CL, Pirila V, Wilkinson DS (1970) Contact dermatitis in the atopic. Acta Derm Venereol (Stockh) 50: 183

Curran WS, Goldman G (1961) Incidence of immediately reacting allergy skin test in a normal adult population. Ann Intern Med 55: 777

Currie JM, Wright RC, Miller OG (1971) The frequency of warts in atopic patients. Cutis 8: 243

Dahl MV, Lynn CK, Quie PG (1978) Neutrophil chemotaxis in patients with atopic dermatitis without infections. Arch Dermatol 114: 544

Dannæus A, Johansson SGO, Foucard T, Öhman S (1977) Clinical and immunological aspects of food allergy in children. I. Estimation of IgG, IgA and IgE antibodies in children with food allergy and atopic dermatitis. Acta Pædiatr Scand 66: 31

David TJ, Longson M (1985) Herpes simplex infections in atopic eczema. Arch Dis Child 60: 338

David TJ, Richmond SJ, Bailey AS (1987) Serological evidence of herpes simplex virus infection in atopic eczema. Arch Dis Child 62: 416

De Besche A (1923) Studies on the reactions of asthmatics and on passive transference of hypersusceptibility. Am J Med Sci 166: 265

De Graciansky P (1966) Eczéma constitutionnel. Soc Med Hop Paris 114: 765

Derbes VJ, Caro MR (1957) Localized eczema induced by house dust extract injections. Arch Dermatol 75: 804

De Shazo RD, Hase T, Wright DG, Diem JE (1982) Evidence for histamine-mediated inhibition of monocyte chemotaxis in atopic dermatitis. J Allergy Clin Immunol 69: 429

Desmons F, Delmas-Marsalet Y, Goudemand J (1976) HLA antigens and atopic dermatitis. J Allergol Immunopathol 4: 29

Dessaint JP, Capron A, Joseph M, Bazin H (1979) Cytophilic binding of IgE to the macrophage II. Immunologic release of lysosomal enzyme from macrophages by IgE and anti-IgE in the rat: a new mechanism of macrophage activation. Cell Immunol 46: 24

De Week AL, Stadler B, Knutti-Müller J (1986) Regulation of IgE by lymphoid cell derived factors. In: Ring J, Burg G (eds) New trends in allergy. II. Springer, Berlin Heidelberg New York, p 16

Dobson RD (1963) In: Discussion of Vanderberg JJ, Epstein WL. Experimental nickel sensitivity. J Invest Dermatol 41: 416

Dolovitch J, Hargreave FE, Chalmers R, Shier KJ, Gauldie Bienenstock J (1973) Late cutaneous responses in isolated IgE-dependent reactions. J Allergy Clin Immunol 52: 38

Dorsch W (1988) IgE and common allergic diseases. Allergy 43 (Suppl 5): 38

Dorsch W, Ring J (1981) Induction of late cutaneous reactions by skin blister fluid from allergen tested and normal skin. J Allergy Clin Immunol 67: 117

Dreborg S (1985) Application of allergen research to diagnosis and immunotherapy. In: Björksten B, Weeke B (eds) Ann Meet. Europ Acad Allergol Clin Immunol Allergy, Vol 40 (Suppl 4): 50

Dupuy PF, Poulter LW, Zachary CB, MacDonald DM (1985) Cell mediated immune mechanisms in atopic dermatitis (abstract). Br J Dermatol 13: 763

Dvorak AM, Mihm MC, Dvorak HF (1976) Degranulation of basophilic leukocytes in allergic contact dermatitis reactions in man. J Immunol 116: 687

Eberhartinger C, Landes E (1960) Zur Frage der Bedeutung der Bakterien bei der Dermatitis eccematosa. Arch Klin Exp Dermatol 212: 17

Edfors-Lubs ML (1971) Allergy in 700 twin pairs. Acta Allergol 26: 249

Edgren G (1943) Prognose und Erblichkeitsmomente bei Ekzema infantum. Eine klinisch-statistische Untersuchung von Allergieerscheinungen. Acta Pædiatr Scand 30 (Suppl 2): 1

Eichenberger ME (1963) Über Vorkommen, Verlauf, Testresultate und Therapie der Neurodermitis. Inaugural Dissertation, Juris, Zürich

Einarsson R (1985) Biochemical and immunochemical methods for purification, characterization and standardization of allergen extract. In: Björksten B, Weeke B (eds) Allergy 40 (Suppl 4) Munsksgaard, Copenhagen, p 35

Elliott ST, Hanifin JM (1979) Delayed cutaneous hypersensitivity and lymphocyte transformation: dissociation in atopic dermatitis. Arch Dermatol 115: 36

Elsayed S, Apold J, Aas K, Bennich H (1976) The allergenic structure of allergen M from cod. I. Tryptic peptides of fragment TMI. Int Arch Allergy Appl Immunol 52: 59

Elsayed S, Titlestad K, Apold J, Aas K (1980) A synthetic hexapeptide derived from allergen M imposing allergenic and antigenic reactivity. Scand J Immunol 12: 171

Engel A, Hagström IC, Salen EB (1934) Unspezifische desensibilisierende Behandlung bei allergischen Zuständen. Acta Med Scand (Suppl 59): 444

Engman MF, Wander WG (1921) The application of cutaneous sensibilisation to diseases of the skin. Arch Dermatol Syph 3: 223

Epstein S (1956) Contact dermatitis due to nickel and chromium: observations on dermal delayed (tuberculin-type) sensitivity. Arch Dermatol 73: 236

Epstein S (1965) Neomycin sensitivity and atopy. Dermatologica 130: 280

Epstein S, Moharejin AH (1964) Incidence of contact sensitivity in atopic dermatitis. Arch Dermatol 90: 284

Epstein S, Palacek M (1951) Studies in infantile eczema. Clinical and statistical observations on the allergic background of 247 consecutive cases of infantile atopic dermatitis. Ann Allergy 9: 421

Eriksson G (1965) A non-specific effect of pollen distinguishable from the anaphylactic behaviour. Acta Derm Venereol (Stockh) 45: 247

Eriksson NE, Formgren H, Svenonius E (1982) Food hypersensitivity in patients with pollen allergy. Allergy 37: 437

Falk E, Bolle R (1983a) IgE antibodies to house dust mite in patients with scabies. Br J Dermatol 102: 283

Falk E, Bolle R (1983b) In vivo demonstration of specific immediate hypersensitivity to scabies mite. Br J Dermatol 103: 367

Faure MR, Nicolas JF, Thivolet J, Gaucherand MA, Czernielewski JM (1982) Studies on T cell subsets in atopic dermatitis: human T-cell subpopulations defined by specific monoclonal antibodies. Clin Immunol Immunopathol 22: 139

Feinberg M (1939) Seasonal atopic dermatitis. Arch Dermatol Syph 40: 200

Feinberg SN, Becker RJ, Slavin RG, Reinberg AR, Sparks DB (1962) The sensitizing effects of emulsified pollen antigens in atopic subjects naturally sensitive to an unrelated antigen. J Allergy 33: 285

Ferguson AC, Salinas FA (1984) Elevated IgG immune complexes in children with atopic eczema. J Allergy Clin Immunol 74: 676

Finn R, Harvey MM, Johnson PM, Verbov JL, Barnes RMR (1985) Serum IgG antibodies to gliadin and other dietary antigens in adults with atopic eczema. Clin Exp Dermatol 10: 222

Firer MA, Hoskins CS, Hill DJ (1982) Cow's milk allergy and eczema patterns of the antibody response to cow's milk in allergic skin disease. Clin Allergy 12: 385

Fischer T, Rystedt I (1985) False-positive, follicular and irritant patch test reactions to metal salts. Contact Dermatitis 12: 93

Fjelde A, Kopeczka B (1967) Cell transformation and histogenic effects in blood leucocyte cultures of atopic dermatitis patients. Acta Derm Venereol (Stockh) 47: 168

Forsbeck M, Hovmark A, Skog E (1976) Patch testing, tuberculin testing and sensitization with dinitrochlorbenzene and nitrosodimethylaniline of patients with atopic dermatitis. Acta Derm Venereol (Stockh) 56: 135

Föström L, Goldyne ME, Winkelmann RK (1975) IgE in human eccrine sweat. J Invest Dermatol 64: 156

Frajman M, Gonzalez L, Alvaredo A et al. (1987) Cellular immunity and IgE levels in atopic patients. Allergy 42: 81

Frankland AL (1968) The pathogenesis of asthma, hay fever and atopic diseases. In: Gell PGH, Coombs RRA (eds) Clinical aspects of immunology, 2nd edn. Blackwell, Oxford, p 648

Freedman S, Sellars W (1959) Food sensitivity. A study of 150 allergic children. J Allergy 30: 42

Freeman GL, Johnson S (1964) Allergic diseases in adolescence. I. Description of survey: prevalence of allergy. Am J Dis Child 107: 549

Friedman SJ, Schroeter AL, Homburger HA (1985) IgE antibodies to Staphylococcus aureus. Arch Dermatol 121: 869

Fries JH (1959) Components of milk and their significance to the allergic child. Ann Allergy 17: 1

Fritz KA, Norris DA, Morris RL, Weston WL (1980) ADCC effector function in patients with atopic dermatitis. J Am Acad Dermatol 3: 167

Fuchs O (1960) Ergebnisse der Kutan- und Intrakutantestungen beim endogenen Ekzem. Ärztl Fortbild 54: 1050

Fulton R, Thivolet J, Garcier F, Gaucherand M (1981) Les sous-populations de lymphocytes T helper et suppressor étudiés par les anticorps monocloneaux dans diverses dermatoses. Ann Dermatol Venereol 108: 243

Furukawa CT, Altman LC (1978) Defective monocyte and polymorphous leukocyte chemotaxis in atopic disease. J Allergy Clin Immunol 61: 288

Gabrielsen TO, Brandtzæg P (1985) Enzyme-linked immunosorbent assay (ELISA) for isotype-specific quantitation of antibodies to Staphylococcus aureus in patients with atopic dermatitis. Acta Derm Venereol [Suppl] (Stockh) 114: 61

Ganpule M, Garrets M (1971) Molluscum contagiosum and sarcoidosis: report of a case. Br J Dermatol 85: 587

Geha RS, Leung DYM (1986) Cellular abnormalities in patients with elevated serum IgE levels. J Allergy Clin Immunol 78: 995

Geha RS, Twarog F, Rappaport J, Parkman R, Rosen S (1980) Increased serum IgE levels following allogeneic bone marrow transplantation. J Allergy Clin Immunol 66: 78

Geha RS, Reinherz E, Leung DYM, McKee KT, Schlossman S, Rosen FS (1981) Deficiency of suppressor T cells in the hyperimmunoglobulinaemia E syndrome. J Clin Invest 68: 783

Gerrard JW, Horne S, Vickers P, McKenzie JWA, Goluboff N, Carson JZ, Maningas CS (1974) Serum IgE levels in parents and children. J Pediatr 85: 660

Giannetti A (1987) Viral skin diseases in atopic dermatitis. In: Happle R, Grosshans E (eds) Pediatric dermatology. Springer, Berlin Heidelberg New York, p 110

Glaser J (1965) The prevention of eczema. J Pediatr 66 (2): 262

Gleich GJ (1982) The late phase of immunoglobulin E-mediated reaction – a line between anaphylaxis and common allergic disease? J Allergy Clin Immunol 70: 160

Gleich GJ, Adolphson CR, Yunginger JW (1980) The mini-RAST: comparison with other varieties of the radioallergosorbent test for the measurement of immunoglobulin E antibodies. J Allergy Clin Immunol 65: 20

Goertler E, Schnyder UW (1975) Zur Erbprognose der Neurodermitis atopica. Hautarzt 26: 18

Goldman AS, Anderson DW, Sellers WA, Saperstein S, Kniker WJ et al. (1963) Milk allergy. I. Oral challenge with milk and isolated milk proteins in allergic children. Pediatrics 32: 425

Gondo A, Saeki N, Tokuda Y (1986) Challenge reactions in atopic dermatitis after percutaneous entry of mite antigen. Br J Dermatol 115: 485

Gondo A, Saeki N, Tokuda Y (1987) IgG4 antibodies in patients with atopic dermatitis. Br J Dermatol 117: 301

Good RA, Kelly WD, Rotstein I, Varco RL (1962) Immunologic deficiency diseases. Progress in allergy, vol 6. Karger, Basel, p 187

Gottlieb BR, Hanifin JM (1974) Circulating T cell deficiency in atopic dermatitis (abstract). Clin Res 22: 159

Gottlieb PM, Stupniker S, Askovitz ST (1960) The reproducibility of intradermal skin tests, a controlled study. Ann Allergy 18: 949

Goverman J, Hunkapiller T, Hood LA (1986) A speculative view of the multicomponent nature of T cell antigen recognition. Cell 45: 475

Grove DI, Reid JG, Forbes IJ (1975) Humoral and cellular immunity in atopic eczema. Br J Dermatol 92: 611

Grulee CG, Sanford HN (1936) Influence of breast and artificial feeding on infantile eczema. J Pediatr 9: 223

Guilhou JJ, Clot J, Bousquet J, Teot M, Meynadier J (1978) Étude in vitro de l'immunité cellulaire dans l'eczéma constitutionnel et dans l'eczéma de contact. Ann Dermatol Venereol 105: 513

Gupta S, Frenkel R, Rosenstein M, Grieco MH (1975) Lymphocyte subpopulations, serum IgE and total eosinophil counts in patients with bronchial asthma. Clin Exp Immunol 22: 438

Gurevitch AW, Heiner DC, Reisner R (1973) IgE in atopic dermatitis and other common dermatoses. Arch Dermatol 107: 712

Gustafsson D, Danielsson D (1981) In vitro diagnosis of atopic allergy in children. Allergy 43: 105

Halpern SR, Sellars WA, Johnson RB, Anderson DW, Saperstein S, Reisch JS (1973) Development of childhood allergy in infants fed breast, soy or milk. J Allergy Clin Immunol 51: 139

Hammar H (1977) Provocation with cow's milk and cereals in atopic dermatitis. Acta Derm Venereol (Stockh) 57: 159

Hampton SF, Cooke RA (1941) The sensitivity of man to human dander, with particular reference to eczema (allergic dermatitis). J Allergy 13: 63

Hanifin JM (1986) Staphylococcal colonization, infection and atopic dermatitis, association not etiology (Editorial). J Allergy Clin Immunol 78: 563

Hanifin JM, Rajka G (1980) Diagnostic features of atopic dermatitis. Acta Derm Venereol [Suppl] (Stockh) 92: 44

Hanifin JM, Rogge JL, Bauman RH (1980) Chemotaxis inhibition by plasma from patients with atopic dermatitis: dissociation in atopic dermatitis. Acta Derm Venereol [Suppl] (Stockh) 92: 52

Hannuksela M (1980) Results of food testing in atopic dermatitis. Acta Derm Venereol [Suppl] (Stockh) 92: 87

Hannuksela M, Lahti A (1977) Immediate reactions to fruits and vegetables. Contact Dermatitis 3: 79

Hansel FK (1953) Clinical allergy. Mosby, St Louis, p 129

Hansen LA, Ahlstedt S, Carlsson B, Fahlström SP (1977) Secretory IgA antibodies against cow's milk proteins in human milk and their possible effect in mixed feeding. Int Arch Allergy Appl Immunol 54: 457

Hard S (1950) Hypersensitivity to horse serum provoked by anticatarrh vaccine. Acta Allergol 3: 129

Harnack K, Lenz U (1970) Familienprognose beim endogenen Ekzem. Dermatol Wochenschr 156: 530

Harvald B, Hauge M (1956) A catamnestic investigation of Danish twins. Dan Med Bull 3: 150

Hashem N, Hirschhorn K, Sedlis E, Holt E (1963) Infantile eczema: evidence of autoimmunity to human skin. Lancet II: 269

Haskins K, Kubo R, White J, Pigeon M, Kappler J, Marrack P (1983) The major histocompatibility complex-restricted antigen receptors on T cells. J Exp Med 157: 1149

Hattevig G, Kjellman B, Björksten B, Johansson SGO (1984) Clinical symptoms and IgE responses to common food proteins in atopic and healthy children. Clin Allergy 14: 551

Hauser C, Wütrich B, Matter L, Wilhelm JA, Schopfer K (1985) Immune response to *Staphylococcus aureus* in atopic dermatitis. Dermatologica 170: 114

Haxthausen H (1925) Le prurigo de Besnier. Ann Dermatol Syphiligr 6: 312
Haxthausen H (1957) Interpretation and value of skin tests in atopic dermatitis. Acta Derm
    Venereol (Stockh) Proceedings of the 10th International Congress of Dermatology vol 3,
    p 6
Haynal A, Schnyder UU (1960) Fünfunddreißig auslesefrei Zwillinge mit Asthma bronchiale,
    Rhinitis atopica und Neurodermitis. Arch Vererbungsforschung Sozialanthropologie
    Rasshygiene 35: 435
Heite HJ, Kleinhans D (1961) Über die Cignolin-Erythemschwelle bei einigen Dermatosen.
    Arch Klin Exp Dermatol 212: 431
Hellerström S, Lidman H (1956) Studies of Besnier's prurigo (atopic dermatitis). Acta Derm
    Venereol 36: 11
Hemady Z, Blomberg F, Gellis S, Rocklin RE (1983) IgE production in vitro by human blood
    mononuclear cells: a comparison between atopic and nonatopic subjects. J Allergy Clin
    Immunol 71: 324
Hénocq E, Bazin JC, Girard J (1966) Les allergènes poussière de maison et squames hu-
    maines. Étude comparative dans l'eczéma atopique. Rev Fr Allergol 6: 213
Hénocq E. Hewitt B, Guerin B (1982) Staphylococcal and human dander IgE antibodies in
    superinfected atopic dermatitis. Clin Allergy 12: 113
Herlin T, Kragballe K (1980) Impaired monocyte cyclic AMP responses and monocyte cyto-
    toxicity in atopic dermatitis. Allergy 35: 647
Hill HR, Quie PG (1974) Raised serum IgE levels and defective neutrophil chemotaxis in
    three children with eczema and recurrent bacterial infections. Lancet I: 183
Hill LW (1934) The value of protein test in infantile eczema. JAMA 103: 1430
Hill LW (1937) Sensitivity to house dust and goose feathers in infantile eczema. J Allergy 9: 37
Hill LW (1955) The treatment of eczema in infants and children. J Pediatr 47: 141
Hill LW, Sulzberger MB (1935) Evolution of atopic dermatitis. Arch Dermatol Syph 32: 451
Hobbs RJ (1968) Immune imbalance in dysgammaglobulinaemia type IV. Lancet I: 110
Hodgkinson GI,, Everall JD, Smith HV (1977) Immunofluorescent patterns in the skin in
    Besnier's prurigo. Br J Dermatol 96: 357
Hoffman DR, Yamamoto FY, Geller B, Haddad Z (1975) Specific IgE antibodies in atopic ec-
    zema. J Allergy Clin Immunol 55: 256
Holti G (1966) Candida allergy. In: Winner HI, Hurley R (eds) Symposium on candida infec-
    tion. Churchill Livingstone, Edinburgh
Hopkins JG, Kesten BM (1935) Allergic eczema initiated by sensitization to foods. Am J Dis
    Child 49: 1511
Horsmanheimo M, Horsmanheimo A (1979) Leukocyte migration inhibition factor in atopic
    dermatitis: induction by concanavalin A in vitro. J Invest Dermatol 72: 128
Hovmark A (1975) An in vitro and in vivo study of cell mediated immunity in atopic dermati-
    tis. Acta Derm Venereol (Stockh) 55: 181
Hovmark A (1977a) An in vitro study of depressed cell-mediated immunity and of T and
    B lymphocytes in atopic dermatitis. Acta Derm Venereol (Stockh) 57: 237
Hovmark A (1977b) Acid napthyl acetate esterase staining of T lymphocytes in human skin.
    Acta Derm Venereol (Stockh) 57: 497
Hovmark A (1979) An in vitro study of IgE production in severe atopic dermatitis. Acta Derm
    Venereol (Stockh) 59: 223
Hsieh KH (1976) Study of E rosettes, serum IgE and eosinophilia in asthmatic children. Ann
    Allergy 37: 383
Huber A, Fartasch M, Diepgen TL, Baurle G, Hornstein OP (1987) Auftreten von Kontaktal-
    lergien beim atopischen Ekzem. Dermatosen 35: 119
Hubscher T, Watson IJ, Godfriend L (1970) Target cells of human ragweed binding antibodies
    in monkey skin. J Immunol 104: 1196
Huntley CC, Lyerly A, Winston-Salem NC (1963) Immune globulin determination on allergic
    children. Am J Dis Child 106: 545
Huriez C (1966) Actualités sur les eczémas. Rev Med Suppl
Husby S, Schultz Larsen F, Ahlstedt S, Svehag SE (1986) Humoral immunity to dietary anti-
    gens in atopic dermatitis. Allergy 41: 386

Hwang KC, Fikrig SM, Friedman HM, Gupta S (1983) Autologous mixed lymphocyte reaction in man. Allergy 38: 113

Inganäs M, Johansson SGO (1981) Influence of alternative protein-A interaction of the precipitation between human monoclonal immunoglobulins and protein-A from *Staphylococcus aureus*. Int Arch Allergy Appl Immunol 65: 91

Inganäs M, Johansson SGO, Bennich H (1981) Anti-IgE antibodies in human serum: occurrence and specificity. Int Arch Allergy Appl Immunol 65: 51

Ishizaka K (1984) Regulation of IgE synthesis. Annu Rev Immunol 2: 159

Ishizaka K, Ishizaka T (1968) Reversed-type allergic reactions by anti-IgE globulin antibodies in humans and monkeys. J Immunol 100: 554

Ishizaka K, Ishizaka T, Holbrook MM (1967) Identification of gamma-E antibodies as a carrier of reaginic activity. J Immunol 99: 1187

Ishizaka K, Ishizaka T, Orange RP, Austen KF (1970) The capacity of human antiglobulin γE to mediate the relase of histamine and slow reacting substance to anaphylaxis (SRS-A) from monkey lung. J Immunol 104: 335

Jadassohn W (1958) Évolution et aspects cliniques des dermatoses atopiques. In: Halpen BN, Holtzer A (eds) Proc 3d Congress Int d'allergologie. Flammarion, Paris, p 605

James J, Warin RF (1971) An assessment of the role of *Candida albicans* and food yeasts in chronic urticaria. Br J Dermatol 84: 227

Jansen CT, Hapalahti J, Hopsu-Havu VK (1973) Immunoglobulin E in the human atopic skin. Arch Dermatol Forsch 246: 229

Janossy G, Duke O, Poulter LW, Panayi G, Bofill M, Goldstein G (1981) Rheumatoid arthritis: a disease of T lymphocyte/macrophage dysfunction. Lancet II: 839

Jarrett EEE (1977) Activation of IgE regulatory mechanisms by transmucosal absorption of antigen. Lancet I: 223

Järvinen KAJ, Pirila V, Björksten F et al. (1979) Unsuitability of bakery work for a person with atopy: a study of 234 bakery workers. Ann Allergy 42: 192

Jensen JR (1985) Reduction of active natural killer cells in patients with atopic dermatitis estimated at the single cell level. Acta Derm Venereol [Suppl] (Stockh) 114: 105

Jensen JR, Cramers M, Thestrup-Pedersen K (1981) Subpopulation of T lymphocytes and non-specific suppressor cell activity in patients with atopic dermatitis. Clin Exp Immunol 45: 118

Jensen JR, Sand TT, Jörgensen AS, Thestrup-Pedersen K (1984) Modulation of natural killer cell activity in patients with atopic dermatitis. J Invest Dermatol 82: 30

Jillson OF (1957) Allergic dermatitis produced by pathogenic and saprophytic fungi. Ann Allergy 15: 14

Jillson OF, Curwan WL, Alexander BR (1959) Problems of contact dermatitis in the atopic individual with reference to neomycin and ragweed sensitivity. Ann Allergy 17: 215

Johansson SGO (1981) The clinical significance of IgE. In: Franklin EC (ed) Clinical immunology update. Elsevier, New York, p 123

Johansson SGO (1984) Anti-IgE antibodies in human serum (Editorial). J Allergy Clin Immunol 77: 555

Johansson SGO (1986) IgE and allergic diseases. In: Ring J, Burg G (eds) New trends in allergy. II. Springer, Berlin Heidelberg New York, p 39

Johansson SGO, Bennich H (1967a) Immunological studies of an atypical (myeloma) immunoglobulin. Immunology 13: 381

Johansson SGO, Bennich H (1967b) Studies on a new class of human immunoglobulins. I. Immunological properties. Nobel symposium 3. Gamma globulin. Structure and control of biosynthesis. Almqvist and Wiksell, Stockholm, p 193

Johansson SGO, Bennich H, Wide L (1968) A new class of immunoglobulins in human serum. Immunology 14: 265

Johansson SGO, Bennich H, Berg T, Högman C (1970) Some factors influencing the serum IgE level in atopic diseases. Clin Exp Immunol 6: 43

Johansson SGO, Juhlin L (1970) Immunoglobulin E in "healed" atopic dermatitis and after treatment with corticosteroids and azathioprine. Br J Dermatol 82: 10

Johnson EE, Irons JS, Patterson R, Roberts M (1974) Serum IgE concentration in atopic dermatitis. J Allergy Clin Immunol 54: 94

Jones HE, Lewis CW, McMarlin SL (1973a) Allergic contact sensitivity in atopic dermatitis. Arch Dermatol 107: 217

Jones HE, Rinaldi MG, Chai H, Kahn G (1973b) Apparent cross-reactivity of airborne molds and the dermatophytic fungi. J Allergy Clin Immunol 52: 346

Jones HE, Inouye JC, McGerity JL, Lewis CW (1975) Atopic disease and serum immunoglobulin-E. Br J Dermatol 92: 17

Juhlin L, Johansson SGO, Bennich H, Högman C, Thyresson N (1969) Immunoglobulin E in dermatoses. Arch Dermatol 100: 12

Juto P, Strannegard Ö (1979) T-lymphocytes and blood eosinophils in early infancy in relation to heredity for allergy and type of feeding. J Allergy Clin Immunol 64: 38

Juto P, Engberg S, Winberg J (1978) Treatment of infantile atopic eczema with a strict elimination diet. Clin Allergy 8: 493

Kaaber K (1976) Occurrence of malignant neoplasms in patients with atopic dermatitis. Acta Derm Venereol (Stockh) 56: 445

Kaliner M (1984) Hypotheses on the contribution of late phase allergic responses to the understanding and treatment of allergic diseases. J Allergy Clin Immunol 73: 311

Kaufman HS (1971) Allergy in the newborn: skin test reactions confirmed by the Prausnitz-Küstner test at birth. Clin Allergy 1: 363

Kaufman HS, Frick OL (1976) The development of allergy in infants of allergic parents. A prospective study concerning the role of heredity. Ann Allergy 37: 410

Kalveram KJ (1985) Neue Entwicklungen bei RAST-Untersuchungen und ihre Beurteilung. Z Hautkr 61: 1363

Kapp A, Gillitzer R, Kirchner H, Schöpf E (1987) Production of interferon and lymphoproliferative response in whole blood cultures derived from patients with atopic dermatitis. Arch Dermatol Res 279: S55

Kapp A, Kemper A, Schöpf E, Deicher H (1986) Detection of circulating immune complexes in patients with atopic dermatitis and psoriasis. Acta Derm Venereol (Stockh) 66: 121

Kazmierowski JA, Peizner DS, Hanifin JM, Wuepper KD (1981) Atopic dermatitis: identification of IgE-containing immune complexes during active disease (abstract). J Invest Dermatol 76: 310

Keller P (1924) Beitrag zu den Beziehungen von Asthma und Ekzem. Arch Dermatol Syph 148: 82

Kerr RM, Wilson MR, Anicetti VR, Lehrer SB, Butcher BT, Salvaggio JE (1981) An approach to fungal antigen relationships by radioallergosorbent test inhibition. J Allergy Clin Immunol 67: 194

Kesten B (1954) Allergic eczema. New York State Medicine 54: 2441

Khan A, Sellers WA, Pflanzer J, Hill JM, Thometz D, Haenke J (1976) Asthma and T-cell immunodeficiency: improvement with transfer factor and immunopeptide. 1. Ann Allergy 37: 267

Kim CW, Schöpf E (1976) A comparative study of nickel hypersensitivity by the lymphocyte transformation test in atopic and nonatopic dermatitis. Arch Dermatol Res 257: 57

King TP (1980) Purification and characterization of atopic allergens. Allergy 35: 169

Kind LS, Banovitz J, Menzel A, Nilsson B (1967) A factor in pollen which enhance vascular permeability. J Allergy 39: 17

Kjellman B, Petterson R (1983) The problem of furred pets in childhood atopic disease. Allergy 38: 65

Kjellman NIM (1976) Predictive value of high IgE levels in children. Acta Paediatr Scand 65: 465

Kjellman NIM, Johansson SGO (1979) Soy versus milk in infants with a bi-parental history of atopic disease: development of atopic disease in immunoglobulins from birth to four years of age. Clin Allergy 9: 347

Kjellman NIM, Johansson SGO, Roth A (1976) Serum IgE levels in healthy children quantified by a sandwich technique (PRIST). Clin Allergy 6: 51

Klareskog L, Tjernlund U, Forsum V, Peterson PA (1977) Epidermal Langerhans' cell express Ia antigens. Nature 268: 248

Klene U, Gollnick H, Bauer R, Orfanos CE (1986) Subpopulationen peripherer T-Lymphozyten (Th/Ts) bei atopischer Dermatitis und bei Psoriasis. Hautarzt 37: 17

Kletter B, Gerry J, Freier S, Noah Z, Davis MA (1971) Immunoglobulin E antibodies to milk proteins. Clin Allergy 1: 249

Kligman AM, Wooding WM (1967) A method for measurement and evaluation of irritants on human skin. J Invest Dermatol 49: 78

Kohler PF, Farr RS (1967) Quantitative comparison of immunoglobulins in atopic (reaginic) individuals: higher D levels in atopic sera. J Allergy 39: 311

Korting HG (1958) Das endogene Ekzem. In: Gottron HA, Schönfeld W (eds) Dermatologie und Venereologie, vol 3/1. Thieme, Stuttgart, p 549

Kragballe K, Borregaard N (1981) Mechanisms of decreased antibody-dependent cell mediated cytotoxicity by monocytes and neutrophiles in atopic dermatitis. Acta Derm Venereol (Stockh) 61: 11

Kragballe K, Herlin T, Jensen JR (1980) Impaired monocyte-mediated cytotoxicity in atopic dermatitis. Arch Dermatol Res 269: 21

Krain LS, Terasaki PI (1973) HLA-antigens in atopic dermatitis. Lancet I: 1059

Kramer MS, Moroz B (1981) Do breast-feeding and delayed introduction of solid foods protect against subsequent atopic eczema? J Pediatr 98: 546

Kusaimi NT, Trentin JJ (1982) Natural cell-mediated cytotoxic activity in the peripheral blood of patients with atopic dermatitis. Arch Dermatol 118: 568

Lahti A, Björksten F, Hannuksela M (1980) Allergy to birch pollen and apple and cross reactivity of the allergens studied with the RAST. Allergy 35: 297

Lammintausta K, Kalimo K, Havu VR (1982) Contact allergy in atopics who perform wet work in hospital. Derm Beruf Umwelt 30: 184

Langeland T (1982a) A clinical and immunological study of allergy to hen's egg white. II. Antigens in hen's egg white studied by crossed immunoelectrophoresis (CIE). Allergy 37: 323

Langeland T (1982b) A clinical and immunological study of allergy to hen's egg white. III. Allergens in hen's egg white studied by crossed radio-immunoelectrophoresis (Crie). Allergy 37: 521

Langeland T (1983) A clinical and immunological study of allergy to hen's egg white. I. A clinical study of egg allergy. Clin Allergy 13: 371

Langeland T, Braathen LR, Borck M (1989) Studies on atopic patch tests. Acta Derm Venereol (Suppl 144) (Stockh) (in press)

Lea T, Braathen LR, Moen T (1980) Class and subclass distribution of specific antibodies to codfish allergen in a patient with atopic allergy. Acta Derm Venereol [Suppl] (Stockh) 92: 73

Leiferman KM, Peterson EA, Fujisawa T, Gray BH, Gleich GJ (1989) Differences between atopic dermatitis and the IgE-mediated neutrophil degranulation in atopic dermatitis (abstract) J invest Dermatol 92: 469

Lemanske RF, Guthman DA, Kaliner M (1983) The biologic activity of mast cell granules. VII. The effect of anti-neutrophil antibody-induced neutropenia on rat cutaneous late phase reactions. J Immunol 131: 929

Leskowitz S, Lowell FC (1961) A comparison in the immune and physiologic response of normal and allergic individuals. J Allergy 32: 152

Leung DYM, Geha RS (1986) Immunoregulatory abnormalities in atopic dermatitis. Clin Rev Allergy 4: 67

Leung DYM, Rhodes AR, Geha RS (1981) Enumeration of the T cell subsets in atopic dermatitis using monoclonal antibodies. J Allergy Clin Immunol 67: 450

Leung DYM, Parkman R, Feller J, Wood N, Geha RS (1982) Cell mediated cytotoxicity against skin fibroblasts in atopic dermatitis. J Immunol 128: 1736

Leung DYM, Bhan AK, Schneeberger EE, Geha RS (1983) Characterization of the mononuclear cell infiltrate in atopic dermatitis using monoclonal antibodies. Dermatologica 169: 330

Lever RS, Lesko MJ, MacKie RM, Parrott DM (1985) Natural killer cell activity in atopic dermatitis: a sequential study. Clin Allergy 15: 479

Lever RS, Turbitt M, Sanderson A, MacKie R (1987) Immunophenotyping of the cutaneous infiltrate and of the mononuclear cells in the peripheral blood in patients with atopic dermatitis. J Invest Dermatol 89: 4

Lichtenstein ML, Osler AO (1964) Studies on the mechanism of hypersensitivity phenomena. IX. Histamine release from human leukocytes by ragweed pollen antigen. J Exp Med 120: 507

Lind P, Löwenstein H (1983) Identification of allergens in *Dermatophagoides pteronyssinus* mite body extract by crossed immunoelectrophoresis with two different antibody pools. Scand J Immunol 17: 263

Lind P, Weeke R, Löwenstein H (1984) A reference allergen preparation of house dust mite *D. pteronyssinus,* produced from whole mite culture. A part of the DAS/76 study. Comparison with allergen preparations from other raw materials. Allergology 39: 259

Lindblad JH, Farr J (1961) The incidence of positive intradermal reactions and the demonstration of skin sensitizing antibody to extracts of ragweed and dust in humans without history of rhinitis or asthma. J Allergy 32: 392

Livingood CS, Pillsbury DM (1949) Specific sensitivity to foods as factors in various types of eczematous dermatitis. Arch Dermatol Syph 60: 1090

Lobitz WC, Honeyman JF, Winkler NW (1972) Suppressed cell-mediated immunity in two adults with atopic dermatitis. Br J Dermatol 86: 317

Lobitz WC, Jillson OF (1958) Anecdotes of an agnostic allergist. Arch Dermatol 78: 458

Löwenstein H, Lind P, Weeke B (1985) Identification and clinical significance of allergenic molecules of cat origin. Part of the DAS/76 study. Allergy 40: 430

Luckasen JR, Sabad A, Goltz RW, Kersey JH (1974) T and B lymphocytes in atopic eczema. Arch Dermatol 110: 375

Lynfield YL (1974) Skin diseases in twins. Arch Dermatol 110: 722

MacKie RM, Dick HM (1979) A study of HLA antigen distribution in families with atopic dermatitis. Allergy 34: 19

MacKie RM, Cobb SJ, Cochran REI, Thomson J (1979) Total and specific IgE levels in patients with atopic dermatitis: correlation between prick testing, clinical history of allergy and in vitro quantification of IgE during clinical exacerbation and remission. Clin Exp Dermatol 4: 187

Magnusson B (1954) Human dander and atopic dermatitis. Acta Allergol 7: 294

Malten KE (1968) The occurrence of hybrids between contact allergic eczema and atopic dermatitis (and vice versa) and their significance. Dermatologica 136: 395

Malten KE (1971) Nickel-allergic contact dermatitis and atopy. Dermatologica 142: 113

Marcussen PV (1959) Specificity of patch test with 5% nickel sulphate. Acta Derm Venereol (Stockh) 39: 187

Marghescu S (1985) Patch test reactions in atopic patients. Acta Derm Venereol [Suppl] (Stockh) 114: 113

Marsh DG, Mayers DA, Bias WB (1981) The epidemiology and genetics of atopic allergy. N Eng J Med 305: 1551

Martinez JD, Santos J, Stechschulte DJ, Abdon NI (1979) Nonspecific suppressor cell function in atopic subjects. J Allergy clin Immunol 64: 385

Massicot JG, Ishizaka K (1986) Workshop on measurement of in vitro IgE synthesis and regulation of IgE snythesis. J Allergy Clin Immunol 77: 544

Mathew DJ, Norman AP, Taylor B, Turner MW, Soothill JF (1977) Prevention of eczema. Lancet I: 321

Maunsell K, Wraith DG, Cunnington AM (1968) Mites and house-dust allergy in bronchial asthma. Lancet I: 1267

McGeady SJ, Buckley RH (1975) Depression of cell-mediated immunity in atopic eczema. J Allergy Clin Immunol 56: 393

McGeady S, Saraclar Y, Mansmann HC (1976) Normal T-cell numbers found in atopic children. J Allergy Clin Immunol 57: 194

Meara RH (1955) Skin reactions in atopic eczema. Br J Dermatol 67: 60

Meneghini CL, Bonifazi E (1985) Correlation between clinical and immunological findings in atopic dermatitis. Acta Derm Venereol [Suppl] (Stockh) 114: 10

Menné T (1978) The revalence of nickel allergy among women. An epidemiological study in hospitalized female patients. Dermatosen 26: 123

Miadonna A, Tedeschi A, Leggieri E, Cottini M, Menni S, Froldi M, Zanussi C (1985) Characterization of T cell subsets in patients with atopic dermatitis using OKT monoclonal antibodies. Ann Allergy 54: 321

Michaelsson G (1973) Decreased phagocytic capacity of the neutrophil leukocytes in patients with atopic dermatitis. Acta Derm Venereol (Stockh) 53: 279

Michel FB, Bousquet J, Greillier P, Robinet-Levy M, Coulomb Y (1980) Comparison of cord blood immunoglobulin E concentration and maternal allergy for the prediction of atopic diseases in infancy. J Allergy Clin Immunol 65: 422

Mihm MC, Soter NA, Dvorak HF, Austen KF (1976) The structure of normal skin and the morphology of atopic eczema. J Invest Dermatol 67: 305

Minor JD, Tolber SG, Frick OL (1980) Leukocyte inhibition factor in delayed onset food allergy. J Allergy Clin Immunol 66: 314

Mitchell EB, Chapman MD, Pope FM, Crow J, Jouhal SS, Platt-Mills TAE (1982) Basophils in allergen induced patch test sites in atopic dermatitis. Lancet I: 127

Mitchell EB, Crow J, Williams G, Platt-Mills TAE (1986) Increase in skin mast cells following chronic house dust mite exposure. Br J Dermatol 114: 65

Miyachi S, Lessof MH, Kemeny DM, Green IA (1979) Comparison of the atopic background between allergic and non-allergic beekeepers. Int Arch Allergy Appl Immunol 58: 160

Mizoguchi M, Furusawa S, Okitsu S, Yoshino K (1985) Macrophage-derived interleukin-1 activity in atopic dermatitis. J Invest Dermatol 84: 303

Möller H, Svensson A (1986) Metal sensitivity: positive history but negative test indicates atopy. Contact Dermatitis 14: 57

Momma K (1965) Immunochemical semiquantitative estimation of gamma M and gamma A immunoglobulin in healthy and diseased children. 3. Immunoglobulin levels in infectious diseases and liver cirrhosis. Acta Pediatr Jpn 7: 1

Moretta L, Ferrarini M, Mirgari MC, Moretta A, Webb SR (1976) Subpopulations of human T cells identified by receptors for immunoglobulins and mitogen responsiveness. J Immunol 117: 2171

Motala C, Potter PC, Weinberg EG, Malherbe D, Hughes J (1986) Anti-*Staphylococcus aureus*-specific IgE in atopic dermatitis. J Allergy Clin Immunol 78: 583

Murray AB (1983) The frequency and severity of cat allergy versus dog allergy in children. J Allergy Clin Immunol 72: 145

Musso E, Brun F, Hunziker N (1959) Un allergène pour decèler l'atopie. Acta Allergol 13: 174

Mustakallio KK (1966) Antistaphylolysin (Asta) level of the blood in relation to barrier function of the skin. Ann Med Exp Biol Fenn 44 (Suppl): 7

Nexmand PH (1948) Clinical studies of prurigo Besnier. Rosenkilde and Bagger, Copenhagen

Niermann H (1964) Zwillingsdermatologie. Springer, Berlin Göttingen

Nilzén Å (1958) Experimental background of some abnormal vascular reactions in atopic dermatitis and significances of skin tests in man. In: Halpern BN, Holtzer A (eds) Proc 3d Congrès International d'Allergologie. Flammarion, Paris, p 635

Norris PG, Schofield O, Camp RDR (1988) A study of the role of house dust mite in atopic dermatitis. Br J Dermatol 118: 435

Norrlind R (1946) Prurigo Besnier (atopic dermatitis). Acta Derm Venereol Suppl 13 (Stockh)

Numata T, Mizuno N, Yoshida K, Toda T (1973) Serum IgE level and white dermographia in atopic dermatitis, atopic skin and in infantile eczema. 8th Int Congr Allergol, Tokyo. Excerpta Medica, Amsterdam, p 16

Oddoze L (1959) Note statistique du prurigo de Besnier en France. Acta Allergol 13: 410

Ogawa M, Berger PA, McIntyre OR, Clendenning WE, Ishizaka K (1971) IgE in atopic dermatitis. Arch Dermatol 103: 575

Ogden BE, Krueger GG, Hill HR (1979) Lymphocyte suppressor activity in atopic eczema. Clin Exp Immunol 35: 269

Öhman S (1971) Immunoglobulin E in atopic dermatitis. Thesis. Offset Center, Uppsala

Öhman S, Johansson SGO (1974) Allergen-specific IgE in atopic dermatitis. Acta Derm Venereol (Stockh) 54: 283

Öhman S, Juhlin L, Johansson SGO (1972) Immunoglobulins in atopic dermatitis. In: Charpin J, Boutin C, Aubert J, Frankland AW (eds) Allergology. Proceedings of the 8th European congress of Allergology. Excerpta Medica, Amsterdam, p 119

O'Keefe E, Rackemann F (1929) Asthma. JAMA 92: 883

O'Loughlin S, Diaz-Perez JL, Gleich GJ, Winkelmann RK (1977) Serum IgE in dermatitis and dermatosis. Arch Dermatol 113: 309

Oprée W, Krause H, Stockberg H (1972) Genetic aspects of serum IgE levels in atopic families. Acta Allergol 27: 247

Ortiz F (1968) Serum levels of immunoglobulin A (IgA) in atopic patients. Allergie Asthma 14: 116

Osborne ED, Murray PF (1953) Atopic dermatitis. A study of its natural course and of wool as a dominant allergenic factor. Arch Dermatol Syph 68: 619

Österballe O, Weeke B (1979) A new lancet for skin prick testing. Allergy 34: 209

Paganelli R, Levinsky RJ, Atherton DJ (1981) Detection of specific antigen within circulating immune complexes: validation of the assay and its application to food antigen-antibody complexes formed in healthy and food-allergic subjects. Clin Exp Immunol 46: 44

Palacios J, Fuller EW, Blaylock WK (1966) Immunological capabilities with atopic dermatitis. J Invest Dermatol 47: 484

Parish WE (1967) Release of histamine and slow-reacting substance with mast cells. Changes after challenge of human lung sensitized passively with reagin in vitro. Nature 215: 738

Parish WE (1970) Short-term anaphylactic IgG antibodies in human sera. Lancet II: 591

Parish WE (1981) The clinical relevance of heat stable short term sensitizing anaphylactic IgG antibodies (IgG S-TS) and of related activities of IgG4 and IgG2. Br J Dermatol 105: 223

Parish WE, Champion RH (1973) Atopic dermatitis. In: Rook A (ed) Recent advances in dermatology, vol 3. Churchill Livingstone, London

Pass R, Larsen WG, Lobitz WC jr (1966) The cultured lymphocytes of atopic patients. Ann Allergy 24: 426

Pauly CR, Artis WM, Jones HE (1978) Atopic dermatitis, impaired cellular immunity and molluscum contagiosum. Arch Dermatol 114: 391

Pepys J (1969) Hypersensitivity diseases of the lungs due to fungi and organic dust. Monographs in Allergy, vol 4. Karger, Basel New York

Pepys J, Chan M, Hargreaves FM (1968) Mites and house-dust allergy. Lancet I: 1270

Perlman F (1958) Insects as inhalant allergens. Considerations on aerobiology, biochemistry, preparation of material and clinical observations. J Allergy 29: 302

Petersen M, Goos M, Küster W, Sterry W (1986) Genetics of atopy (abstract). J Invest Dermatol 86: 332

Peterson RDA (1965) Immunological responses in infantile eczema. J Pediatr 66 (2): 225

Pigatto PD, Polenghi MM, Altomare GF (1987) Occupational dermatitis in bakers: a clue for atopic contact dermatitis. Contact Dermatitis 16: 263

Prahl P (1981) Allergens in cow hair and dander. Allergy 36: 561

Prausnitz C, Küstner H (1921) Studien über die Überempfindlichkeit. Zentralbl Bakteriol Parasitenkd Infektionskr Hygiene 86: 160

Prince HE (1961) Molds and bacteria in the etiology of respiratory diseases. XX. Studies with mold extracts produced from cultures grown in modified synthetic media. Ann Allergy 19: 259

Prystowski SD, Allen AA, Smith RW, Nonomura JH, Odom RB, Akers WA (1979) Allergic contact hypersensitivity to nickel, neomycin, ethylenediamine and benzocaine. Arch Dermatol 107: 217

Quinti I, Brozek C, Geha RS, Leung DYM (1984) Circulating IgG antibodies to IgE in atopic syndromes. Clin Research 32: 146A

Rachelefsky GS, Opelz G, Mickey MR, Kiuchi M, Terasaki PI, Siegel SC, Stiehm RE (1976) Defective T-cell function in atopic dermatitis. J Allergy Clin Immunol 57: 569

Rademecker M, Maldague MP (1981) Depression of neutrophil chemotaxis in atopic individuals. An H_2 histamine receptor response. Int Arch Allergy Appl Immunol 65: 144

Rajka G (1960) Prurigo Besnier (atopic dermatitis) with special reference to the role of allergic factors. I. The influence of atopic hereditary factors. Acta Derm Venereol (Stockh) 40: 285

Rajka G (1961) Prurigo Besnier (atopic dermatitis) with special reference to the role of allergic factors. II. The evaluation of skin reactions. Acta Derm Venereol (Stockh) 41: 1

Rajka G (1962) Discussion to Blank: The structure, biochemical and physiological defense mechanisms of the skin. In: Pillsbury DM, Livingsod CS (eds) Proceedings of the 12th International Congress of Dermatology Washington, vol 1. Excerpta medica, Amsterdam, p 480

Rajka G (1963) Studies in hypersensitivity to molds and staphylococci in prurigo Besnier (atopic dermatitis). Acta Derm Venereol [Suppl] (Stockh) 13: 54

Rajka G (1967) Delayed dermal and epicutaneous reactivity in atopic dermatitis (Prurigo Besnier). I. Delayed reactivity to bacterial and mold allergens. Acta Derm Venereol (Stockh) 47: 158

Rajka G (1968) Delayed dermal and epidermal reactivity in atopic dermatitis (prurigo Besnier). III. Further studies with bacterial and viral allergens. Acta Derm Venereol (Stockh) 48: 186

Rajka G (1975) Atopic dermatitis. Saunders, London

Rajka G (1980) Itch and IgE in atopic dermatitis. Acta Derm Venereol [Suppl] (Stockh) 92: 38

Rajka G, Barlinn C (1979) On the significance of the trichophytin reactivity in atopic dermatitis. Acta Derm Venereol (Stockh) 59: 45

Räsänen L, Lehto M, Reunala T, Jansen C, Lehtinen M, Leinikki P (1987) Langerhans' cell and T lymphocyte functions in patients with atopic dermatitis with disseminated cutaneous herpes simplex virus infection. J Invest Dermatol 89: 15

Ratner B, Collins-Williams C (1958) Protein skin reactivity in infantile and childhood eczema. Am J Dis Childr 96: 184

Ratner B, Untracht S (1952) Egg allergy in children. Am J Dis Child 83: 309

Reinherz EL, Schlossman SF (1980) Regulation of the immune response-inducer and suppressor T lymphocyte subsets in human beings. N Engl J Med 303: 370

Reinhold U, Wehrmann W, Bauer R, Kreysel HW (1986) Defizit natürlicher Killerzellen (NK-Zellen) im peripheren Blut bei atopischer Dermatitis. Hautarzt 37: 438

Reitamo S, Visa K, Kähonen K, Käyhkö K, Stubb S, Salo OB (1986) Eczematous reactions in atopic patients caused by epicutaneous testing with inhalant allergens. Br J Dermatol 114: 303

Ring J (1985) Beeinflussung des RAST durch Glukokortikoide. Hautarzt 36: 645

Ring J, Lutz J (1983) Decreased release of lysosomal enzymes from peripheral leukocytes of patients with atopic dermatitis. J Am Acad Dermatol 8: 378

Ring J, Przybilla B, Senner H (1987) In vitro IgE Sekretion in Lymphozytenkulturen von Patienten mit atopischem Ekzem und Kontrollpersonen. Allergologie 10: 211

Ringden O, Persson U, Johansson SGO (1983) Are increased levels a signal of an acute graft-versus-host reaction? Immunol Rev 71: 57

Rocha C, Maubeuge J de, Sarfati M, Song M, Delespesse G (1984) Characterization of cellular infiltrates in ski lesions of atopic eczema by means of monoclonal antibodies. Dermatologica 169: 330

Rogge L, Hanifin JM (1976) Immunodeficiencies in severe atopic dermatitis. Arch Dermatol 112: 1391

Rola-Pleszczynski M, Blanchard R (1981) Abnormal suppressor cell function in atopic dermatitis. J Invest Dermatol 76: 279

Rost AG (1929) Über Erfahrungen mit der allergenfreien Kammer nach Storm van Leeuwen, insbesondere in der Spätperiode der exsudativen Diathese. Arch Dermatol Syph 155: 297

Rost G, Marchionini A (1932) Asthma-Eksem, Asthma-Prurigo und Neurodermitis als allergische Hautkrankheiten. Würz Abh Gesamtgeb Prakt Med 27: 10

Rostenberg A, Solomon L (1968) Infantile eczema and systemic disease. Arch Dermatol 98: 41

Rostenberg A, Solomon LM (1971) Atopic dermatitis and infantile eczema. In: Sherman WB (ed) Immunological diseases, 2nd edn, vol II. Little and Brown, Boston, p 920

Rostenberg A, Sulzberger MB (1937) Some results of patch tests: compilation and discussion of cutaneous reactions to about 500 different substances as elicited by over 10,000 tests in approximately 1000 patients. Arch Dermatol Syph 35: 433

Rothberg RM, Farr RS (1965) Anti-bovine serum albumin and anti-alpha lactalbumin in the serum of children and adults. Pediatrics 35: 571

Rowe AH (1946) Dermatitis of the hands due to atopic allergy to pollen. Arch Dermatol Syph 53: 437

Rowe AH, Rowe AH (1951) Atopic dermatitis in infants and children. J Pediatr 39: 80

Rowntree S, Platt-Mills TAE, Cogswell J, Mitchell EB (1987) A subclass IgG4-specific antigen-binding radioimmunoassay (RIA): comparison between IgG and IgG4 antibodies to food and inhaled antigens in adult atopic dermatitis after desensitization treatment and during development of antibody responses in children. J Allergy Clin Immunol 80: 622

Rudzki E, Moskalewska K, Maciejowska E (1965) Bakterienallergie bei Hautkrankheiten. III. Bakterienallergie bei Ekzeme, Urticara and Prurigo. Arch Klin Exp Dermatol 223: 243

Ruiz-Moreno C (1959) Alimentary and gastro-intestinal allergy. In: Jamar JM (ed) Textbook of allergy. Blackwell, Oxford, p 481

Rystedt I (1985) Contact sensitivity in adults with atopic dermatitis in childhood. Contact Dermatitis 13: 1

Salvaggio JE, Cavanaugh JJA, Lowell FC, Leskowitz S (1964) A comparison of the immunologic response of normal and atopic individuals to intranasally administered antigen. J Allergy 35: 62

Sampson H (1983) Role of immediate food hypersensitivity in the pathogenesis of atopic dermatitis. J Allergy Clin Immunol 71: 473

Sampson HA (1988) The role of food allergy and mediator release in atopic dermatitis. J Allergy Clin Immunol 81: 635

Sampson H, Albergo R (1984) Comparison of results of skin tests, RAST and double-blind, placebo-controlled food challenges in children with atopic dermatitis. J Allergy Clin Immunol 74: 26

Sampson HA, Jolie PI (1984) Increased plasma histamine concentrations after food challenges in children with atopic dermatitis. N Engl J Med 311: 372

Saraclar Y, McGeady SJ, Mansmann HC (1977) Lymphocyte subpopulations of atopic children and effect of therapy upon them. J Allergy Clin Immunol 60: 301

Saryan JA, Leung DYM, Geha RS (1983) Induction of human IgE synthesis by a factor derived from T cells of patients with hyper IgE states. J Immunol 130: 242

Sauder DN, Dinarello CA, Morhenn VB (1984) Langerhans' cell production of interleukin-1. J Invest Dermatol 82: 605

Saurat JH, Woodley D, Helfer N (1985) Cutaneous symptoms in primary immunodeficiencies. Curr Probl Dermatol 13: 50

Schnyder UW (1957) The importance of intracutaneous tests in various types of constitutional neurodermitis. Int Arch Allergy Appl Immunol 11: 64

Schnyder UW (1960) Neurodermitis–Asthma–Rhinitis. Karger, Basel

Schnyder UW (1972) Zur Humangenetik der Neurodermitis atopica. Arch Dermatol Forsch 244: 345

Schnyder UW, Borelli S (1965) Neurodermatitis constitutionalis sive atopica. In: Miescher C, Storck H (eds) Entzündliche Dermatosen. II. Springer, Berlin Heidelberg New York, p 228 (Handbuch der Haut- und Geschlechtskrankheiten, vol II/1)

Scholtz S, Ziegler E, Wüster H, Braun-Falco O, Albert ED (1977) HLA family studies in patients with atopic dermatitis. Monogr Allergy 11: 44

Schöpf E, Boehringer D (1974) IgE and cell-mediated immunity in atopic dermatitis. J Dermatol 1: 333

Schöpf E, Kapp A (1987) Chemiluminescence response of polymorphonuclear leukocytes in atopic dermatitis. Int Arch Allergy Appl Immunol 82: 380

Schöpf E, Kapp A, Kim CW (1978) T cell function in atopic dermatitis. Controlled examination of Concanavalin A dose-response relations in cultured lymphocytes. Arch Dermatol Res 262: 37

Schopfer K, Baerlocher K, Price P et al. (1979) Staphylococcal IgE antibodies, hyperimmunoglobulinaemia E and Staphylococcus aureus infections. N Engl Med J 300: 835

Schröder H, Thalberg K, Lundberg A (1985) New techniques in specific IgE antibody measurement. Allergy 40 (Suppl 4): 14

Schubert H, Berova N, Czernielewski A, Hegyi E et al. (1987) Epidemiology of nickel allergy. Contact Dermatitis 16: 122

Schultz Larsen F (1985) Atopic dermatitis. Etiological studies based on a twin population. Lægeforeningens, Copenhagen

Schultz Larsen F, Holm NV, Henningsen K (1986) Atopic dermatitis. A genetic-epidemiologic study in a population based twin sample. J Am Acad Dermatol 15: 487

Schultz Larsen F, Jörgensen AS, Grunnet N (1985) Natural killer cell function in atopic dermatitis. Clin Exp Dermatol 10: 104

Schur S, Hyde JS, Wypich JL (1974) Egg-white sensitivity in atopic eczema. J Allergy Clin Immunol 54: 174

Schuster DL, Bongiovanni BA, Peterson DL, Barbaro JF, Wong DTO, Levinson AL (1980) Selective deficiency of a T cell subpopulation in active atopic dermatitis. J Immunol 124: 1662

Schwartz M (1952) The heredity in bronchial asthma. Acta Allergol (Suppl 2)

Secher L, Permin H, Juhl F (1978) Immunofluorescence of the skin in allergic diseases: an investigation of patients with contact dermatitis, allergic vasculitis and atopic dermatitis. Acta Derm Venereol (Stockh) 58: 117

Sedlis E (1965) Some challenge studies with foods. J Pediatr 66: 153–274

Sedlis E, Prose PH, Holt LE (1966) Infantile eczema. Postgrad Med J 40: 63

Shakib F, Morrow Brown H, Readhead R et al. (1985) IgE and IgG4 antibodies to bovine milk fat globule membrane in atopic eczema patients: a study of their occurrence, relevance and antigenic specificity. Clin Allergy 15: 265

Shelley WB, Juhlin L (1977) Selective uptake of contact allergens by the Langerhans' cells. Arch Dermatol 113: 187

Shohat B, Metzker A, Trainin N (1980) Cell-mediated immunity and the in vitro effect of thymic humoral factor (THF) on blood lymphocytes of children with atopic dermatitis. Clin Immunol Immunopathol 15: 646

Siemens HW (1924) Die Zwillingspathologie. Springer, Berlin Heidelberg New York

Silberberg I (1973) Apposition of mononuclear cells to Langerhans' cells in contact allergic reactions. An ultrastructural study. Acta Derm Venereol (Stockh) 53: 1

Sillevis Smith JH, Bos JD, Hulsebosch HJ, Krieg SR (1986) In situ immunophagotyping of antigen presenting cells and T cell subsets in atopic dermatitis. Clin Exp Dermatol 11: 159

Silvennoinen-Kassinen S (1981) The specificity of a nickel sulphate reaction in vitro: a family study and a study of chromium-allergic subjects. Scand J Immunol 13: 231

Simon FA (1944) On the allergen in human dander. J Allergy 15: 338

Simon FA (1949) Allergy to human dander in infantile eczema. In: Progr Allergy 2: 246

Simon FA, Rackemann FM (1934a) The development of hypersensitiveness in man. I. Following intradermal injection of the antigen. J Allergy 5: 439

Simon FA, Rackemann FM (1934b) The development of hypersensitiveness in man. II. Absorption of antigen through nasal mucous membrane. J Allergy 5: 451

Skog E (1960) Primary irritant and eczematous reaction induced in patients with dermatoses. Acta Derm Venereol (Stockh) 50: 183

Skog E, Thyresson N (1953) The occupational significance of some common contact allergens. Acta Derm Venereol (Stockh) 33: 65

Snyderman R, Rogers E, Buckley RH (1977) Abnormalities of leukotaxis in atopic dermatitis. J Allergy Clin Immunol 60: 121

Solomon LM, Telner P (1966) Eruptive molluscum contagiosum in atopic dermatitis. Can Med Assoc J 95: 978

Sonck CE, Widholm O (1954) Zur Frage der Antistreptolysin- und Antistaphylolysintiter bei einigen Hautkrankheiten. Z Haut Geschlechtskr 17: 175

Soothill JF (1974) Immunodeficiency and allergy. In: Brostoff I (ed) Clinical immunology-allergy in paediatric medicine, vol 1. Blackwell, Oxford, p 21

Spaich D, Ostertag M (1936) Untersuchungen über allergische Erkrankungen bei Zwillingen. Z Menschl Vererb Konstitutionsl 19: 731

Spiegelberg HL (1986) IgE receptors in lymphocytes. In: Ring J, Burg G (eds) New trends in allergy II. Springer, Berlin Heidelberg New York, p 33

Stanworth DR (1957) The use of gel-precipitation technique in the identification of horse dandruff antigen and in the study of serological relationship between horse dandruff and horse serum proteins. Int Arch Allergy Appl Immunol 2: 170

Stanworth DR (1963) Reaginic antibodies. Adv Immunol 3: 181

Steigleder GK (ed) (1979) Kölner RAST symposium, 1979. Grosse, Berlin

Steigleder GK (ed) (1981) Kölner RAST symposium, 1981. Grosse, Berlin

Stingl G, Gazze LA, Czarneski N, Wolff K (1981) T cell abnormalities in atopic dermatitis patients: imbalance in T cell subpopulations and impaired generation of Con-A induced suppressor cells. J Invest Dermatol 76: 478

Stone SP, Gleich GJ, Muller SA (1976) Atopic dermatitis and IgE. Arch Dermatol 112: 1254

Storck H (1954) Eksemreaktion durch Inhalation des Allergens. Dermatologica 108: 411

Storck H (1955) Eksem durch Inhalation. Schweiz Med Wochenschr 85: 608

Storck H (1961) Le rôle de la prédisposition, du système neurovégétatif et de l'allergie dans le prurigo de Besnier. Arch Belg Dermatol 17: 95

Storck H (1979) Geklärtes und ungeklärtes der dermatologischen Immunologie. Hautarzt 30: 62

Storck H, Schnyder UW, Schwartz K (1960) Neurodermitis disseminata mit Verschlimmerung im Sommer. Aufflammen nach Inhalation von Pollenallergenen. Dermatologica 121: 150

Strannegård IL, Strannegård Ö (1977) Increased sensitivity of lymphocytes from atopic individuals to histamine-induced suppression. Scand J Immunol 6: 1225

Strannegård IL, Strannegård Ö (1980) Natural killer cells and interferon production in atopic dermatitis. Acta Derm Venereol [Suppl] (Stockh) 92: 48

Strannegård IL, Lindholm L, Strannegård Ö (1976) Studies of T lymphocytes in atopic children. Int Arch Allergy Appl Immunol 50: 684

Strannegård Ö, Strannegård IL (1978) T lymphocyte numbers and function in human IgE-mediated allergy. Immunol Rev 41: 149

Strannegård Ö, Strannegård IL, Rystedt I (1985) Viral infections in atopic dermatitis. Acta Derm Venereol [Suppl] (Stockh) 114: 121

Strauss MB (1960) Allergens. In: Prigal SJ (ed) Fundamentals of modern allergy. McGraw Hill, New York

Strauss J, Kligman AM (1957) Relationship of atopic allergy and dermatitis. Arch Dermatol 75: 806

Sulzberger MB (1936) The relative importance of specific skin hypersensitivity in adult dermatitis. JAMA 106: 1000

Sulzberger MB (1940) Dermatologic allergy. Thomas, Springfield

Sulzberger MB, Spain WC, Sammis F, Shahon HF (1932) Studies in hypersensitiveness in certain dermatoses (disseminated type). J Allergy 3: 423

Swainson JA, Wilson PB, Dore P, Pumphrey RSH (1985) Evidence for circulating complexes containing IgE in patients with atopic dermatitis. Int Arch Allergy Appl Immunol 76: 237

Swineford O, Holman J (1949) Studies on bactrial allergy. III. Results of 3680 cutaneous tests with 34 crude polysaccharide and nucleoprotein fractions of 14 different bacteria. J Allergy 20: 420

Tada T (1975) Regulation of reaginic antibody information in animals. Progr Allergy 19: 122

Tada T, Ishizaka K (1970) Distribution of E-forming cells in lymphoid tissues of the human and monkey. J Immunol 104: 377

Takahashi I, Aliyama T, Yamamura M, Sasaoka K, Anan S (1977) Evaluation of RAST in atopic dermatitis. J Dermatol 4: 217

Takigawa M, Tamamori T, Horiguchi D, Sakamoto T, Yamada M (1989) Fc$_\varepsilon$ receptor positive cells in atopic dermatitis. Acta Derm Venereol (suppl 144) (Stockh) (in press)

Tanaka V, Tanaka M, Anan S, Yoshida H (1989) Immunohistochemical studies on dust mite antigen in the positive reaction site of the patch test. Acta Derm Venereol (Suppl 144) (Stockh) (in press)

Taylor B, Norman AP, Orgel HA, Stokes CR, Turner MW, Soothill JF (1973) Transient IgA deficiency and pathogenesis of infantile atopy. Lancet II: 111

Thestrup Pedersen KK, Ellegård J, Thulin H, Zachariae H (1977) PPD and mitogen responsiveness of patients with atopic dermatitis. Clin Exp Immunol 27: 118

Thulin H, Hanifin JM, Bryant R (1980) Leucocyte adherence in atopic dermatitis: diminished responses to histamine and isoproterenol. Acta Derm Venereol (Stockh) 60: 235

Ting S, Dunsky EH, Lavker RM, Zweiman B (1980) Patterns of mast cell alterations and in vivo mediator release in human allergic skin reactions. J Allergy Clin Immunol 66: 417

Tovey ER, Chapman MD, Wells CW, Platt-Mills TAE (1981) The distribution of dust mite allergen in houses of patients with asthma. Am Rev Respir Dis 124: 630

Tuft L (1949) Importance of inhalant allergens in atopic dermatitis. J Invest Dermatol 12: 211

Tuft L, Heck VM (1952) Studies in atopic dermatitis. IV. Importance of seasonal inhalant allergen, especially ragweed. J Allergy 23: 528

Turk JL (1970) Contribution of modern immunological concepts to an understanding of diseases of the skin. Br Med J II: 363

Turner MW, Brostoff J, Wells RS, Stokes CR, Soothill F (1977) HLA in eczema and hay fever. Clin Exp Immunol 27: 43

Uehara M (1980) Tuberculin reaction in atopic dermatitis. Acta Derm Venereol [Suppl] (Stockh) 92: 70

Uehara M (1986) Heterogeneity of serum IgE levels in atopic dermatitis. Acta Derm Venereol (Stockh) 66: 404

Uehara M, Ofuji S (1974) The leukocyte migration test in atopic dermatitis. Acta Derm Venereol (Stockh) 54: 279

Uehara M, Ofuji S (1976) Patch test reactions to human dander in atopic dermatitis. Arch Dermatol 112: 951

Uehara M, Takahashi C, Ofuji S (1975) Pustular patch test reactions in atopic dermatitis. Arch Dermatol 111: 1154

Uno H, Hanifin JM (1980) Langerhans' cells in acute and chronic epidermal lesions of atopic dermatitis, observed by L-dopa histofluorescence, glycol methacrylate thin section and electron microscopy. J Invest Dermatol 75: 52

Van Arsdal PP, Motulsky AG (1959) Frequency and hereditability of asthma and allergic rhinitis in college students. Acta Genet Stat Med 9: 101

Van der Bijl WJF (1960) Studies on the technique of skin testing in allergy. Thomas, Springfield

Varelzidis A, Wilson AB, Meara RH, Turk L (1966) Immunoglobulin levels in atopic eczema. Br Med J II: 925

Vaughan W (1929) The interpretation of borderline allergic reactions. K Lab Clin Med 14: 433

Vestey JP, Howie SEM, Norval M, Maingay JP, Neill WA (1988) Immune response to herpes simplex virus in patients with facial herpes simplex and those with eczema herpeticum. Br J Dermatol 118: 775

Viander M, Uksila J, Lassila O, Jansen CT (1982) Natural killer cell activity in atopic dermatitis. Arch Dermatol Res 274: 283

Vogel F, Dorn H (1964) Krankheiten der Haut und ihrer Anhanggebiete. In: Becker PE (ed) Humangenetik, vol 14. Thieme, Stuttgart, p 346

Vogel F, Matulsky AG (1979) Human genetics. Problems and approaches. Springer, Berlin Heidelberg New York

Voorhorst R (1962) Basic facts of allergy. Stenfert Kroese, Leiden

Voorhorst R, Spieksma FTM, Varekamp H, Leupen MJ, Lyklema AW (1967) The house dust mite (dermatophagoides pteronyssinus) and the allergens it produces. Identity with the house dust allergen. J Allergy 39: 325

Wahlberg JE, Skog E (1971) Nickel allergy and atopy. Threshold of nickel sensitivity and immunoglobulin E determinations. Br J Dermatol 85: 97

Wahn U, Herold U, Danielsen K, Löwenstein H (1982) Allergoprints in horse allergic children. Allergy 37: 335

Watt TL, Baumann RR (1968) Nickel earlobe dermatitis. Arch Dermatol 98: 155

Wells GC (1956) Effects of nickel on the skin. Br J Dermatol 68: 237

Werner M (1972) Panel on food allergy. In: Allergology. Proc 8th Europ Cong of Allergy Excerpta Medica, Amsterdam, p 370

White MI, Noble WC (1985) The cutaneous reaction to staphylococcal protein A in normal subjects and patients with atopic dermatitis or psoriasis. Br J Dermatol 113: 179

Wide L, Porath J (1966) Radioimmunoassay of proteins with the use of Sephadex-coupled antibodies. Acta Biochem Biophysic 130: 257

Wide L, Bennich H, Johansson SGO (1967) Diagnosis of allergy by an in-vitro test or allergen antibodies. II: 1105

Wide L, Aronsen T, Fagerberg E, Zetterstrom Ö (1972) Radioimmunoassay of allergen-specific IgE. In: Charpin J, Boutin C, Aubert J, Frankland AW (eds) Allergology. Proceedings of the 8th European Congress of Allergology. Excerpta Medica, Amsterdam, p 85

Wiener AS, Zieve I, Fries JH (1936) The inheritance of allergic disease. Ann Eugenics 7: 141

Willemze R, De Graaff-Reitsma CB, Crossen J, Van Vloten WA, Meijer CJLM (1983) Characterization of T cell subpopulations in skin and peripheral blood of patients with cutaneous T cell lymphomas and benign inflammatory dermatoses. J Invest Dermatol 80: 60

Williams RC, Griffiths RW, Emmons JD, Field RC (1972) Naturally occurring human antiglobulin with specificity for IgE. J Clin Invest 51: 955

Wilson HTH (1956) Nickel dermatitis. Br J Dermatol 68: 229

Wittig HJ, Beloit F, Filippi ID, Royal G (1980) Age-related serum immunoglobulin E levels in healthy subjects and in patients with allergic disease. J Allergy Clin Immunol 66: 305

Wraith DG, Merrett J, Roth A, Yman L, Merrett TG (1979) Recognition of food-allergic patients and their allergens by the RAST technique and clinical investigation. Clin Allergy 9: 25

Wütrich B (1974) Allergenspezifische IgE im Radioallergosorbenttest bei Neurodermitis. Hautarzt 25: 603

Wütrich B (1975) Zur Immunpathologie der Neurodermitis constitutionalis. Huber, Bern

Wütrich B (1987) Neuere Aspekte zur Diagnostik und Therapie der Nahrungsmittelallergie. Allergologie 9: 370

Wütrich B, Baumann E, Fries RA, Schnyder UW (1981) Total and specific IgE (RAST) in atopic twins. Clin Allergy 11: 147

Wütrich B, Benz A, Skvaril F (1983) IgE and IgG4 levels in children with atopic dermatitis. Dermatologica 166: 229

Wütrich B, Kopper E, Virchow C (1973) IgE-Bestimmung bei Neurodermitis und anderen Dermatosen. Hautarzt 24: 381

Yman L (1985) New developments in serum IgE measurement. Allergy 40 (Suppl 4): 10

Yocum MW, Strong DM, Lakin JD (1976) Competent cellular immunity in allergic rhinitis patients with elevated IgE. J Allergy Clin Immunol 57: 384

Young E, Bruynzeel-Koomen C, Berrens L (1985) Delayed type hypersensitivity in atopic dermatitis. Acta Derm Venereol [Suppl] (Stockh) 114: 77

Young E, Pepper M, Everard J, Shaw S, Wilkinson DM (1986) Attitudes to additives – a preliminary report. Br J Dermatol (Suppl 30): 36

Yunginger JW, Jones RT, Gleich GJ (1976) Studies on alternaria allergens. II. Measurements of the relative potency of commercial *Alternaria* extracts by the direct RAST inhibition. J Allergy Clin Immunol 58: 405

Zachary CB, Allen MH, MacDonald DM (1985a) In situ quantification of T-lymphocyte subsets and Langerhans' cells in the inflammatory infiltrate of atopic eczema. Br J Dermatol 112: 149

Zachary CB, Poulter LW, MacDonald DM (1985b) Cell mediated immune responses in atopic dermatitis: the relevance of antigen-presenting cells. Br J Dermatol (Suppl 114): 77

Zakon SJ, Taub SJ (1938) The inhalation of house and horse danders as an etiologic factor in atopic dermatitis. J Allergy 9: 523

Zetterstrom Ö, Osterman K, Machado L, Johansson SGO (1981) Another smoking hazard: raised serum IgE concentration and increased risk for occupational allergy. Br Med J 283: 1215

Zezschwitz KA (1957) Antistreptolysintiterbestimmungen bei Dermatosen. Derm Wochenschr 135: 185

Zimmermann T (1987) Reduzierung der Hausstaubmilbenallergens nach Zimmer- und Bettsanierung. Untersuchung mit einem Teststreifensystem (Acarex). Allergologie 10: 31

6 Pathomechanism: Cells and Mediators

6.1 Mast Cells and Histamine

From this immense field only some details with putative roles in AD will be discussed.

6.1.1 Mast Cells

Mast cells participate in inflammatory and immunological reactions, particularly of the immediate type, but also in nonimmunological mechanisms. Mast cells are present in high concentrations in the skin – $7225-12\,000/mm^2$, depending on the histological technique used (Mikhail and Miller-Milinska 1964; Soter et al. 1978) – and in an increased number in AD (Levi et al. 1959; Mikhail and Miller-Milinska 1964). This was convincingly demonstrated by Mihm et al. (1976), particularly in chronic forms of the disorder. Increased number of mast cells were demonstrated in lichenified lesions of AD patients with personal history of respiratory atopy (Sugiura et al. 1989). The number of basophils in the peripheral circulation (Rorsman 1958) or in the skin (Mihm et al. 1976) of AD patients are normal.

Activated by IgE, anaphylatoxins, chemical and physical stimuli, drugs, and other factors, mast cells participate in inflammation by expulsing their granules, which release biologically active mediators, or by secreting these mediators. Among them histamine is doubtlessly the major agent in inflammatory and immunoregulatory processes, particularly in the initial phase, subsequently being followed by mast cell-secreted chemotactic factors which attract inflammatory cells to the area of inflammation (for review, see Wintroub and Soter 1983). Mast cell mediators also include prostaglandins, leukotrienes/slow-reacting substance (LTC_4, LTD_4, LTE_4), kinins, platelet activating factor (PAF), and several proteoglycans (e.g., heparin), as well as enzymes (e.g., trypsin, chymotrypsin, phospholipase A_2). High affinity IgE Fc receptors on mast cells bind IgE, and antigen elicits a cross-linking of two Fc receptors, which induces the mediator release. The number of IgE receptors is higher in atopics (Feltkamp-Vroom 1977); in the rat it was maximally $30\,000/cell$ (Conrad et al. 1975), while on human basophils it was $40\,000-100\,000/cell$ (Ishizaka et al. 1973). For a review of the mast cell, see Czarnetzki (1986).

6.1.2 Histamine

There is well-known evidence that histamine is a mediator of type I reactivity, and reports relevant to AD include the following: By intramuscular injections of histamine Williams (1938) produced a rise in skin temperature which was restricted to the face and neck in normal persons but was greatest in the flexures in AD patients. Nilzén (1958), using the Code technique, found higher histamine levels in the antecubital fossae in similar patients, this finding being confirmed by Johnson et al. (1960) and by Juhlin (1967); the latter author visualized the histamine in the skin by its forming a fluorescent complex with o-phthalaldehyde. However, macroscopically symptom-free skin in AD and also in various types of eczema has the same histamine content. In addition, Winkelmann (1966), using a perfusate technique, readily obtained histamine release from the skin of most AD patients, but this was unrelated to the severity of the skin disease.

On the other hand normal skin histamine levels were registered by Ruzicka and Glück (1983). Higher histamine levels were more infrequently found, mostly in severe cases, by Ring and O'Connor (1979) and Ring (1983); these levels returned to normal during remission or after food challenge (Sampson and Jolie 1984). Urinary histamine excretion is normal in AD (Overgaard Petersen et al. 1979).

Among earlier relevant studies were those by Möller and Rorsman (1958), using intracutaneous injections, and Eilard and Hellgren (1961), employing iontophoresis; in both studies histamine was administered to AD patients and each group reported diminished exudation.

The histaminopexic capacity of the blood, according to Parrot and Laborde (1963), is low in contact dermatitis and in AD, but it increases parallel to improvement in the skin condition. The cardinal effects of histamine with relevance to AD are its pruritogenic action carried out via H_1 receptors and its vasodilative/vascular permeability-increasing property on venules, which is mediated by both H_1 and H_2 receptors (Greaves et al. 1977). Furthermore, it cannot be ignored that stress induces histamine generation (Reimann et al. 1981).

An important discovery was that mast cells (and basophils) release histamine and other mediators more easily, i. e., usually there is an increased releasability in atopy (Conroy et al. 1977; Lichtenstein et al. 1978), including AD (Ring and O'Connor 1979; Butler et al. 1985; Marone et al. 1986). In this context Lebel et al. (1980) registered that there was a group of high, and another of low, responders among AD children. Ring and his group (Ring et al. 1986) systematically studied the conditions of the histamine releasability in AD by measuring anti-IgE-induced histamine release from basophils in vitro. The factors influencing this reaction are shown in Table 6.1.

The enhancing effect of cholinergic stimuli found by Ring et al. in their studies is a subject for debate (Schmutzler et al. 1979; Kaliner 1984; Butler et al. 1985). It is of further interest that substance P, present in the nervous system, stimulated histamine release from mast cells (Ebertz et al. 1985). The cyclic nu-

Table 6.1. Factors influencing histamine releasability

Nerval influence (autonomic, endorphins, neuropeptides)
Cyclic nucleotide system (cAMP/cGMP)
Arachidonic acid metabolites
Negative feedback
Age
Sex
Microbial infection
Disease

cleotide system will be discussed below (see Sect. 6.3). The role of arachidonic acid metabolites (see Sect. 6.4) seems to be important, since histamine release from basophils is:

1. *Enhanced* by cyclooxygenase inhibitors (indomethacin, acetylsalicylic acid), increasing age (Marone et al. 1983), female sex (Ring et al. 1986), and viral infections (Ida et al. 1977)
2. *Inhibited* by PGE_2, lipoxygenase inhibitors, eicosatetraenoic acid or pheni-done (Sauer et al. 1987a), or cyclooxygenase plus eicosatetraenoic acid (Sobotka et al. 1979)

Histamine release can also be studied on basophils after adding antigens which showed a good parallelism to RAST values (Sauer et al. 1987b), by Ca-iono-phore, by C5a, or after adding the lectin Con A as a divalent substance able to combine with cell-bound IgE. It is believed, however, that histamine releasabil-ity is neither of greater differential diagnostic nor of pathomechanistic signifi-cance in AD/atopy (Kownatzki and Grüninger 1987).

6.1.3 Histamine Inhibition

The inhibitory role of histamine (in high concentrations) on its own release, i. e., negative feedback, shown in the quoted histamine-release experiments, in-dicates an important immunoregulatory role for histamine. This inhibitory ef-fect predominantly occurs via H_2 receptors on the surface of T-lymphocytes having these receptors (mast cells, basophils, etc. also have H_2 receptors on their surface). Subsequent to histamine influence the H_2 receptor possibly acts by producing, via interleukin-1, a histamine-suppressor factor (HSF). This re-sults in an inhibitory effect on both T- and B-lymphocytes, expressed in less proliferation, reduced production of lymphokines, and dampening of other lymphocyte functions, including B-cell immunoglobulin production (Rocklin et al. 1980; Beer and Rocklin 1984). These authors also suppose the participation of lymphocyte-produced histamine-releasing factor, acting on mast cells and basophils, in this regulation. The negative feedback is also present in atopy (Ring et al. 1986) although the number of H_2 receptor-bearing cells and HSF production are less here, as an expression of an immunoregulatory defect (Beer et al. 1982; Matloff et al. 1983).

The inhibitory effect of histamine through H_2 receptors also includes eosinophil chemotaxis (while the latter is stimulated when histamine acts via H_1 receptors).

6.2 Eosinophils and Their Products

Mast cells and eosinophils have complex interactions which may include both antagonism and cooperation. Eosinophilic chemotactic factor (ECF, presumably identical with LTB_4) of mast cells attracts eosinophils, and on the other hand, the eosinophil enzyme histaminase inactivates histamine. Prostaglandins originating from eosinophils inhibit basophil degranulation and slow reacting substance from basophils (i. e., LTC_4, LTD_4, and LTE_4) is inhibited by arylsulfatase.

Eosinophils even act as phagocytes of antigen: they ingest and remove IgE from the sites of allergic reaction (Parish 1972; Parish and Champion 1973) and antigen-antibody complexes. Eosinophils are also attracted by C5a and lymphokines. Although ECF levels were not detected in AD sera (Czarnetzki et al. 1979), the demonstration that eosinophil granule proteins are involved in the mechanism of AD was of great interest. The major basic protein (MBP, which causes the release of histamine from basophils and rat mast cells), was found outside the eosinophils in all 18 investigated AD patients' biopsies. The predominating fibrillar pattern was similar to that of onchocerciasis. This indicated that, although the number of eosinophils in skin infiltrates of AD is low, eosinophil involvement is probable in this disease (Gleich et al. 1976; Leiferman et al. 1985). The role of eosinophils is further confirmed by the observation that even eosinophilic cationic protein (ECP) (which also causes histamine release from rat mast cells) can be demonstrated in AD. Investigation of patch test reactions to mites and grass pollen via a monoclonal antibody technique against ECP revealed that activated eosinophils appeared early in the dermis and, according to electron microscopic studies, were in close contact to Langerhans' cells, suggesting interaction between these two cells (Bruynzeel-Koomen et al. 1988). MBP was further demonstrated to be a prominent feature of late cutaneous reaction (see Sect. 5.8) since it appears in such reactions after 3 h and persists until 48 h (Leiferman et al. 1986).

In a clinical context eosinophilia not infrequently is found in normal individuals, provoked possibly by nonimmunological stimuli; it consequently is of rather limited value in differential diagnosis. The total eosinophil count in the blood in cases of AD has been found to be raised by different groups of authors (Wagner and Pürschel 1962; de Graciansky 1966; Mustakallio 1966; Stüttgen et al. 1968), but these values can show considerable variations during the course of the disease.

Hellerström and Lidman (1956) compared blood eosinophil counts in AD patients on their admission to and discharge from hospital; they concluded that there is a good correlation between blood eosinophilia and activity of the disease. Higher eosinophil counts in the blood have also been reported in infants and children with AD (Huriez 1966). In an attempt to correlate the occurrence of eosinophilia in the blood and in nasal secretions with different stages of AD, Voorhorst et al. (1963) found the following: in the infantile phase, eosinophilia is present only in the blood; during childhood it occurs both in the blood and in nasal secretions; later, it decreases in both. A good correlation exists between respiratory symptoms and nasal secretion eosinophilia, and it is possible that the latter heralds respiratory allergic symptoms (Girard 1972). Counts of eosinophils taken from denuded skin have been shown to correlate well with results of skin tests and with seasonal symptoms in patients with concomitant AD and respiratory atopic manifestations (Felarca and Lowell 1971).

6.3 Cyclic Nucleotides

From the vast literature some points of view which are of relevance for AD have been selected:

6.3.1 Introduction

It was Ahlqvist (1948) who first demonstrated that α- and β-adrenergic receptors are present in various organs and that each type reacts differently to catecholamines: α-Receptors have the greatest affinity to epinephrine, less to norepinephrine, and least to isoproterenol whereas β-receptors have the greatest affinity to isoproterenol, less to epinephrine, and least to norepinephrine.

Later it was discovered that both receptors can be subclassified into groups 1 and 2. β-Receptors are: inhibited by, for example, practolol. The β_2-receptor is particularly stimulated by epinephrine and inhibited by butoxamine. On the membranes of leukocytes and monocytes, β_2-receptors are present, with 1000–2000 receptors/cell (Williams et al. 1976).

Stimulation of α-receptors causes responses such as vasoconstriction (except in skeletal muscle) and glycogenolysis, as well as inhibition of histamine release, antibody response, and T cell cytolytic activity. The adrenoceptors were studied by radioactive binding of their ligands (agonists and antagonists) (for technical details see the review of Hoffman and Lefkowitz 1980, and of Djurup 1981).

The investigations of the nature of the β-receptors on the membrane of mononuclear cells or granulocytes were focused on its coupling to the enzyme adenylate cyclase, which mediates most effects of the receptor stimulation. Via a guanine nucleotide-sensitive regulatory protein, adenylate cyclase is activated and catalyzes the synthesis from adenosine triphosphate (ATP) to cyclic 3,5-adenosine monophosphate (cAMP) (Sutherland and Robison 1966). The raised intracellular concentration of cAMP then activates a protein kinase which phosphorylates various regulatory enzymes and proteins and ultimately inhibits mediator release.

The number of β-receptors may be influenced by various factors, e. g., after long stimulation they decrease in number and/or the cAMP response is downregulated (desensitization). The molecular mechanism of α-receptors is less known; Ca^2-ions are probably the second messenger for α_1-receptor stimulation.

The cyclic guanine monophosphate (GMP) in cells has an effect antagonistic to that of cAMP and a balance between these was postulated (Ignarro 1973; Goldberg et al. 1974). The concept of the importance of a cAMP/GMP regulatory system, primarily modulating the mediator responses, has, however, received less general support in recent years.

6.3.2 Conditions in Atopy/AD

Szentivanyi (1966, 1968) postulated that a basic event in atopy is a β-adrenergic hyposensitivity or a functional imbalance between β- and α-adrenoceptors (β-blockade theory). The β/α ratio in normals is about 7, whereas in asthmatics, for example, it is only approximately 0.8. Szentivanyi et al. (1980) also postulated an interconversion from β- to α-receptors, while Venter et al. (1980) explained the reduction of β-receptors as being attributable to autoantibodies against the receptors.

According to this concept the consequence of β-receptor impairment is an excess activation of α-receptors by catecholamines; this α-adrenergic hyperresponsiveness leads to increased liberation of histamine and other mediators, which plays an important part in the mechanism of AD. In accordance with this view, β-agonists did not produce the expected inhibition of DNA synthesis in cultured skin cells in AD patients (Carr et al. 1973); further, the β-agonist effect resulted in low leukocytic cAMP levels (Reed et al. 1976). A normal number, but a reduced affinity, of β-receptors to the antagonist ^{125}I-hydroxybenzyl-pindolol was demonstrated in AD by Pochet et al. (1980). There were, however, reports of diminished response in AD cells to other mediators as well, such as histamine (Busse and Lantis 1979) and PGE_1 (Parker et al. 1977).

Hanifin and his group systematically investigated the evidence of a broader regulatory effect. They did not find any abnormalities of β-receptors in AD (Galant et al. 1979), and this was confirmed by Ruoho et al. (1980).

Safko et al. (1981) were able to show that, in addition to isoproterenol, other adenylate cyclase-activating agents such as histamine and PGE_1, in low concentration, desensitized normal leukocytes to subsequent stimuli from these agonists.

In other words, a lower cAMP level was demonstrated on normal leukocytes, thus simulating atopic conditions and creating a model technique. In a further series of investigations, it was shown that the increase of cAMP-specific phosphodiesterase (PDE) activity, demonstrable on leukocytes (Chan et al. 1982; Grewe et al. 1982) and particularly on monocytes (Holden et al. 1985; 1986), was responsible for the low cAMP values found in AD.

The normal PDE activity demonstrated previously in AD by Mier and Urselmann (1970) and Holla et al. (1972), which contrasted with their results, was explained by differences in concentrations used in the experiments. The validity of the concept of increased PDE activity was confirmed by further results:

1. A correlation between high PDE activity and Con A-stimulated histamine release (Butler et al. 1983 a)
2. A correlation between PDE and spontaneous mononuclear IgE synthesis (Cooper et al. 1985)
3. The reversal of the former findings after application of the PDE inhibitor Ro 20-1724 (Cooper et al. 1985), pointing to blocking of B cells
4. Decreased cAMP responsiveness of mononuclear cells in a canine model (Butler et al. 1983 b)

Based on these experimental findings and the detection of high PDE activity in cord leukocytes in neonates of atopic mothers or fathers (Heskel et al. 1984; McMillan et al. 1985), the Hanifin group created the concept that elevated PDE activity may be a primary gene-associated defect and a marker for AD. These children also showed a tendency, during the observation period of 18 months, to develop atopic symptoms (Hanifin 1987). The molecular basis of the increase in PDE activity in AD leukocytes was further investigated and the role of an impaired protein kinase-C phosphorylation was focused on (Chan et al. 1986; Trask et al. 1988). It is also of importance that increased PDE values were found in patients with AD in remission and also in allergic rhinitis (Grewe et al. 1982; Hanifin 1986).

Other authors have also studied the effect of cyclic nucleotides in AD. Herlin and Kragballe (1980) reported impaired monocyte function associated with abnormal cAMP responses to agonist stimulation. Hovmark and Åsbrink (1981) observed increased IgE synthesis after applying a β-receptor blocker (propranolol).

Archer et al. (1983) found defective cAMP responsiveness of AD lymphocytes to isoproterenol, histamine, and PGE_2. Crespi et al. (1982) reported normal catecholamine levels in AD – in contrast to an earlier demonstration of reduced levels by Solomon and Wentzel (1963) – and an impairment of the β-receptor mediated amylase secretion of the parotis. Ring et al. (1981) showed an increased GMP response to cholinergic stimuli in AD and observed that the intracellular level of either cAMP or GMP in AD was identical to that in controls.

The in vivo studies of Archer et al. (1984) are not consistent with the β-adrenergic impairment in AD, since AD patients and healthy persons had the same reduction of the histamine-elicited cutaneous response by a β-agonist (salbutamol) and by the predominantly adrenergic agonist norepinephrine (acting probably by vasoconstriction). A reduction of antigen-elicited skin test response by pretreatment with a β-adrenergic agent (isoproterenol) had been reported previously by Shereff et al. (1973). Archer et al. (1987) reported no differences between AD patients and controls in terms of adrenomedullary function as assessed by the plasma levels of cAMP and catecholamines, including after histamine infusion and standing or after epinephrine infusion. By contrast Schwartz et al. (1987) reported an elevation of plasma cAMP levels in AD.

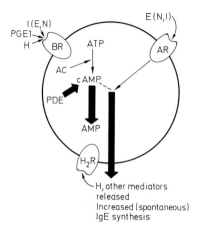

Fig. 6.1. Simplified view on the role of cyclic nucleotides in AD. *I*, isoproterenol; *N*, norepenephrine; *E*, epinephrine; *BR*, beta-receptor; *AR*, adrenergic receptor; *H2R*, H_2-receptor; *AC*, adenylate cyclase; *H*, histamine; for other abbreviations, see text. *Single arrow*, weak stimulation; *thick arrow*, strong stimulation; *broken arrow*, weak inhibition

6.3.3 Concluding Remarks

The major consequences of raised PDE and reduced cAMP activity in AD are:

1. Increased (in vitro) IgE synthesis and mediator release (a feedback mechanism via H_2-receptors may subsequently lead to the opposite effects).
2. On a broader basis, the mast cell is also involved in AD via the inhibitory effect of cAMP on histamine release. The possible consequence of this mechanism may be histamine releasability in mast cells and impaired functions in leukocytes.
3. The use of PDE-inhibiting drugs like theophylline and caffeine not only in asthma but also in AD, based among other things on the statement of Archer et al. (1984) of an anti-inflammatory effect of β-agonists.

Some major aspects of the role of cyclic nucleotides in AD are depicted in Fig. 6.1.

6.4 Eicosanoids

The "eicosanoids" include arachidonic acid-derived proinflammatory substances produced mainly by neutrophils, eosinophils, and macrophages, which have vasoactive and chemotactic effects on leukocytes. Skin 5-lipoxygenase activity results in the end metabolites of leukotrienes, whereas cyclooxygenase activity leads to the major products of prostaglandins and thromboxanes. LTC_4 (a component of slow reacting substance) induced wheals after intradermal injection (Juhlin and Hammarström 1982). Similarly, Soter et al. (1983) observed an urticarial response to LTC_4, LTD_4, and LTE_4. After applying LTB_4, a transient erythema and wheal appeared, followed in 3–4 h by induration consisting predominantly of neutrophils. This reaction was enhanced by PGD_2 or, according to the studies of Camp et al. (1983), by PGE_2. Czarnetzki (1983) found an increased monocyte response to LTB_4 chemotaxis in AD (and in psoriasis). By challenge of mononuclear cells, including by anti-IgE, as well as by radioim-munological analysis of skin suction blister content, a marked elevation of LTB_4 was demonstrated in lesional AD skin. This did not show any correlation with the severity of the disease or with LTB_4 serum levels (Ruzicka et al. 1984; Ruzicka 1986).

6.4.1 Prostaglandins

A group of substances with various, in part antagonistic, biological effects are released in cutaneous inflammation (Greaves et al. 1971). PGE_1 and PGE_2 elic-it, after intracutaneous injection, local edema and a dark persistent erythema (Solomon et al. 1968; Camp et al. 1983). PGD_2 also induces a wheal and flare reaction (Soter et al. 1983). In atopic skin 20 min after injection of PGE_1, the reaction is subnormal; however, a normal erythematous response subsequently develops (Juhlin and Michaelsson 1969). The PGE_2 content of skin suction blisters in AD was not different to that in controls (Ruzicka et al. 1984). On the other hand it was shown that lesional and perilesional AD skin contained ele-vated concentrations of PGE_2 (Kragballe and Fogh, 1989). PGE_1 and PGE_2 are not real pruritogenic agents, but these substances potentiate itch induced by, for example, histamine (see Sect. 3.1).

6.5 Complement

Complement components in the peripheral blood of AD patients have been studied by a number of authors. The C3 levels were mostly found to be within normal limits (Fontana et al. 1962 Beard et al. 1981), although increased values were detected by Kaufman et al. (1968) and by Kapp and Schöpf (1985). C3 split products were also demonstrated in the sera of AD patients (Ring et al. 1979) and were found to be somewhat elevated (Kapp et al. 1983; Kapp and Schöpf 1985). Furthermore, decreased levels of C3c were shown by Wütrich et al. (1972).

Of other components, decreased C2 values were observed via immunologi-cal tests by Giannetti (1980), while using a radioimmunodiffusion technique in-creased levels of C4 and C1 INA were reported in AD patients as compared to healthy persons (Kapp and Schöpf 1985). The total serum hemolytic activity (CH 50) was found to be decreased (Yamamoto 1975; Ring et al. 1979).

In the skin, complement-bearing lymphocytes were detected by Cormane et al. (1974) and confirmed by other authors (Hodgkinson et al. 1977; Secher et al. 1978), especially in severe cases of AD (Ring et al. 1978).

An explanation for the diverging reports of complement components in the blood may lie in differences in techniques or in the fact that infections and therapy were not always considered. One can, however, conclude that the com-plement system probably participates in the inflammatory process in AD. Complement activating factors, including immune complexes, may be responsi-ble for the local complement consumption, with subsequent increased produc-tion (Kapp and Schöpf 1985).

6.6 Other Mediators

Other mediator substances with some relevance to AD are briefly mentined below.

6.6.1 Acetylcholine

Scott (1962), using a fluorimetric method, found that the amount of acetylcholine is 15 times higher than normal in AD skin and that it parallels the severity of the dermatitis although it remains high in remissions; by contrast the amounts in other eczemas are only five times greater than normal, and then only during an active phase. According to Scheidegger (1966), acetylcholinesterase is increased in AD skin. Blood levels of acetylcholine in children with AD or asthma were found by Chlebarov (1972) to be elevated parallel to the severity of the disease; serum cholinesterase levels were, however, normal. Analogous to the situation in asthma (Tiffenau 1958), bronchial sensitivity is increased in patients with AD plus respiratory atopy, and Gottesfeld (1964) postulated that this is also the case in patients with "pure" AD; however, parenteral administration of acetylcholine was shown to produce no abnormal general reactions. There was no difference between AD patients and controls in general responsiveness to cholinergic stimuli, nor to sympathetic ones, i. e., the autonomic functins were normal (Murphy et al. 1984).

Acetylcholine has, otherwise, several areas of relevance in AD: in influencing histamine release (see Sect. 6.1), in sweating and vasomotor reactions (see Chap. 7), and in cyclic nucleotide metabolism (see above). Cholinergic urticaria in association with AD was mentioned in Sect. 2.14.3.

6.6.2 Kinins

Kinins, which are vasodilatory substances activated in various physiological and pathological states (for review see Müller-Esterl and Fritz 1981), are suspected of being mediators of type I reactivity, although to date this has not definitely been proved. Michaelsson (1969) found the reaction to intracutaneously administered kallikrein, a kinin-releasing enzyme, to be reduced in AD, and, after similar administration of bradykinin, which has been assumed to release catecholamines (Rocha de Silva 1964), there is usually no flare around the wheal, which leaves an area of blanching when it disappears. In the same report, Michaelsson noted that both of these abnormal reactions tend to revert to normal as the dermatitis resolves. Blood kininogens are increased in severe cases of AD, but this seems to be a secondary phenomenon as total plasma kininogens are also increased in other extensive chronic skin inflammations (Winkelmann 1971, 1984).

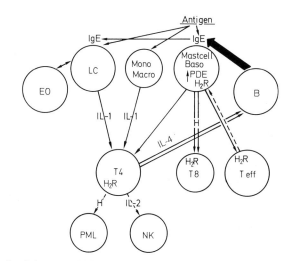

Abbreviations:
B, B cell;
Baso, Basophil leukocyte;
Eo, Eosinophil;
H_2R, H_2 receptor;
Lc, Langerhans cell;
Macro, Macrophage;
Mono, Monocyte;
NK, Natural killer cell;
PDE, Phosphodiesterase;
PML, Polymorphonuclear cell;
T 4, T helper cell;
T 8, T suppressor/cytotoxic cell;
T eff, T effector cell

Fig. 6.2. Some schematically visualized data on relations between cells and mediators in AD

6.6.3 Miscellaneous

Serotonin: The vasodilatatin in AD skin produced by intracutaneous injection of serotonin is less than normal according to Clendenning et al. (1959).

Lymphokines: For some data on interferons in AD, see Sect. 5.7.6; for orientation some more widely known relations are schematically presented in Fig. 6.2.

Monokines: Macrophages, including monocytes and Langerhans' cells, produce the T-cell activating interleukin-1 (IL-1), which is reduced in AD (Mizoguchi et al. 1985; Räsänen et al. 1987) (see Sect. 5.7.3).

The level of IL-2 receptors, released from T cells and a B cell subpopulation, is elevated in AD (Kapp et al. 1988) and a down-regulation is demonstrable with clinical improvement (Reusch et al. 1989).

High production of the T cell product IL-4, in first hand regulating IgE synthesis (Snapper et al. 1989) of B cells and low IFN-gamma values in AD were reported by Wierenga et al. (1989). Furthermore a possible dysregulation of IFN-gamma, related to increased IgE and IgG4 production was found by Reinhold et al. (1988) and Wehrmann et al. (1989).

References

Ahlqvist RP (1948) A study of the adrenotropic receptors. Am J Physiol 153: 586
Archer CB, Morley J, MacDonald DM (1983) Impaired lymphocyte cyclic adenosine monophosphate response in atopic eczema. Br J Dermatol 109: 559
Archer CB, Paul W, Morley J, MacDonald DM (1984) Actions of locally administered adrenoceptor agonists on histamine-induced cutaneous responses in atopic eczema. Clin Exp Dermatol 9: 358
Archer CB, Dalton N, Turner C, MacDonald DM (1987) Investigations of adrenomedullary function in atopic dermatitis. Br J Dermatol 116: 793

Beard LJ, Thong YH, Turner TW (1981) The immunologic status of children with atopic dermatitis. Acta Pædiatr Scand 70: 551

Beer DJ, Rocklin RE (1984) Histamine-induced suppressor cell activity. J Allergy Clin Immunol 73: 439

Beer DJ, Rosenwasser IJ, Dinarello CA, Rocklin RE (1982) Cellular interactions in the generation and expression of histamine-induced suppressor activity. Cell Immunol 69: 101

Bruynzeel-Koomen CAFM, van Wichen DF, Spry C, Venge P, Bruynzeel P (1988) Active participation of eosinophils in patch test reactions to inhalant allergens in patients with atopic dermatitis. Br J Dermatol 118: 229

Busse WW, Lantis SOH (1979) Decreased H_2 histamine granulocyte response in active atopic eczema. J Invest Dermatol 73: 184

Butler JM, Chan SC, Stevens S, Hanifin JM (1983a) Increased leukocyte histamine release with elevated cyclic AMP-phosphodiesterase activity in atopic dermatitis. J Allergy Clin Immunol 71: 490

Butler JM, Peters JE, Hirshman CA, White CR, Margolin LB, Hanifin JM (1983b) Pruritic dermatitis in asthmatic Basenji-Greyhound dogs: a model for human atopic dermatitis. J Am Acad Dermatol 8: 33

Butler JM, Eberth M, Chan SC, Stevens SR, Szobieszozuk D, Hanifin JM (1985) Basophil histamine release in atopic dermatitis and its relationship to disordered cyclic nucleotide metabolism. Acta Derm Venereol [Suppl] (Stockh) 114: 55

Camp RDR, Coutts A, Greaves MW, Kay AB, Walport MJ (1983) Responses of human skin to intradermal injection of leukotrienes C4, D4 and B4. Br J Pharmacol 80: 497

Carr RH, Busse WW, Reed CE (1973) Failure of catecholamines to inhibit epidermal mitosis in vitro. J Allergy Clin Immunol 55: 255

Chan SC, Grewe SR, Hanifin JM (1982) Functional desensitization associated with elevated cAMP phosphodiesterase in human mononuclear leukocytes. J Cyclic Nucleotide Res 8: 211

Chan SC, Trask DM, Sherman SD, Hanifin JM (1986) Histamine agonist-stimulated protein kinase C-phosphorylation of a 61 K monocyte protein with characteristics of atopic cyclic AMP-phosphodiesterase (abstract). J Invest Dermatol 86: 468

Chlebarov S (1972) Acetylcholinspiegel im Blut und Serum-Cholinesteraseaktivität bei Kindern mit Neurodermitis constitutionalis mit und ohne Asthma bronchiale. Arch Dermatol Forsch 244: 338

Clendenning WE, de Oreo GA, Stoughton RB (1959) Serotonin. Arch Dermatol 69: 503

Conrad DH, Bazib H, Sehon AH, Froese A (1975) Binding parameters of the interaction between rat IgE and rat mast cell receptors. J Immunol 114: 688

Conroy MC, Adkinson NF, Lichtenstein LM (1977) Measurement of IgE on human basophils, relation to serum IgE and anti-IgE induced histamine release. J Immunol 118: 1317

Cooper KD, Kang K, Chan SC, Hanifin JM (1985) Phosphodiesterase inhibition by Ro-20-1724 reduces hyper-IgE synthesis by atopic dermatitis cells in vitro. J Invest Dermatol 84: 477

Cormane RH, Husz S, Hamerlinck F (1974) Immunoglobulin and complement bearing lymphocytes in allergic contact dermatitis and atopic dermatitis (eczema). Br J Dermatol 90: 592

Crespi H, Armando I, Tumilasci O, Levi G, Massimo J, Barontini M, Perec C (1982) Catecholamine levels in parotid secretion in children with chronic atopic dermatitis. J Invest Dermatol 78: 493

Czarnetzki BM (1983) Incresed monocyte chemotaxis toward leukotriene B_4 and platelet activating factor in patients with inflammatory dermatoses. Clin Exp Immunol 54: 486

Czarnetzki BM (1986) Urticaria. Springer, Berlin Heidelberg New York Tokyo, p 6

Czarnetzki BM, Kalveram KJ, Dirkmeier U (1979) Serum eosinophil chemotactic factor levels in patients with bullous pemphigoid, drug reactions and atopic eczema. J Invest Dermatol 73: 163

De Graciansky P (1966) Eczema constitutionnel. Soc Med Hopit Paris 117: 765 (Hopitaux de Paris)

Djurup R (1981) Adrenoreceptors: molecular nature and role in atopic diseases. Allergy 36: 289

Ebertz JM, Kettelkamp NS, Hirshman CA, Uno J, Hanifin JM (1985) Substance P-induced histamine release in human cutaneous mast cells (abstract). J Invest Dermatol 84: 350

Eilard U, Hellgren L (1961) Skin sensitivity to histamine in eczema and psoriasis. Int Arch Allergy Appl Immunol 26: 81

Felarca AB, Lowell FC (1971) Accumulation of eosinophils and basophils at skin sites in relation to intensity of skin reactivity and symptoms in atopic disease. J Allergy 48: 125

Feltkamp-Vroom TM (1977) Mast cells in atopic and non-atopic subjects. Scand J Respir Dis 58: 8

Fontana VJ, Sedlis E, Prose PH, Messina VP, Holt LE (1962) Complement titer, C-reactive protein and electrophoretic serum protein patterns in eczematous children. NY State J Med 62: 2801

Galant SP, Underwood S, Allred S, Hanifin JM (1979) Beta-adrenergic receptor binding polymorphonuclear leukocytes in atopic dermatitis. J Invest Dermatol 72: 330

Giannetti A (1980) High frequency of hereditary complement defects in association with atopic diseases. Acta Derm Venereol [Suppl] (Stockh) 92: 77

Girard JP (1972) Biological measurements of atopy. In: Charpin J et al. (eds) Allergology. Proc 8th European Congress on Allergy. Excerpta Medica, Amsterdam, p 133

Gleich GJ, Loegering DA, Mann KG, Maldonado JE (1976) Comparative properties of the Charcot-Leyden crystal protein and the major basic protein from human eosinophils. J Clin Invest 57: 633

Goldberg ND, Haddox MK, Dunham E, Lopez C, Hadden JW (1974) The yin yang hypothesis of biological control: opposing influences of cyclic GMP and cyclic AMP in the regulation of cell proliferation and other biological processes. Control of animal cells. Cold Spring Harbor, New York, p 609

Gottesfeld G (1964) Acetylcholin- und Histamine-Bronchospasmus bei Neurodermitikern und Kontrollen. Int Arch Allergy Appl Immunol 2 (Suppl): 52

Greaves M, Marks R, Robertson I (1977) Receptors for histamine in human skin blood vessels: a review. Br J Dermatol 97: 225

Greaves MW, Sondergaard J, McDonald-Gibson W (1971) Recovery of prostaglandins in healthy subjects and in patients with urticaria and atopic dermatitis in human cutaneous inflammation. Br Med J II: 258

Grewe SR, Chan SC, Hanifin JM (1982) Elevated leukocyte cyclic AMP-phosphodiesterase in atopic disease: a possible mechanism for cyclic AMP-agonist hyporesponsiveness. J Allergy Clin Immunol 70: 452

Hanifin JM (1986) Pharmacophysiology of atopic dermatitis. Clin Rev Allergy 4: 43

Hanifin JM (1987) Veränderte Phosphodiesterase-Aktivität der Leukozyten bei atopischem Ekzem. Hautarzt 38: 258

Hellerström S, Lidman H (1956) Studies of Besnier's prurigo (atopic dermatitis). Acta Derm Venereol (Stockh) 36: 11

Herlin T, Kragballe K (1980) Impaired monocyte cyclic AMP responses and monocyte cytotoxicity in atopic dermatitis. Allergy 35: 337

Heskel NS, Chan SC, Thiel ML, Stevens SR, Casperson LS, Hanifin JM (1984) Elevated umbilical cord blood leukocyte cyclic adenosine monophosphate-phosphodiesterase activity in children with atopic parents. J Am Acad Dermatol 11: 422

Hodgkinson GI, Everall D, Smith HV (1977) Immunofluorescent patterns in Besnier's prurigo. Br J Dermatol 96: 357

Hoffman BB, Lefkowitz RJ (1980) Alpha-adrenergic receptor subtypes. N Engl J Med 302: 1390

Holden CA, Chan SC, Hanifin JM (1985) Adenylate cyclase activity in mononuclear leukocytes from patients with atopic dermatitis. Acta Derm Venereol [Suppl] (Stockh) 114: 149

Holden CA, Chan SC, Hanifin JM (1986) Monocyte localisation of elevated cAMP phosphodiesterase activity in atopic dermatitis. J Invest Dermatol 87: 372

Holla SWJ, Hollman EPMJ, Mier PD, Staak WJBM van den, Urselmann E, Warndorff JA (1972) Adenosine 3′:5′-cyclic monophosphate phosphodiesterase in skin. II. Levels in atopic dermatitis. Br J Dermatol 86: 147

Hovmark A, Åsbrink E (1981) Effects of a beta-receptor blocking agent (Propranolol) on synthesis of IgE in vitro by peripheral blood lymphocytes from atopic patients. Allergy 36: 391

Huriez C (1966) Actualités sur les eczémas. Rev Med (Suppl)

Ida S, Hooks SJ, Siraganian RP, Notkins AL (1977) Enhancement of IgE-mediated histamine release from human basophils by viruses: role of interferon. J Exp Med 145: 892

Ignarro LJ (1973) Neutral protease release from human leukocytes regulated by neurohormones and cyclic nucleotides. Nature 245: 151

Ishizaka T, Ishizaka K, Conrad DH, Froese A (1978) A new concept of triggering mechanisms of IgE-mediated histamine release. J Allergy Clin Immunol 61: 320

Ishizaka T, Soto CS, Ishizaka K (1973) Mechanisms of passive sensitization III. Number of IgE molecules and their receptor sites on human basophil granulocytes. J Immunol 111: 500

Johnson HH, de Oreo GA, Lascheid WP, Mitchell F (1960) Skin histamine levels in chronic atopic dermatitis. J Invest Dermatol 34: 237

Juhlin L (1967) Localisation and content of histamine in normal and diseased skin. Acta Derm Venereol 47: 383

Juhlin L, Hammarström S (1982) Effects of intradermally injected leukotriene C_4 and histamine in patients with urticaria, psoriasis and atopic dermatitis. Acta Derm Venereol (Stockh) 49: 251

Juhlin L, Michaelsson G (1969) Cutaneous vascular reactions to prostaglandins in healthy subjects and in patients with urticaria and atopic dermatitis. Acta Derm Venereol (Stockh) 49: 251

Kaliner M (1984) Hypotheses on the contribution of late-phase allergic responses to the understanding and treatment of allergic disease. J Allergy Clin Immunol 73: 311

Kapp A, Schöpf E (1985) Involvement of complement in atopic dermatitis. Acta Derm Venereol [Suppl] (Stockh) 114: 152

Kapp A, Piskorski A, Schöpf E (1988) Elevated levels of interleukin 2 receptor in sera of patients with atopic dermatitis and psoriasis. Br J Dermatol 119: 707

Kapp A, Russwurm R, Schöpf E (1983) Aktivierung des Komplementsystems bei Patienten mit Neurodermitis atopica-Bestimmung von C3a in plasma. Z Haut Geschlechtskr 149: 100

Kaufman HS, Frick OL, Fink D (1968) Serum complement in young children with atopic dermatitis. J Allergy 42: 1

Kownatzki E, Grüninger G (1987) Bedingungen der anti-IgE-induzierten Histaminfreisetzung aus den isolierten Leukozyten von Normalpersonen und Patienten mit atopischer Dermatitis, allergischer Rhinitis und Psoriasis. Allergologie 10: 86

Kragballe K, Fogh K (1989) Prostaglandin E 2 and leukotriene B4 in atopic dermatitis. Acta Dermatovenereol (Suppl 144) (Stockh) (in press)

Lebel B, Venencie PY, Saurat JH, Soubrane C, Paupe J (1980) Anti-IgE induced histamine release from basophils in children with atopic dermatitis. Acta Derm Venereol [Suppl] (Stockh) 92: 57

Leiferman KM, Ackerman SJ, Sampson HA, Haugen HS, Venencie PY, Gleich GJ (1985) Dermal deposition of eosinophile-granule major basic protein in atopic dermatitis. Comparison with onchocerciasis. N Engl J Med 313: 282

Leiferman KM, Haugen HS, Gleich GJ (1986) Evidence for eosinophil degranulation in the late phase of the immediate wheal and flare skin reaction (abstract). J Invest Dermatol 86: 488

Levi L, Meneghini C, Rantuccio F (1959) Activité cholinesterasique: pouvoir histaminolitique et dosage de l'histamine dans la peau des sujets sains et atteint de certaines dermatoses allergiques. Acta Allergol 13: 332

Lichtenstein LM, Marone G, Thomas LT, Malveaux FJ (1978) The role of basophils in inflammatory reactions. J Invest Dermatol 71: 65

Marone G, Poto S, Colombo M, Quattrin S, Condorelli M (1983) Histamine release from human basophils in vitro: effects of age of cell donor. Monogr Allergy 18: 139

Marone G, Giugliano R, Lembo G, Ayala F (1986) Human basophil releasability. II. Changes in basophil releasability in patients with atopic dermatitis. J Invest Dermatol 87: 19

Matloff SM, Kiselis IK, Rocklin RE (1983) Reduced production of histamine-induced suppressor factor (HSF) by atopic mononuclear cells and decreased prostaglandin E₂ output by HSF-stimulated atopic monocytes. J Allergy Clin Immunol 72: 359

McMillan JC, Heskel NS, Hanifin JM (1985) Cyclic AMP-phosphodiesterase activity and histamine release in cord blood leukocyte preparations. Acta Derm Venereol [Suppl] (Stockh) 114: 24

Michaelsson G (1969) Cutaneous reactions to kallikrein and prostaglandins in healthy and diseased skin. Thesis, Uppsala University, Sweden

Mier PD, Urselmann E (1970) The adenyl cyclase of skin. Br J Dermatol 83: 364

Mihm MC, Soter NA, Dvorak HF, Austen KF (1976) The structure of normal skin and the morphology of atopic eczema. J Invest Dermatol 67: 305

Mikhail GR, Miller-Nilinska A (1964) Mast cell population in human skin. J Invest Dermatol 43: 249

Mizoguchi M, Furusawa S, Okitsu S, Yoshino K (1985) Macrophage-derived interleukin-1 activity in atopic dermatitis. J Invest Dermatol 84: 303

Möller H, Rorsman H (1958) Studies on vascular permeability factors with sodium fluorescein. II. The effect of intracutaneously injected histamine and serum in patients with atopic dermatitis. Acta Derm Venereol (Stockh) 38: 243

Müller-Esterl W, Fritz H (1981) Kallikreins, kinins and allergy. In: Ring J, Burg G (eds) New trends in allergy. Springer, Berlin Heidelberg New York, p 81

Murphy GM, Smith SE, Smith SA, Greaves MW (1984) Autonomic function in cholinergic urticaria and atopic eczema. Br J Dermatol 110: 581

Mustakallio KK (1966) Antistaphylolysin (ASta) level of the blood in relation to barrier function of the skin. Ann Med Exp Biol Fenniæ 44 (Suppl): 7

Nilzén A (1958) Experimental background of some abnormal vascular reactions in atopic dermatitis and significance of skin tests in man. In: Holpern BN, Holtzer A (eds) Proc 3ème Congrès International d'Allergologie Flammarion, Paris, p 635

Overgaard Petersen H, Thormann J, Zachariæ H (1979) Urinary histamine and atopic dermatitis. Arch Dermatol Res 264: 193

Parish WE (1972) Eosinophilia. III. The anaphylactic release from isolated human basophils of a substance that selectively attracts eosinophils. Clin Allergy 2: 381

Parish WE, Champion RH (1973) Atopic dermatitis. In: Rook A (ed) Recent advances in dermatology, vol 3. Churchill Livingstone, Edinburgh, p 193

Parker CW, Kennedy S, Eisen AZ (1977) Leukocyte and lymphocyte cyclic AMP response in atopic eczema. J Invest Dermatol 68: 302

Parrot JL, Laborde C (1963) Le pouvoir histaminopexique du serum sanguin. Son absence chez les sujets allergiques. Presse Med 71: 1267

Pochet P, Delespesse G, de Maubeuge J (1980) Characterization of β-adrenergic receptors on intact circulating lymphocytes from patients with atopic dermatitis. Acta Derm Venereol [Suppl] (Stockh) 92: 26

Räsanen L, Lehto M, Reunala T, Jansen C, Leinikki P (1987) Decreased monocyte production of interleukin-1 and impaired lymphocyte proliferation in atopic dermatitis. Arch Dermatol Res 279: 215

Reed CE, Busse WW, Lee TP (1976) Adrenergic mechanisms and the adenyl cyclase system in atopic dermatitis. J Invest Dermatol 67: 333

Reimann HJ, Meyer HJ, Wendt P (1981) Stress and histamine. In: Ring J, Burg G (eds) New trends in allergy. Springer, Berlin Heidelberg New York, p 50

Reinhold U, Pawelec G, Wehrmann W, Herold M, Vernet P, Kreysel HW (1988) Immunoglobulin E and immunoglobulin G subclass distribution in vivo and relationship to in vitro generation if interferon-gamma and neopterin in patiens with severe atopic dermatitis. Int Arch Allergy Appl Immunol 87: 120

Reusch MK, Mielke V, Christophers S, Sterry W (1989) I1-2 receptor down-regulation of T cells correlates with the clinical improvement of psoriasis and atopic dermatitis during treatment with cyclosporin A (Cy-A) (Abstract) J Invest Derm Dermatol 92: 506

Ring J (1983) Plasma histamine concentration in atopic eczema. Clin Allergy 13: 545

Ring J, Lutz J (1983) Decreased release of lysosomal enzymes from peripheral leukocytes of patients with atopic dermatitis. J Am Acad Dermatol 8: 378

Ring J, O'Connor R (1979) In vitro histamine and serotonin release studies in atopic dermatitis. Int Arch Allergy Appl Immunol 58: 322

Ring J, Senter T, Cornell RC, Arroyave CM, Tan EM (1978) Complement and immunoglobulin deposits in the skin of patients with atopic dermatitis. Br J Dermatol 99: 459

Ring J, Senter T, Cornell RC, Arroyave CM, Tan EM (1979) Plasma complement and histamine changes in atopic dermatitis. Br J Dermatol 100: 521

Ring J, Mathison DA, O'Connor R (1981) In vitro cyclic nucleotide responsiveness of leukocytes and platelets in patients suffering from atopic dermatitis. Int Arch Allergy Appl Immunol 65: 1

Ring J, Sedlmaier F, von der Helm D, Mayr T, Walz U, Ibel H, Riepel H, Przybilla B, Reimann HJ, Dorsch W (1986) Histamine and allergic diseases. In: Ring J, Burg G (ed) New trends in allergy. II. Springer, Berlin Heidelberg New York, p 44

Rocha de Silva M (1964) Chemical mediators of the acute inflammatory reaction. Ann N Y Acad Sci 116: 899

Rocklin RE, Beard J, Gupta S, Good RA, Melmon KL (1980) Characterization of the human blood lymphocytes that produce histamine-induced suppressor factor. Cell Immunol 51: 226

Rorsman H (1958) Basophil leukocytes in urticaria, asthma and atopic dermatitis. Acta Allergol 12: 205

Ruoho AE, De Clerque JL, Busse WW (1980) Characterization of granulocyte beta adrenergic receptors in atopic eczema. J Allergy Clin Immunol 66: 46

Ruzicka T (1986) Lipoxygenase activity in cutaneous inflammation. In: Ring J, Burg G (eds) New trends in allergy. II. Springer, Berlin Heidelberg New York, p 90

Ruzicka T, Glück T (1983) Cutaneous histamine levels and histamine releasability from the skin in atopic dermatitis and hyper-IgE syndrome. Arch Dermatol Res 275: 14

Ruzicka T, Simmet T, Peskar BA, Ring J (1984) Skin levels of arachidonic acid-derived inflammatory mediators and histamine in atopic dermatitis and psoriasis. J Invest Dermatol 86: 105

Safko MJ, Chan SC, Cooper KD, Hanifin JM (1981) Heterologous desensitization of leukocytes: a possible mechanism of beta adrenergic blockade in atopic dermatitis. J Allergy Clin Immunol 68: 215

Sampson H, Jolie PL (1984) Increased plasma histamine concentrations after food challenges in children with atopic dermatitis. N Engl J Med 311: 372

Sauer RR, Sauer CI, Merk H, Steigleder GK (1987a) Einfluß des 5-Lipoxygenasehemmers Phenidon auf die antigenbedingte Histaminfreisetzung in vitro. Z Hautkr 62: 1175

Sauer RR, Sauer CI, Merk H, Steigleder GK (1987b) Erfahrungen mit der antigenbedingten Histaminfreisetzung (HF) in vitro aus Leukozytensuspensionen und Vollblut. Vergleich der Ergebnisse von Histaminfreisetzung, Hauttest und RAST. Z Hautkr 62: 1164

Scheidegger JP (1966) Acetylcholinesterasegehalt normaler und neurodermitischer Haut. Arch Klin Exp Dermatol 226: 265

Schmutzler W, Poblete-Freundt G, Rauch K, Schoenfeld W (1979) Response to immunological or cholinergic stimulation on isolated mast cells from man, guinea pig and rat. Monogr Allergy 14: 288

Schwarz W, Bock G, Hornstein OP (1987) Plasma levels of cyclic nucleotides are elevated in atopic eczema. Arch Dermatol Res 279: 59

Scott A (1962) Acetylcholine in normal and diseased skin. Br J Dermatol 74: 317

Secher L, Permin H, Juhl F (1978) Immunofluorescence of the skin in allergic diseases: an investigation of patients with contact dermatitis, allergic vasculitis and atopic dermatitis. Acta Derm Venereol (Stockh) 58: 117

Shereff RH, Harwell W, Lieberman P, Rosenberg EW (1973) Effect of beta adrenergic stimulation and blockade on immediate hypersensitivity skin test reactions. J Allergy Clin Immunol 52: 328

Snapper CM, Finkelman FD, Paul WE (1989) Differential regulation of IgG1 and IgE synthesis by interleukin 4. J Exp Med 167: 183

Sobotka AG, Marone G, Lichtens LM (1979) Indomethacin, arachidonic acid metabolism and basophil histamine release. Monogr Allergy 14: 285

Solomon L, Wentzel HE (1963) Plasma catecholamines in atopic dermatitis. J Invest Dermatol 41: 401

Solomon LM, Juhlin L, Kirschenbaum MS (1968) Prostaglandin on cutaneous vasculature. J Invest Dermatol 51: 282

Soter NA, Mihm MC, Dvorak HF, Austen HF (1978) Cutaneous necrotizing venulitis: a sequential analysis of the morphologic alterations occurring after mast cell degranulation in a patient with a unique syndrome. Clin Exp Immunol 32: 46

Soter NA, Lewis RA, Corey EJ, Austen JF (1983) Local effects of synthetic leukotrienes (LTC$_4$, LTD$_4$, LTE$_4$ and LTB$_4$) in human skin. J Invest Dermatol 80: 115

Stüttgen G, Knoblich I, Schmidthaus H (1968) Zahl und Morphe basophiler Leucocyten, deren Korrelatin zu eosinophilen Leucocyten, Immunoglobulinen und Blutkörperchen-Senkungsgeschwindigkeit bei Dermatosen. Hautarzt 19: 388

Sugiura H, Hirota Y, Uehara M (1989) Heterogenous distribution of mast cells in lichenified lesions of atopic dermatitis. Acta Derm Venereol (Suppl 144) (Stockh) (in press)

Sullivan TJ, Parker KL, Stenson W, Parker CW (1975) Modulation of cyclic AMP in purified mast cells. I. Response to pharmacologic, metabolic and physical stimuli. J Immunol 114: 1473

Sutherland EW, Robison GA (1966) The role of cyclic-3′,5′-AMP responses to catecholamines and other hormones. Pharmacol Rev 18: 145

Szentivanyi A (1966) The biomechanical pharmacology of adrenergic reactions as related to the pathogenesis of bronchial asthma. Ann Allergy 24: 253

Szentivanyi A (1968) The beta adrenergic theory of the atopic abnormality in bronchial asthma. J Allergy 42: 203

Szentivanyi A, Heim O, Schultze P, Szentivanyi J (1980) Adrenoceptor binding studies with (^{3}H) Dihydroalprenolol and (^{3}H) Dihydroergocryptine on membranes of lymphocytes from patients with atopic disease. Acta Derm Venereol (Stockh) Suppl 92: 19

Tiffenau R (1958) Hypersensibilité cholinergique et histaminique pulmonaire de l'astmatique. Acta Allergol 12: 187

Trask DM, Chan SC, Sherman SE, Hanifin JM (1988) Altered leucocyte protein kinase activity in atopic dermatitis. J Invest Dermatol 90: 526

Venter JC, Fraser CM, Harrison LC (1980) Autoantibodies to β_2-adrenergic receptors: a possible cause of adrenergic hyporesponsiveness in allergic rhinitis and asthma. Science 207: 1361

Voorhorst R, Grosfeld JCM, de Vries J, Kuiper JP (1963) Development of atopics syndrome in group of patients with (atopic) constitutional dermatitis. Acta Allergol 18: 56

Wagner G, Pürschel W (1962) Klinisch-analytische Studie zum Neurodermitisproblem. Dermatologica 125: 1

Wehrmann W, Reinhold U, Pavelec G, Vernet P, Kreysel HW (1989) In vitro generation of IFN-ga, a and in vivo Fce/Rl/CD 23 positive lymphocytes in relationship to IgE and IgG subclasses in patients with severe atopic dermatitis. Acta Derm Venereol (Suppl 144) (Stockh) (in press)

Wierenga EA, Snoek M, Jansen HM, de Groot C, Bos JD, Chretien I, de Vries JE, Kapsenberg ML (1989) High allergen-specific IgE levels are associated with imbalanced interleukin 4 and interferon-gamma production by functional allergen-specific helper CD4? T lymphocytes (abstract). J invest Dermatol 92: 541

Williams DH (1938) Skin temperature reaction to histamine in atopic dermatitis (disseminated neurodermitis). J Invest Dermatol 1: 119

Williams L, Snyderman T, Lefkowitz RJ (1976) Identification of beta-adrenergic receptors in human lymphocytes by(-)[^{3}H]alperenol binding. J Clin Invest 57: 149

Winkelmann RK (1966) Nonallergic factors in atopic dermatitis. J Allergy 37: 29

Winkelmann RK (1971) Molecular inflammation of the skin. J Invest Dermatol 57: 197

Winkelmann RK (1984) Total plasma kininogen in psoriasis and atopic dermatitis. Acta Derm Venereol (Stockh) 64: 261

Wintroub BU, Soter NA (1983) Biology of the mast cell and its role in cutaneous inflammation. In: Gigli IN, Miescher PA, Müller-Eberhard HJ (eds) Immunodermatology. Springer, Berlin Heidelberg New York, p 57

Wütrich B, Storck H, Grob P, Schwarz-Speck M (1972) Zur Immunpathologie der Neurodermitis. Arch Dermatol Forsch 244: 327

Yamamoto K (1975) Immunoglobulin, complement and fibrinolytic enzyme system in atopic dermatitis. Mod Probl Paediatr 17: 30

7 Pathomechanism: The Altered Skin

The immunological characteristics of atopy and the inflammatory changes of AD occur in skin which is altered in many respects although being of normal appearance clinically. This coincides with the author's definition of AD as being "a specific dermatitis in the abnormally reacting skin of the atopic," and gave rise to the introduction of the definition "symptom-free skin" (see Chap. 1). The alterations in the symptom-free skin in AD include several structural and/or functional changes which may be of primary, and frequently of nonimmunological, character, or secondary to immunological and pathophysiological changes present in the disease.

7.1 Itch

Itch as the major symptom of AD has already been discussed in Chap. 3. Here, it is again stressed that the itch threshold is lowered in the symptom-free skin of AD patients (see Table 3.4). According to the author's view this is a basic trait and can explain the action of several factors on the AD skin. It is, however, possible that it is secondary to histamine releasability.

7.2 Alteration of Skin Structure and Some Consequences

Al-Jaberi and Marks (1984) carried out an important study on the noninvolved horny layer of patients with different forms of dermatitis in the quiescent phase. The study included morphological and physiological tests on 22 AD patients. In the test of barrier function and sensitivity to irritants, minimum blister time [after applying ammonium hydroxide according to Frosch and Kligman (1977)] was clearly reduced, although similar to that in other dermatitic conditions. AD patients had the lowest mean corneocyte values and the greatest epidermal thickness. The basal layer/granular layer ratio also showed the greatest increase in AD patients. In other words, a functional abnormality of the symptom-free skin was demonstrated in all types of dermatitis but was particularly pronounced in AD, where a defective barrier function was also present.

Via electron microscopy Werner et al. (1987) noted an increase in membrane coating granules in the transition zone between stratum granulosum and corneum in the dry skin of AD patients. This impairment of the granules (Odland's bodies) in the keratinocytes of the upper layers indicates a maturation defect or changes in lipid production correlated with a defective barrier function. As a consequence of defective barrier function, staphylococcal colonization on the symptom-free skin is higher than on normal skin (see Sect. 2.9.1 and Table 2.5). Furthermore, as discussed in Sect. 5.6.2, the majority of experiments showed that contact irritants provoke reactions more easily on the symptom-free skin of AD patients than on the skin of healthy persons.

7.2.1 Epidermodermal Changes

Mihm et al. (1976) and Soter and Mihm (1980) reported their findings in the clinically normal skin of AD. They found traces of hyperkeratosis and epidermal hyperplasia, intercellular edema, alterations in venules, occasional fibrosis and focal demyelinization of cutaneous sensory nerves. These authors were also able to observe a slight dermal infiltrate consisting primarily of lymphocytes. According to data on the involved skin, these lymphocytes may be assumed to be mostly T helper cells (see Chap. 4). These findings clearly show that the symptom-free skin of AD patients differs from normal skin. Of great importance are the findings of Barker et al. (1988) that surface IgE was also found on dendritic cells in symptom-free skin; if confirmed, this may constitute an important differential diagnostic trait.

7.3 Water Exchange

Water exchange is an important skin function and a valuable indicator of the barrier function located in the stratum corneum. It is necessary to distinguish between sweating and loss of fluid through the skin as insensible perspiration. The measurement of sweat secretion is usually via pharmacological stimulation, administering small amounts of the physiological sweat stimulator acetylcholine or its synergists, like methacholine, into the skin via intracutaneous injection or iontophoresis. Sweating has to be blocked by an anticholinergic drug when one measures transepidermal water loss (TWL, also abbreviated TEWL). The quantitative registration of water loss has been studied by means of several techniques. These include (a) measurement of the changes in nitrogen or dry air before and after contact with the skin via gravimetry (Grice and Bettley 1967), electric hygrometry (Baker and Kligman 1967), or electric water analyzer (Meeco; Gasselt and Vierhout 1963), and (b) determination of the flux of water vapor from the test site with an evaporimeter (Nilsson 1977).

The water content of the stratum corneum is independent of the TWL (Triebkorn et al. 1983) and can be studied using various methods. These include spectroscopic methods (infrared: Gloor et al. 1981; Potts et al. 1985; photoacoustic: Kölmel et al. 1985), surface contour analysis (Marks and Nicholls 1981: the skin surface structure is related to the water content of stratum corneum), and measurement of the electrical properties of the skin. These properties include conductance, resistance, and impedance [total electric opposition to alternate current, also including the capacitance, i.e., the capacity of taking/holding an electric charge (Tagami et al. 1980)]. Several such devices have been used in order to study the water content of the stratum corneum in AD.

The consequence of using these different techniques is that methodological problems dominate these studies. The techniques are often not comparable, give inter- and even intraindividual variations, and measure different qualities and different layers of the stratum corneum. In addition, several conditions have to be considered in relation to these measurements: conditions such as ambient temperature and relative humidity (several authors noted differences between studies carried out in winter and autumn), the skin site and its condition, e.g., thickness of the stratum corneum (barrier damage in inflammation; microcirculation) (Bettley and Grice 1965; Spruit and Herweyer 1967; Thiele and Senden 1967; Spruit and Malten 1969; Grice et al. 1971; Hattingh 1972), and the quality and quantity of skin lipids strongly influencing the skin barrier (Elias 1981). All of these considerations are also relevant in the investigation of AD.

7.3.1 Sweat Secretion

It has already been mentioned that AD patients frequently judge their disease by the severity of their pruritus, and they often mention spontaneously in their clinical history that their skin itches when sweating is induced by high temperature or excitement. They usually report that during a moderately but not excessively hot summer, they feel moore comfortable, sweating more freely without intense pruritus, and that their skin is less dry in winter (see also Sect. 9.1); this is a good illustration of the great significance of sweat disturbances in AD.

In thermal sweating, sweat glands of the skin surface participate, whereas in emotional sweating, also of importance in AD, palmoplantar, axillary, and forehead glands are primarily involved and sweating may be generalized if elicited by very intense stimuli. In attempting to explain sweat disturbances in AD, Sulzberger et al. (1947, 1953), Sulzberger and Herrmann (1954), and Sulzberger et al. (1959) stressed that sweat secretion is unimpaired, an observation supported by the glycogen content of sweat secretory cells (Cormia and Kuykendall 1955). Their theory was a follows: deficient sebaceous gland activity leads to a reduction in the surface lipids of the dry keratotic AD skin, and this in turn promotes not only a rapid and excessive absorption of sweat droplets by the stratum corneum (pseudoanhidrosis), producing periostial edema, but also parakeratotic plugging of the sweat duct ostium. This poral closure precludes sweat evaporation, and consequently minute intracutaneous "injections" of sweat pass through the duct wall into the epidermis or the dermis, wherein irritants, allergens, or both, present in the sweat, may induce pruritus, urticaria, or a condition resembling miliaria with a subsequent sweat retention syndrome. Clinically, a relative humidity higher than 60% is helpful if there is keratotic plugging, whereas dry heat is beneficial if periporal edema is present. The Sulzberger group, in reports of their studies, also emphasized the mutual relationships between sweat and sebum, and between the aqueous and lipid phases on the skin surface (Herrmann and Prose 1951; Herrmann et al. 1953).

The theory of Sulzberger and his associates has become predominant, despite the failure of thorough histological investigations to demonstrate either frank miliaria or obvious extravasations of sweat into the tissues (Prose 1965), and despite an inability to show that allergens present in sweat play any pathogenic role on reaching the tissues. It has, however, been shown that sweat does in fact contain various proteins, mainly from the blood, and can produce urticaria, especially in AD (Stüttgen and Atzwanger 1961).

Herrmann (1972) emphasized that a clinical equivalent of miliaria rubra, in the form of itchy papulovesicles, is not infrequently observed in patients with AD and that some patients regularly develop this complication. This was not, however, confirmed by Lobitz (1958 a).

Evidence of pseudoanhidrotic conditions was produced by Gordon and Maibach (1968) in the form of sudorometer recordings demonstrating an accumulation of sweat droplets under the stratum corneum of symptom-free skin which had been stripped with Scotch tape. Using acetylcholine peripherally, to influence the cerebral centers, Korting (1954) demonstrated that whereas hypohidrosis is usually found in AD patients on areas without active skin lesions, hyperhidrosis is present in the flexures and in some cases, given the relevant stimuli, also on other areas such as the forehead, around the mouth, and on the sides of the face. In studies with a resistance hygrometer on children with AD, Rovensky and Saxl (1964) showed that a sweat response to thermal, psychological, or exertional stimuli occurs on lichenified areas but not on the adjacent skin; they postulated that this is due to a lowered excitation threshold in the sudomotor nerves in affected skin.

Warndorff (1970, 1972 a, b) used a Meeco electrolytic water analyzer on the volar surface of the forearm to record the reactivity to acetylcholine in AD patients. He found that a) the "sensitivity" (the threshold response to repeatedly administered acetycholine) showed differences between cases of AD and controls only in males, and b) that the "productivity" (the sweat production, which is also shown by color indicator of the test method) was higher in AD patients than in normal controls; in summer, however, there was no statistical difference between male AD cases and the controls, owing to increased sweating by the latter. The observed disturbances of sweating were independent of the state of the skin disease, but Warndorff (1972 b) found them only in the "eczematous," not in the "subacute prurigo," group of AD patients. The best explanation of these changes is given in the theory of Szentivanyi (1968), which postulates incresed sensitivity of the parasympathetic part of the autonomic nervous system due to sympathetic blockade. Furthermore, Warndorff (1972 b) suggested that sweating after the administration of epinephrine may depend on stimulation of the dark cells in the secretory part of the sweat gland, and that isoproterenol appears to have an indirect stimulatory action on sweat production as its action is inhibited by scopolamine. However, in the light of animal experiments, he concluded that α-receptors as well as β-receptors may be represent in the sweat gland (because sweating can be elicited by epinephrine and can be blocked by α-adrenergic receptor inhibitors) (Warndorff 1972 b). Hemels (1970) injected acetylcholine before and after administering the β-blocking drug propranolol and observed an increased sweat response in controls but not in AD patients; these results were not confirmed by Foster et al. (1971). Work in our department (Thune and Kocsis 1975) showed that terbutaline (a $β_2$-agonist) induced sweating in AD patients but this was no different from that induced in normal subjects. It could be partly inhibited by propranolol and abolished by atropine. The epinephrine-evoked sweat response was also only partly inhibited by the α-blocker phentolamine. These findings pointed to the role of th β-receptor mechanism as being in some way related to cholinergic receptors. There were also higher sweating values in winter than in late autumn, in accordance with Warndorff's (1970) report. Cotton et al. (1971) noted no difference in heat-induced sweat between atopics and normals whereas in further studies Kaliner (1976) found an increased sweat response to methacholine in respiratory atopics. Murphy et al. (1984), in the counting of sweat glands by the plastic impression method (Thomson and Sutarman 1953; Clubley et al. 1978), were unable to register any differences in the acetylcholine sweat responses of AD patients and controls. The sweat pore density on fingertips, studied by a similar fingerprint technique, was identical in atopics and controls; however, in AD a flattening of the epidermal ridges was noted (Bachmann et al. 1987). Kiistala (1983), registering methacholine-induced sweat response by evaporimetry, found normal reactivity in AD. In further studies she observed that sweat loss was reduced in AD, particularly in dry skin (R. Kiistala, personal communication). Using the chemical spot test and optical measurements to analyze sweat, Cotton et al. (1971) found no difference between atopics and nonatopics. Furthermore, no difference was observed in the glucose metabolism of isolated sweat glands from atopic and from normal subjects by Cotton and van Rossum (1973).

The importance of sweat training has been shown by the experience of AD patients who find that they improve clinically after sweat training in a dry sauna, and who learn to suppress sweating that would lead to pruritus (a process of automatic learning) (Miller 1969); furthermore, Kuyper and Cotton (1972) have used an instrument to condition palmar sweating. After exposure to dry heat, parotid secretion is decreased in nonatopic persons, but in AD patients it is increased and does not parallel sweat secretion (Stüttgen et al. 1966). When considered collectively there are rather contradictory findings regarding sweat productioin in AD. From a clinical point of view, however, the itch-eliciting role of sweating in AD is generally accepted.

7.3.2 Transepidermal Water Loss

Since Blank demonstrated (1952) that the cause of the dry, brittle skin (chapping) is not a low lipid but a low moisture content, several investigators have studied the role of water exchange from the stratum corneum in AD. Holz-

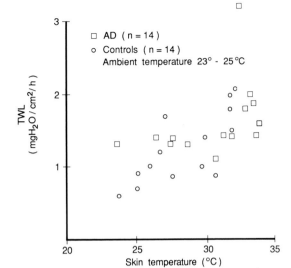

Fig. 7.1. The TWL measured on the backs of the hands by a Meeco electrolytic water analyzer in patients with AD and controls

mann et al. (1961) found higher water loss from the antecubital flexure in AD, even if this skin area was involved. Shahidullah et al. (1969), using an electrolytic hygrometer, noted a parallelism between TWL and the activity of the dermatitis, including five subjects with AD. The symptom-free skin showed variable TWL values. On the other hand, Baker (1971) did not find any differences between AD patients and controls when measuring water loss on the forearm. Using the Meeco apparatus, the author (Rajka 1974a) investigated water loss through both epidermis and eccrine glands on the symptom-free, and in some cases mildly involved, skin of the backs of the hands of 14 patients with AD. An increase in the TWL was found in AD (see Fig. 7.1). Simultaneous measurements of TWL and of skin surface lipids were made on the hands (see Sect. 7.3.3) and the qualitative changes demonstrated in skin lipids were assumed possibly to play a role in increased TWL, by influencing water-binding substances (Rajka 1974b). These findings were verified by Abe et al. (1978), by electrohygrometry in children with AD, but no inverse correlation was found between TWL and casual lipids (although a reduced level of sebaceous lipids was observed). Using the evaporimeter on the dry skin of AD patients, Finlay et al. (1980) found increased TWL but reduced electrical resistance, despite the belief, accepted since Blank's (1952) report, that the latter is increased. This was confirmed by infrared spectroscopic studies by Gloor et al. (1981) and by earlier similar findings by Lawler et al. (1960) on reduced electrical impedance. Increased TWL was also found by Werner and Lindberg (1985) by use of the evaporimeter in both dry noneczematous skin and clinically normal-looking skin.

Whereas, according to the above-mentioned studies, the TWL was mostly found to be increased in involved and symptom-free skin, judgment of the water content of the stratum corneum in AD has differed. According to Finlay et al. (1980) and Gloor et al. (1981) the water content is in fact higher in AD. On the other hand, Werner et al. (1981) found reduced water binding capacity in noneczematous skin of AD patients by weighing the water content of skin biopsies and calculating the water desorption. In later experiments Werner (1986) applied a new instrument, the Corneometer CM 420, based on electrical capacitance, influenced by the high dielectric content of water. Using this method the water content of the deep layers of stratum corneum could be measured. A lower water content was detected in dry skin, whereas the symptom-free AD skin did not differ from the skin of healthy controls. Kölmel et al. (1985) could, not, however, detect any differences between dry AD skin and normal skin by the photoacoustic method.

In dry scaly hand eczema, reduced water-holding capacity was registered (Tagami et al. 1980; Blickmann and Serup 1987). Relatively few exact data exist on water-binding substances in the corneum, but urea is probably one of them. The beneficial effect of urea-containing preparations applied on hyperkeratotic dry skin (Swanbeck 1968) supports the theory that, in AD, the amount of skin constituents responsible for keeping the skin soft and pliable is reduced.

7.3.3 Sebum Excretion

The skin of AD patients is generally very dry, and this is especially so when there is associated xerosis, as is often the case (see Sect. 2.13).

In addition to deficient secretion of eccrine sweat in this disease, it is postulated that sebum output is low, for, as was mentioned in Chap. 4, there are not only fewer sebaceous glands but also fewer secretory cells in these glands in infantile AD than in normal skin.

The author has used the paper-absorbent method of Strauss and Pochi (1961), as modified by Cunliffe and Shuster (1969), to estimate, in adult AD patients, the sebum secretion rate not only on the forehead but also on the hands, which is an area with obvious clinical relevance to the disease. An appreciable quantitative reduction in the sebum secretion rate is shown in the results presented in Table 7.1, and the results of qualitative lipid estimation in AD and in contact dermatitis from the few published reports and the author's study (Rajka 1974 a) are shown in Table 7.2.

Although the age and sex of the patients investigated are significant, it is important, when comparing the different estimations, carefully to take into consideration the site tested and the method used, as the values for the "epidermal lipids" (free fatty acids and cholesterol) are higher when lipid solvents are used (Downing 1968; Cotterill et al. 1971) than when the absorbent paper technique is employed (Cunliffe et al. 1971). Thus, the author estimated the lipids on the symptom-free skin of the backs of the hands of AD patients by the absorbent technique and found that those from sebaceous glands (wax esters, triglycerides, and squalene) were decreased, whereas epidermal lipids were correspondingly increased; this was in agreement with the results of studies of epidermal lipids on the forearm of such patients by Mustakallio et al. (1967). Furthermore, Wheatley (1965) has pointed out that skin surface lipids in AD are deficient in constituents derived from sebaceous glands. Various other methods of

Table 7.1. Sebum excretion on the back of the hand collected by the gravimetric technique of Strauss and Pochi (1961) (as modified by Cunliffe and Shuster 1969)

Patient material	n	Mean ± SEM	Significance of differences
Men, 16–39 years, with AD	15	0.152 ± 0.031	
Controls (men 16–39 years)	9	0.339 ± 0.056	$0.05 > P > 0.01$
Women, 16–39 years, with AD	20	0.136 ± 0.018	
Controls (women 16–39 years)	12	0.283 ± 0.064	$0.001 > P$

Table 7.2. Skin surface (and epidermal[b]) lipid analyses in AD and contact dermatitis by thin-layer chromatography

	AD: hands[a] (n=16)	Controls: hands[a] (n=24)	AD: forearm skin[b]	Controls: forearm skin[b]	Contact dermatitis: hands[c]	Contact dermatitis: back[d]	Controls: back[d]
Triglycerides	19.7	24.6	7.2	13.4	Elevated	34.58	36.32
Diglycerides	14.6	14.6	11.4	14.1			
Free fatty acids	25.1	21.7	11.3	8.5	Reduced	12.60	14.13
Cholesterol	8.9	3.7	20.9[e]	16.5[e]		4.22	4.32
Cholesterol esters			6.0[f]	8.0[f]	Reduced		
Wax esters	22.2	25.6			Elevated	17.77	18.95
Squalene	7.1	9.8	2.2	1.5	Reduced	14.02	12.99
Phospholipids			3.6[g]	6.8[g]	Elevated		

[a] Author's investigations young persons; matched controls; lipids collected by absorbent paper (Rajka 1974a)
[b] Mustakallio et al. (1967): young persons; controls: males; suction blister method
[c] Vallechi, Tinti, and Panconesi quoted by Gloor et al. (1972)
[d] Gloor et al. (1972): both sexes; matched controls; lipid solvent method
[e] Sterols
[f] Sterol esters
[g] Referring only to phosphatidylethanolamine for forearm skin and back; the analysis also includes other substances

analyzing skin surface lipids have, in recent years, been added to the previously usual method of removal via solvents. An optical density technique, observing alterations in the light transmission of glass plates or crystals after contact with fat, has been described (Schaefer and Kuhn-Bussius 1970). This photometric principle was exploited in the lipometer method (St Leger et al. 1979) and in its modification (Cunliffe et al. 1980). Another relatively simple instrument is the Sebumeter (Kesseler et al. 1985), which also uses photometry in order to measure surface lipids removed by the pressure of a plastic layer. Kligman et al. (1986) introduced a sebum-sensitive film (Sebutape) for visualizing and measuring the sebaceous secretion.

According to the studies of Ead et al. (1977) the facial skin of AD patients showed no difference in sebum secretion when compared with normal skin. On the other hand, Wirth et al. (1981) could, by kinetic studies, for the first time show that the number of sebaceous glands per skin area is reduced in AD, which is convincing proof of the reduction of sebum secretion in AD, previously shown by other techniques.

7.3.4 Skin Dryness

In contrast to the clinical term, which is primarily based on visual observation
and reflects the relation to ichthyosis (see Sect. 2.6.1), the pathophysiology of
dry skin is complex. In the more conventional view, dry skin is influenced by
the water and lipid content of the skin. An important research contribution regarding dry skin was the report by Finlay et al. (1980). By measuring cohesion
between corneocytes, they found disturbances of epidermal functions in AD,
i. e., increased cohesion and increase in epidermal thickness, an indication of
keratinization disturbances. The altered cohesion of the dry skin has recently

Table 7.3. Possible causes and mechanisms of dry skin in AD

Major causes:

Lowered humidity
Lowered ambient temperature
Epidermal cell damage (due to lipid solvents, friction, etc.)

Major mechanisms:	*References:*
A. Disturbances of water content:	
Increased TWL	Shahidullah et al. 1969; Rajka 1974 a; Abe et al. 1978; Finlay et al. 1980; Werner and Lindberg 1985
Increased hydration of stratum corneum/Low electrical impedance	Lawler et al. 1960; Finlay et al. 1980; Gloor et al. 1981
Reduced hydration of stratum corneum/deficiency of water-binding substances?	Tagami et al. 1980; Werner et al. 1980; Werner 1985
B. Disturbances of epidermal functions:	
Disturbances of keratinization/epidermal hyperplasia	Finlay et al. 1980
Increased cohesion between corneocytes	Finlay et al. 1980
C. Disturbances of sebaceous gland functions:	
Reduction in number of sebaceous glands	Prose 1965; Wirth et al. 1981
Reduction of cell proliferation in sebaceous glands	Wirth et al. 1981
Reduction of sebaceous lipid secretion	Wheatley 1965; Mustakallio et al. 1967; Rajka (1974 b); Abe et al. 1978

Possibilities of combination:

Interaction between A-B-C	
e. g., Between water/lipids	Rajka 1974 a, b
Not between water/lipids	Abe et al. 1978
Association with follicular keratosis/ichthyosis	
Association with inflammatory changes	

Consequences/correlations to dry skin:

Impaired barrier function
Increased colonization of *Staph. aureus*

been confirmed by Piérard (1986). Based on the majority of the contributions, the data are summarized in Table 7.3.

There are, however, objections to the assumption that the dry skin really is dry, i. e., has less water content (see Finlay et al. 1980, in Table 7.3). Analogously, in the dry skin of the aged the stratum corneum has not a lower but a greater water content and the TWL is in fact reduced (Kligman 1979). Probably Piérard (1987) is correct in pointing out that the term "dry skin" is a misnomer, which may be understood as a sum of changes in lipids and hydration, unrelated to the condition, which also includes rough or smooth qualities of the stratum corneum, and which may be studied by densitometry, computer image analysis, or cohesometry.

7.4 Paradoxical Vascular Responses

Clinicians have long been aware of the paleness of the skin of AD patients, and of facial skin in particular, and they have frequently interpreted this as evidence of a vasoconstrictor tendency in this disease. However, it is still undecided as to how much of this pallor may be attributed to peripheral vasoconstriction and how much to the characteristically thickened epidermis. Nevertheless, there are several well-documented vascular phenomena in AD which are attributable to the behavior of small blood vessels (see also Sect 10.1).

7.4.1 White Dermographism

White dermographism, produced by a medium strength mechanical stroking, which on the skin of healthy subjects elicits redness, comprises a white line, without urticaria, which rapidly replaces the initial traumatic erythematous reaction (Ebbecke 1917; Whitfield 1938; Reed et al. 1958) and is best seen on the abnormal skin during an active phase of AD (see Fig. 7.2). It has, however, also been observed on the involved skin in other dermatoses, and in macroscopically normal AD skin. It may be measured by simple instruments (dermo-

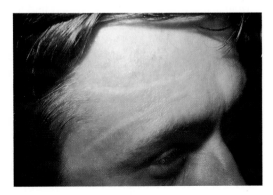

Fig. 7.2. White dermographism on the front in a patient with AD

graphometer, Hornstein et al. (1989). Lobitz and Dobson (1956) regard it as a prognostic sign for disease deterioration. The reaction is most prominent on the arms, legs, and neck. It is based on a non-nerve-mediated mechanism and is not abolished by procaine, adrenolytics, or atropine. A vasoconstrictor mechanism is indicated by the speed with which the blanching occurs, the absence of urticaria, and the failure of antihistamines, which decrease capillary permeability, to interfere with the reaction. Furthermore, evidence of arteriolar constriction in the involved skin of AD patients was found by Ramsay (1969) in photoelectric pulse meter recordings.

Investigating white dermographism by using an epicutaneous labeling technique with ^{133}Xe, Klemp and Staberg (1982) showed blanching and decreased blood flow in six of seven AD patients (although in the remaining patient blood flow was increased and redness was found as in normal subjects). The usual blanching after application of a new anesthetic cream was seen only at the onset in AD patients, and after 15–60 min the reaction became red. This reaction, elicited on dry and eczematous areas, was interpreted as being due to late onset vasodilatation (Juhlin and Rollman 1984).

7.4.2 Nicotinate Reactions

Application to the skin of nicotinic acid esters, in an ointment base or as a solution, may produce either no erythematous response or a white reaction in AD patients (Illig 1952). This implies that a great number of these patients fail to react with the expected erythema, the rubbed area either retaining the normal skin color or blanching (chemical white dermographism). In other cases, only a reduced erythema develops (see Fig. 7.3). This phenomenon has been observed in other conditions (see Table 7.4), and as it is blocked by dihydroergotoxine (Hydergine) but not by local anesthetics, which are characteristic features of the nicotinic effect of acetylcholine (Borelli 1955), it is assumed to represent vasoconstriction. Thune and Rajka (1974) studied reactivity to Trafuril (thurfyl nicotinate) in the symptom-free and involved skin of AD patients, simultaneously measuring the superficial venous vessels by a photoelectric reflection meter (Photovolt 670) and the arteriolar pulse height by photoelectric pulse plethysmography. Reflectometry revealed a certain temporal variability of the vascular response (see Fig. 7.4), which had also been observed by Heite (1961), and different patterns of reactivity were generally demonstrated by both methods (Table 7.5, Fig. 7.5). The Trafuril flush is probably mediated by prostaglandins (Wilkin et al. 1982) and inhibited by prior administration of aspirin (Winkelmann and Wilhelmj 1963); similar inhibition is seen with indomethacin. In sequential skin biopsies, after nicotinate application, first mononuclear and subsequently – beginning after 2 h – neutrophil accumulation was seen, even showing nonimmune leukocytoclasia. In six investigated AD patients no, and in one case a reduced, red reaction was noted, and consequently neutrophil infiltration did not occur (in one case some neutrophils had accumulated). Interestingly, similar events can be provoked by LTB_4 and other leukocyte chemoattractants (English et al. 1987).

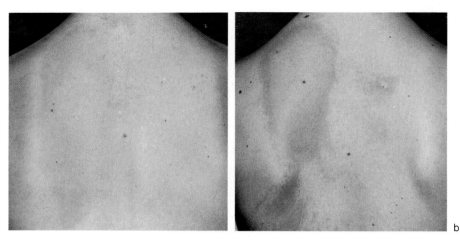

a   b

Fig. 7.3. a Reduced reaction to Trafuril in monovular twin A with AD. **b** Red reaction to Trafuril in monovular twin B with AD

Table 7.4. Atypical reactivity to locally applied nicotinic acid esters

Patient categories	Percentage	Authors
AD	44–100	Illig 1952; Borelli 1955; Stüttgen and Krause 1957; Scott 1958; Murrell and Taylor 1959; Jillson et al. 1959; Rajka 1960; Rothman and Bloom 1958; Callaway 1956
Healthy persons	0–3.3	Callaway 1956; Bolte 1952; Weiss 1956; De Vaillancourt 1954; Solomon and Wentzel 1963
Dermatoses (controls)	1.4–6	Engelhardt 1961; Illig 1952; Callaway 1956; Stüttgen and Krause 1957
Medical diseases (controls)	0.5–4.7	Lyndian 1961; Oka 1953; Engelhardt 1961
Bronchial asthma	8–50	Lyndian 1961; Stüttgen and Krause 1957
Asthma + allergic rhinitis	17.5	Rajka 1960
Rheumatoid arthritis	67–89	Murrell and Taylor 1959; Oka 1953; Saslaw 1955; De Vaillancourt 1954
Rheumatic fever	67–90	Rovensky and Preis 1959
Rheumatoid spondylitis Psoriatic arthritis	69–75	Oka 1953
Pneumonia, tonsilitis	68–89	Weiss 1956
Hepatitis, allergies, "focal sepsis," glomerulonephritis	Occasionally	Stüttgen and Krause 1957
Diabetes mellitus:	50	Murrell and Taylor 1959
with retinopathy	64	Rajka and Östman, unpublished
with nephropathy	50	Rajka and Östman, unpublished
with neuropathy	72	Rajka and Östman, unpublished

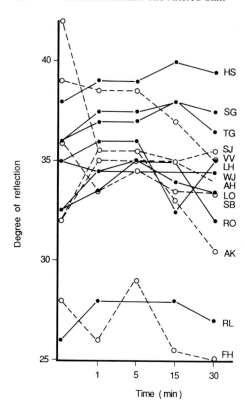

Fig. 7.4. Reflectometric values after Trafuril on the uninvolved forearm in 14 patients with AD, showing increase (⎯) or decrease (---)

7.4.3 Delayed Blanch and Comments

Intracutaneously injected acetylcholine produces a wheal with surrounding erythema, and, in AD patients, an anemic zone which develops 3–30 min later and sometimes persists for more than an hour (Lobitz and Campbell 1953) (see Fig. 7.6). This reaction has the following features:

1. It is abolished by atropine, suggesting that the acetylcholine has a muscarinic effect.
2. It is not affected by local anesthetics.
3. It is found mostly in lichenified lesions in AD (Champion 1963) but also occurs in as many as 50% of atopics with no dermatitis (West et al. 1962).
4. It has been found in 16%, and possibly in 21%, of infants without any relationship to a family history of atopy (Hinrichs et al. 1966).
5. It has also been seen in lichenified plaques of infective or of seborrheic eczema (Engelhardt 1965), and even in 22% of apparently nonatopic persons (Thomsen and Osmundsen 1965).

The interpretation of all the above-mentioned vascular phenomena, and especially of the delayed blanch, is one of the most discussed and as yet undecided

Table 7.5. Some comparable studies on paradoxical vascular reactions in AD

	Paradoxical reactions	Normal reactions	Authors
White dermographism			
1. Involved skin	2/7 blanching/decreased pulsation 5/7 blanching/unchanged/slightly increased pulsation		Ramsay (1969)
	5/7 blanching/decreased blood flow		Klemp and Staberg (1982)
2. Symptom-free skin	1/7 blanching/decreased blood flow	1/7 redness/increased blood flow	
Trafuril			
1. Involved skin	3/6 blanching/decreased pulsation 1/6 blanching/increased pulsation	2/6 redness/increased pulsation	Thune and Rajka (1974)
2. Symptom-free skin	8/14 blanching/increased pulsation	6/14 redness/increased pulsation	
Delayed blanch (via methacholine)			
1. Involved skin	1/6 blanching/unchanged pulsation[a] 3/6 blanching/decreased pulsation[a]	2/6 redness/increased pulsation[a]	Thune and Rajka (1974)
	7/8 blanching/increased pulsation		Ramsay (1969)

[a] Somewhat varying values

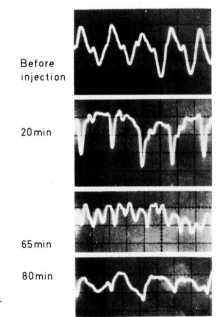

Before injection

20 min

65 min

80 min

Fig. 7.5. Effect of Trafuril on involved skin of AD registered by photoelectric pulse plethysmography (reduced pulse height indicates vasoconstriction)

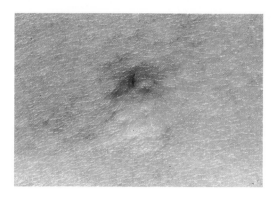

Fig. 7.6. Delayed blanch in a patient with AD

facets of AD. The pallor seems to evidence vasoconstriction, but it is not obvious whether this is due to "true" vasoconstriction or to the blood vessels being narrowed by the surrounding exudative edema, resulting from vasodilatation and increased capillary permeability. It is impossible to mention all the arguments for and against these alternatives or to judge, for example, between the conflicting reports on the local accumulation of intravenously administered dyes (Möller and Rorsman 1958; Kalz and Fekete 1960; Juhlin 1962; Copeman and Winkelmann 1969); however, the majority of these experiments indicate a tendency to vasoconstriction.

Other reports worthy of mention include the following: Lobitz (1958) found no edema after injecting acetylcholine into excised skin. Juhlin (1961 a, b, 1962) advanced a hypothesis that delayed blanch is due to increased liberation of norepinephrine in the skin. He based this theory on his discovery that: (a) smaller quantities of norepinephrine were required to blanch skin of AD patients compared with normal skin; (b) delayed blanch could be induced also in normal persons by acetylcholine if the skin had been pretreated with norepinephrine; (c) the delayed blanch returned to normal if the skin was pretreated with guanethidine, a substance known to deplete norepinephrine deposits in the skin. Norepinephrine stores, tightly or loosely bound, were shown to be increased in AD skin by Solomon et al. (1964), using isotope-labeled norepinephrine. On the other hand, Davis and Lawler (1958) injected acetylcholine into AD skin which they then excised and observed under the capillary microscope; it was found to show capillary dilatation. This has been criticized on the grounds that vasodilatation caused by the previous use of the skin stripping techniques could apparently cause the changes observed. It has already been mentioned that these findings have not been confirmed by Lobitz (1958 b). However, other authors also have pointed out that vasodilatation occurs after administration of acetylcholine even in AD patients. Scott (1962), for example, pretreated skin with hyaluronidase and found a normal erythema response to acetylcholine in AD patients, and he postulated that edema obscured the vasodilatation. The fact that the adrenergic blocker phentolamine does not impair the delayed blanch (Reed and Kierland 1958) also argues against the hypothesis that a vasoconstrictor catecholamine is released. Champion (1963), who stressed the importance of vasoconstriction, found that a weak dilution of mecholyl elicits a delayed blanch but that higher concentrations of the order of 10^{-2} or 10^{-3} M cause edema. Bystryn et al. (1969), using a radioactive iodoantipyrene clearance technique, showed increased blood flow after administering acetylcholine. Thune and Rajka (1974) measured the delayed blanch elicited by methacholine in the involved skin of six patients with AD using simultaneously a photoelectric reflection meter and a pulse plethysmograph; they observed four types of response (Table 7.5; Figs. 7.7, 7.8). Included in Table 7.5 are the observations of Ramsay (1969), who found that after administering methacholine, photoelectric pulse meter recordings taken from erythematous areas of symptom-free and from blanched areas of involved skin of AD patients were identical; this was suggestive of arteriolar dilatation. In addition, this author registered blanching, with decreased or unchanged pulsation, in white dermographism. Table 7.5 thus demonstrates that, in AD, the events following vasodilator stimuli seem to be more complex than was at one time postulated.

Comments: In 100 AD and 20 contact dermatitis patients, the paradoxical vascular reactions were elicited on both involved and symptom-free skin. Such

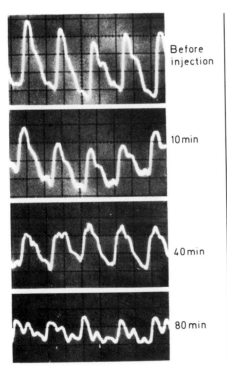

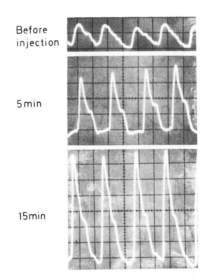

Fig. 7.7. Effect of methacholine on involved skin of AD registered by photoelectric pulse plethysmography. (Reduced pulse height indicates vasoconstriction.)

Fig. 7.8. Effect of methacholine on symptom-free skin of AD registered by photoelectric pulse plethysmography. (Increased pulse height indicates vasodilatation.)

reactions were only detected on eczematous areas in both conditions and on the dry skin of AD patients, which points to their nonspecific secondary role in AD (Uehara and Ofuji 1977). This report is in agreement with data on the occurrence of paradoxical reactions in other types of eczema, although the frequency was higher than most investigators report (see, e. g., Table 7.4). It is, however, not consistent with several observations that white dermographism and nicotinate reactivity can be elicited on symptom-free AD skin (see, e. g., Table 7.5), though to a lesser degree than on the involved skin. There is a consensus that AD patients primarily do not show redness after vasodilatory stimuli. The mechanism of these nonspecific but characteristic reactions is, however, still under debate and the vasoconstrictive hypothesis has its adversaries. It seems that it is not a question of *either* vasoconstriction *or* edema/ dilatation, because AD subjects may react to both these stimuli (see Table 7.5). The variable responses, indicating impaired vasoregulation, are probably related to disease parameters, particularly to the activity of AD. These responses show no correlation with hereditary factors (Rajka 1960) or with IgE production (Öhman et al. 1972). In a broader sense, the paradoxical vascular responses are related to the effects of pharmacological agents in AD (see Chap. 6). Here the autonomic nervous system may possible play a role.

7.4.4 Further Vascular Changes

7.4.4.1 Vasoconstrictor Tendency in Acral Circulation

A tendency to vasoconstriction in the terminal vasculature of the peripheral circulation (in the extremities) has also been demonstrated, at normal room temperature, in AD patients by using techniques such as photoelectric plethysmography (Blaich 1958), but different findings have been reported (Huff 1955). In addition, AD patients were shown to have a slower peripheral blood flow by Korting and Holzmann (1960), who used a fluorescence method, and to have a reduced total blood flow in extremities free of skin lesions by Klüken and Ullrich (1969). These findings are in keeping with the commonly noted clinical fact that many AD patients have cold hands and feet.

7.4.4.2 Circulation Through Musculature of the Extremities

In contrast to the skin circulation, total blood flow through the capillaries of the limb musculature is normal in AD (Klüken and Ullrich 1969; van Staak and Kuiper 1971), and in this connection it should be noted that only α-receptors are present in skin blood vessels, whereas muscle blood vessels have mostly β-receptors.

7.4.4.3 Cardiovascular Changes in AD

This aspect of the disease was considered first by Storck and his co-workers (Heim and Storck 1961; Konzelmann and Storck 1965). Earlier findings on cardiac function have been amended by the results of modern investigative techniques. The blood pressure after exercise, as measured by the ergometric meth-od or by the Schellong test, seems to be decreased in some cases (Storck et al. 1972). Furthermore, radiological evidence of aortic narrowing was found in about 50% of AD patients studied by Storck et al. (1965).

7.4.4.4 Absence of Flare After Intracutaneously Administered Histamine or Protein Allergens

Observation of this phenomenon is not new, having been mentioned by Roussy and Mosinger (1932), Norrlind (1946), Eyster et al. (1952), and Storck (1955). The flare is connected with certain functions of the nervous system and may be abolished by some lesions of the central nervous system by local anaesthesia or by hypnosis (West et al. 1961); it probably depends on local vasoconstriction, as stroking will abolish histamine flare in AD patients with white dermogra-phism (Reed et al. 1958).

7.4.4.5 Alterations in Reactivity to Changes in Ambient Temperature

The principal changes caused by these general stimuli can be summarized as follows. In a cold room, vasoconstriction tends to be greater in the toes and fingers and less in the antecubital and popliteal fossae in AD patients than in normal persons, whereas in a hot room there is a more delayed vasodilatation in the toes and fingers and a somewhat greater vasodilatation in the flexures in these patients than in normal people; these findings indicate a vasoconstrictor tendency, the flexures excepted, in AD (Eyster et al. 1952; Weber et al. 1955). Modern plethysmographic and fluvographic measurements have confirmed these earlier findings, yet sometimes such paradoxical reactivity as total blood flow in the extremities increasing after exposure to cold and decreasing after heat, or even normal skin circulation, has been recorded (van Staak and Kuiper 1971; Storck et al. 1972; Kocsard et al. 1973). Heyer et al. (1988) applied cold and warm stimuli to the forearms of 21 AD patients and registered the reaction of the contralateral site. Whereas in controls parallel reactions occurred, in AD the changes were slight, indicating a rigid central thermoregulation which had already been stressed by Korting in 1960 and clearly demonstrated by Horn-stein et al. (1989).

7.5 Other Alterations

7.5.1 Pilomotor Reaction

In earlier literature, special consideration was given to increased pilomotor reactivity in AD; this reactivity was said to be increased by cold stimuli, but de-creased by a sympathomimetic substance: oxedrine (Korting 1954). The cur-rently accepted view is that the stimulation of α-adrenergic receptors is respon-sible for pilomotor contractions.

7.5.2 Endocrine Alterations

Readett (1955), by means of formularies, found that one-third of patients with thyrotoxicosis had AD and that 21% of AD patients had thyroid diseases. These unexpected findings were not later confirmed (Schwartz 1966). No convincing evidence has been found for other assumed hormonal dysfunctions in AD.

The circadian cortisol rhythm showed deviations in AD, particularly in healing cases. Lowest values were registered at night when patients awoke suffering from an intense itch (Heubeck et al. 1988). The deviations were interpreted as a possible neuroendocrine dysregulative trait. Similarly, parallelism was shown between urinary cortisol secretion and skin reactivity to histamine and antigens (Lee et al. 1977). Some of the mentioned circulatory abnormalities and others, such as endocrine alterations, are systemic abnormalities more or less present in AD. This supports the impression that the skin should not be considered as an isolated organ.

7.6 Concluding Remarks

According to the findings collected in this chapter there are several alterations in the symptom-free skin of the AD subject. Although sometimes of a secondary character, these findings, shown in Table 7.6, confirm the view expressed in the definition of the disease (see Chap. 8), that the altered skin is a basic trait in the pathomechanism of AD.

Table 7.6. Alterations in symptom-free AD skin

1. Increased itchiness (lower itch threshold)
2. Increased epidermal thickness
3. Impaired barrier function
4. Lowered resistance to contact irritants
5. Increased staphylococcal colonization
6. Increased TWL
7. Coexistence with dry skin
8. Slight dermal lymphocyte infiltrate, alteration in venules
9. IgE on antigen-presenting cells[a]
10. White dermographism[b]
11. Nicotinate white reaction[b]
12. Delayed blanch[b]
13. Acral vasoconstriction
14. Absence of flare after histamine or allergen injection
15. Increased pilomotor reaction

[a] Found by one group
[b] Not unanimously stated

References

Abe T, Ohikido M, Yamamoto K (1978) Studies on skin surface barrier functions: skin surface lipids and transepidermal water loss in atopic skin during childhood. Jap J Dermatol 5: 223

Al-Jaberi H, Marks R (1984) Studies of the clinically uninvolved skin in patients with dermatitis. Br J Dermatol 111: 437

Bachmann Andersen L, Thestrup-Pedersen K (1987) Sweat pore density on the fingertips of atopic patients. Br J Dermatol 117: 225

Baker H (1971) Deperdition d'eau par voie transepidermique. Ann Dermatol Syphiligr 98: 289

Baker H, Kligman AM (1967) Measurement of transepidermal water loss by electrical hygrometry. Arch Derm 96: 441

Barker JNWN, Alegre VA, MacDonald DM (1988) Surface-bound immunoglobulin E on antigen-presenting cells in cutaneous tissue of atopic dermatitis. J Invest Dermatol 90: 117

Bettley FR, Grice KA (1965) A method for measuring transepidermal water loss and a means of inactivating sweat glands. Br J Dermatol 77: 627

Blaich W (1958) Das neuro-vaskuläre Problem der Neurodermitis unter dem Gesichtswinkel funktioneller Prüfungen der terminalen Strombahn. Arch Klin Exp Dermatol 208: 63

Blank JH (1952) Factors which influence water content of stratum corneum. J Invest Dermatol 18: 433

Blichmann C, Serup J (1987) Hydration studies in scaly hand eczema. Contact Dermatitis 16: 155

Bolte O (1952) Hautdurchblutungsproben mit hyperaemisierenden Substanzen als diagnostisches Hilfsmittel. Hautarzt 3: 304

Borelli S (1955) Paradoxe und adequate Hautreaktionen bei der Neurodermitis nach Einwirkung von Pharmaka. Arch f Dermatol 200: 479

Borelli S, Kopecka B (1966) Über das reaktive Verhalten der Hautdurchblutung auf Kälte und Wärmereize bei Kranken mit atopischer konstitutioneller Neurodermitis. Dermatol Wochenschr 152: 1365

Braathen LR, Förre O, Natvig JB, Rajka G (1978) Lymphocyte subpopulations, serum immunoglobulins and complement factors in patients with atopic dermatitis. Br J Dermatol 98: 521

Bystryn JC, Freedman RI, Hyman C (1969) Clearance of iodoantipyrene from metacholine blanched skin in atopics. Arch Dermatol 100: 165

Callaway JL (1956) Dermatologic research: an office procedure? J Invest Dermatol 27: 215

Champion RH (1963) Abnormal vascular reactions in atopic eczema. Br J Dermatol 75: 12

Clubley M, Bye CE, Henson T, Peck AW, Riddington C (1978) A technique for studying the effect of drugs of human sweat gland activity. Eur J Clin Pharmacol 14: 221

Copeman PW, Winkelmann RK (1969) Vascular changes accompanying white dermographism and delayed blanch in atopic dermatitis. Br J Dermatol 81: 944

Cormia FE, Kuykendall V (1955) Studies on sweat retention on various dermatoses. Arch Dermatol 71: 425

Cotterill JA, Cunliffe WJ, Williamson B, Forster RA (1971) A semiquantitative method for the biochemical analysis of sebum. Br J Dermatol 85: 35

Cotton DWK, van Rossum E (1973) Hexokinase, glucose-6-phosphate dehydrogenase and malate dehydrogenase in the isolated sweat glands of normal and atopic subjects. Br J Dermatol 89: 459

Cotton DWK, Sutorius AHM, Urselmann EJM (1971) The fractionation of sweat from atopic and nonatopic subjects. Acta Derm Venereol (Stockh) 51: 189

Cunliffe WJ, Shuster S (1969) The rate of sebum secretion in man. Br J Dermatol 81: 69

Cunliffe WJ, Cotterill JA, Williamson B (1971) Variations in surface lipid composition with different sampling techniques. Br J Dermatol 85: 40

Cunliffe WJ, Kearney JN, Simpson NB (1980) A modified photometric technique for measuring sebum secretion rate. J Invest Dermatol 75: 394

Davis M, Lawler JC (1958) Observations on delayed blanch phenomenon in atopic subjects. J Invest Dermatol 30: 127

De Vaillancourt G de (1954) The cutaneous application of a nicotinic acid cream as diagnostic and in various diseases. Can Med Assoc J 71: 283

Downing DT (1968) Photodensitometry in the thin-layer chromatographic analysis of neutral lipids. J Chromatogr 38: 91

Ead RD, Fairbank RA, Cunliffe WJ (1977) Sebum excretion rate, surface lipid composition and constitutional eczema. Clin Exp Dermatol 2: 361

Ebbecke U (1917) Die lokale vasomotorische Reaktion (LVR) der Haut und der inneren Organe. Pflugers Arch Ges Physiol Mens Tiere 169: 1

Elias PM (1981) Lipids and the epidermal permeability barrier. Arch Dermatol Res 270: 95

Engelhardt A (1961) Hautreaktionen auf Nikotinsäurebenzylester und ihre Bedeutung für die Differentialdiagnostik von Dermatosen. Hautarzt 12: 346

Engelhardt A (1965) Gefäßreaktionen bei verschiedenen Formen des mikrobiell-seborrhoischen Ekzems als nosologischen Ordnungsprinzips. Arch Klin Exp Dermatol 223: 116

English JSC, Winkelmann RK, Louback JB, Greaves MW, MacDonald DM (1987) The cellular inflammatory response in nicotinate skin reactions. Br J Dermatol 116: 341

Eyster WH, Roth GM, Kierland RR (1952) Studies of the peripheral vascular physiology of patients with atopic dermatitis. J Invest Dermatol 18: 37

Finlay AY, Nicholls S, King CS, Marks R (1980) The "dry" non-eczematous skin associated with atopic eczema. Br J Dermatol 102: 249

Foster KH, Haspineall JR, Mollel CL (1971) Effects of propranolol on the response of eccrine sweat glands to acetylcholine. Br J Dermatol 85: 363

Frosch PJ, Kligman AM (1977) Rapid blister formation in human skin with ammonium hydroxide. Br J Dermatol 96: 461

Gasselt HRM van, Vierhout RR (1963) Registration of the insensible perspiration of small quantities of sweat. Dermatologica 127: 255

Gloor M, Heymann B, Stuhlert T (1981) Infrared-spectroscopic determination of the horny layer in healthy subjects and in patients suffering from atopic dermatitis. Arch Dermatol Res 271: 429

Gloor M, Strack R, Geissler H, Friederich HC (1972) Quantity and composition of skin surface lipids and alkaline-resistance in subjects with contact allergy and healthy controls. Arch Dermatol Forsch 245: 184

Gordon BI, Maibach HI (1968) On the mechanism of the inactive eccrine human sweat gland. Arch Dermatol 97: 66

Grice KA, Bettley FR (1967) Skin water loss and accidental hypothermia in psoriasis, ichthyosis and erythroderma. Br Med J 74: 195

Grice K, Sattar H, Sharratt M, Baker H (1971) Skin temperature and transepidermal water loss. J Invest Dermatol 57: 108

Hattingh J (1972) The influence of skin temperature, environmental temperature and relative humidity on transepidermal water loss. Acta Derm Venereol (Stockh) 52: 438

Heim E, Storck H (1961) Vergleichende kreislaufanalytische Untersuchungen bei Atopikern und Kontrollpersonen. Dermatologica 122: 249

Heite HJ (1961) Klinische Untersuchungen zur Spätprognose des Eczema infantum. Arch Klin Exp Dermatol 213: 460

Hemels HGWM (1970) The effect of pranolol on acetylcholine-induced sweat response in atopic and nonatopic subjects. Br J Dermatol 83: 313

Herrmann F (1972) Über Schwitzen bei der Neurodermitis. Arch Dermatol Forsch 244: 344

Herrmann F, Prose RH (1951) Studies on the ether soluble substances on human skin. I. Quantity and replacement sum. J. Invest Dermatol 16: 217

Herrmann F, Prose PH, Sulzberger MB (1953) Studies on the ether soluble substances on the human skin. III. The effect of sweat on the quantity of ether soluble substances on skin. J Invest Dermatol 21: 397

Heubeck B, Schönberger A, Hornstein OP (1988) Sind Verschiebungen des zirkadianen Cortisolrhytmus ein endokrines Symptom des atopischen Ekzems? Hautarzt 39: 12

Heyer G, Schönberger A, Hornstein P (1988) Störungen der Thermoregulation auf externe Kälte und Wärmereize bei Patienten mit atopischem Ekzem. Hautarzt 39: 18

Hinrichs WL, Logan GB, Winkelmann RK (1966) Delayed blanch phenomenon as an indication of atopy in newborn infants. J Invest Dermatol 46: 189

Holzmann H, Korting GW, Oemichen C (1961) Vergleichende Messungen der Feuchtigkeitsabgabe von Herdbezirk und unveränderter Haut bei verschiedener Hautkrankheiten. Arch Klin Exp Dermatol 212: 312

Hornqvist R, Henriksson R, Bäck O (1988) Iontophoretic study of skin vessel reactivity in atopic dermatitis and its correlation to serum IgE levels. J Am Acad Dermatol 18: 269

Hornstein OP (1989) Responses of skin temperature to different stimuli in atopic dermatitis. Acta Dermatovenereol (Suppl 144) (Stockh) (in press)

Hornstein OP (1989) Studies on dermographometry in atopic dermatitis. Acta Dermatovenereol (Suppl 144) (Stockh) (in press)

Huff SE (1955) Observations on peripheral circulation in various dermatoses. Arch Dermatol 71: 575

Illig L (1952) Die Reaktion der Haut des Neurodermitikers auf zwei nikotinsäureesterhaltige Reizstoffe. Dermatol Wochenschr 126: 753

Jillson OF, Curwen WI, Alexander BR (1959) Problems of contact dermatitis in the atopic individual. Ann Allergy 17: 215

Juhlin L (1961 a) Skin reactions to iontophoretically administered epinephrine and norepinephrine in atopic dermatitis. J Invest Dermatol 37: 201

Juhlin L (1961 b) The fate of iontophoretically introduced epinephrine and norepinephrine in patients with atopic dermatitis and normal skin. J Invest Dermatol 37: 251

Juhlin L (1962) Vascular reactions in atopic dermatitis. Acta Derm Venereol 42: 218

Juhlin L, Rollman O (1984) Vascular effects of local anaesthetic mixture in atopic dermatitis. Acta Derm Venereol 64: 439

Kaliner M (1976) The cholinergic nervous system and immediate hypersensitivity. I. Eccrine sweat response in allergic patients. J Allergy Clin Immunol 58: 308

Kalz F, Fekete Z (1960) Studies on the mechanism of the white response and of the delayed blanch phenomenon in atopic subjects by means of Coomassie blue. J Invest Dermatol 35: 135

Kesseler T, Enderer K, Steigleder GK (1985) Die quantitative Analyse der Hautoberflächenlipide mit Hilfe einer Sebumetermethode. Z Hautkr 60: 857

Kiistala R (1983) Stimulated local sweating response in atopic dermatitis (abstract). XVI. International Congress of Dermatology, Tokyo, p 320

Klemp P, Staberg G (1982) Cutaneous blood flow during white dermographism in patients with atopic dermatitis. J Invest Dermatol 79: 243

Kligman AM (1979) Perspectives and problems of cutaneous gerontology. J Invest Dermatol 73: 39

Kligman AM, Miller DL, McGinley KJ (1986) Sebutape: a device for visualizing and measuring human sebaceous secretion. J Soc Cosmet Chem 37: 369

Klüken N, Ulrich B (1969) Vasculare Faktoren bei Neurodermitis constitutionalis. Hautarzt 20: 261

Kocsard E, Ofner F, Broe GA (1973) Paradox temperature response in atopic dermatitis. Dermatologica 146: 8

Kölmel K, Nicolaus A, Giese K (1985) Photoacoustic determination of the water uptake by the upper horny layer of non-eczematous skin in atopic dermatitis. Bioeng Skin 1: 125

Konzelmann M, Storck H (1965) Wirkung von Cholinestern (Metacholin), Histamin, Kältereizen und psychischen Einflüssen auf Haut und Zirkulation von Neurodermitispatienten und Vergleichspersonen. Hautarzt 16: 303

Korting GW (1954) Zur Pathogenese des endogenen Ekzems. Thieme, Stuttgart

Korting GW (1960) Einige Wesenszüge des endogenen Ekzematikers. Dtsch Med Wschr 85: 417

Korting GW, Holzmann H (1960) Zur peripheren Durchströmungsgeschwindigkeit bei endogenen Ekzematikern. Arch Dermatol 210: 575

Kuyper BRM, Cotton DWK (1972) Conditioning of sweating. Br J Dermatol 87: 154

Lawler JC, Davis MJ, Griffith EC (1960) Electrical characteristics of the skin. The impedance of the surface sheath and deep tissues. J Invest Dermatol 34: 301

Lee RE, Smolensky M, Leach CS, McGovern P (1977) Circadian rhythms in the cutaneous reactivity to histamine and selected antigens, including phase relationship to urinary cortisol secretion. Ann Allergy 38: 231

Levi L, Meneghini CL, Rantuccio F (1959) Activité cholinesterasique: pouvoir histaminolitique et dosage de l'histamine dans la peau des sujets sains et atteint de certaines dermatoses allergiques. Acta Allergol 13: 332

Lobitz WC (1958 a) Anecdotes of an agnostic allergist. Arch Dermatol 78: 458

Lobitz WC (1958 b) Discussion to David and Lawler. J Invest Dermatol 30: 127

Lobitz WC, Campbell (1953) Physiologic studies in atopic dermatitis (disseminated neurodermitis). I. The local cutaneous response to intradermally injected acetylcholine and epinephrine. Arch Dermatol 67: 575

Lobitz WC, Dobson RL (1956) Physical and physiological clues for diagnosing eczema. JAMA 161: 1226

Lyndian HH (1961) Der diagnostische Wert der Nikotinsäureester-Reaktion bei allergischen Krankheiten. In: Findeisen DGR, Hansen KV (eds). Aktuelle Allergiefragen, vol 4. Barth, Leipzig, p 389

Marks R, Nicholls SC (1981) Drugs which influence the stratum corneum and techniques for their evaluation. Clin Exp Dermatol 6: 419

Michaelsson G (1969) Cutaneous reactions to kallikrein and prostaglandins in healthy and diseased skin. Thesis, Söderstrom and Finn, Uppsala

Mihm MC, Soter NA, Dvorak HF, Austen KF (1976) The structure of normal skin and the morphology of atopic eczema. J Invest Dermatol 67: 305

Miller NE (1969) Learning of visceral and glandular responses. Science 163: 434

Möller H, Rorsman H (1958) Studies on vascular permeability factors with sodium fluorescein. II. The effect of intracutaneously injected histamine and serum in patients with atopic dermatitis. Acta Derm Venereol (Stockh) 38: 243

Murphy CM, Smith SE, Smith SA, Greaves MW (1984) Autonomic functions in cholinergic urticaria and atopic eczema. Br J Dermatol 110: 591

Murrell TW, Taylor WM (1959) The cutaneous reactions to nicotinic furfuryl. Arch Dermatol 79: 545

Mustakallio KK, Kiistala U, Piha J, Nieminen E (1967) Epidermal lipids in Besnier's prurigo (atopic eczema). Ann Med Exp Biol Fenn 45: 323

Nilsson GE (1977) Measurement of water exchange through skin. Med Biol Eng Comput 15: 209

Norrlind R (1946) Prurigo Besnier (atopic dermatitis). Acta Derm Venereol [Suppl] (Stockh) 13

Öhman S, Juhlin L, Johansson SGO (1972) Immunoglobulins in atopic dermatitis. In: Charpin J, Boutin C, Aubert J, Frankland AW (eds) Allergology. Proceedings of the 8th European Congress of Allergy. Excerpta Medica, Amsterdam, p 119

Oka M (1953) A nicotinic acid ester ("Trafuril") skin test in rheumatic diseases. Acta Med Scand 145: 258

Piérard GE (1987) What does "dry skin" mean? Int J Dermatol 26: 167

Piérard GE (1986) Assessment of environmental "dry skin". Bioeng Skin 2: 31

Potts RO, Gouzek DB, Harris RR, McKie JE (1985) A noninvasive in vivo technique to quantitatively measure water concentration of the stratum corneum using attenuated total-reflectance infrared spectroscopy. Arch Dermatol Res 277: 489

Prose PH (1965) Pathologic changes in eczema. J Pediatr 66 (2): 178

Rajka G (1960) Prurigo Besnier (atopic dermatitis) with special reference to the role of allergic factors. I. The influence of atopic hereditary factors. Acta Derm Venereol (Stockh) 40: 285

Rajka G (1974 a) Transepidermal water loss on the hands in atopic dermatitis. Arch Dermatol Res 251: 111

Rajka G (1974 b) Surface lipid estimation on the back of the hands in atopic dermatitis. Arch Dermatol Res 251: 43

Ramsay C (1969) Vascular changes accompanying white dermographism and delayed blanch in atopic dermatitis. Br J Dermatol 81: 37

Readett MD (1955) Constitutional eczema and thyroid disease. J Invest Dermatol 24: 126

Reed WB, Kierland KP (1958) Vascular reaction in chronically inflamed skin. II. Action of epinephrine and phentolamine (Regitin); action of acetylcholine and metacholine (Mecholyl) and the delayed blanch. Arch Dermatol 77: 181

Reed WB, Kierland RP, Code CF (1958) Vascular reactions in chronically inflamed skin. III. Action of histamine, the histamine releaser 48-80 and monoethanolamine nicotinate. Arch Dermatol 77: 263

Rothman S, Bloom RE (1958) The increased vasoconstrictor tendency in atopic dermatitis. Arch Belg Syphiligr 13: 300

Roussy G, Mosinger M (1932) La réaction cutanée locale à l'histamine. CR Soc Biol (Paris) 109: 103

Rovensky J, Peis A (1959) The significance of the Trafuril test with special reference to atopy and rheumatic fever. A capillaroscopic study. Ann Pediatr (Paris) 193: 289

Rovensky J, Saxl O (1964) Differences in the dynamics of sweat secretion in atopic children. J Invest Dermatol 43: 171

Saslaw MS (1955) Rheumatic fever-diagnosis, prophylaxis and therapy. JAMA 159: 653

Schaefer H, Kuhn-Bussius H (1970) Methodik zur quantitativen Bestimmung der menschlichen Talgsekretion. Arch Klin Exp Dermatol 238: 429

Schwartz HJ (1966) the relationship of thyroid disease and the atopic state. Ann Allergy 24: 234

Scott A (1958) The distribution and behaviour of cutaneous nerves in normal and abnormal skin. Brit J Dermatol 70: 1

Scott A (1962) Acetylcholine in normal and diseases skin. Br J Dermatol 74: 317

Shahidullah M, Raffle EJ, Rimmer AR, Frain-Bell W (1969) Transepidermal water loss in patients with dermatitis. Br J Dermatol 81: 722

Solomon L, Wentzel HE (1963) Plasma catecholamines in atopic dermatitis. J Invest Dermatol 41: 401

Solomon LM, Wentzel HE, Tulsky E (1964) The physiological disposition of C 14 norepinephrine in patients with atopic dermatitis and other dermatoses. J Invest Dermatol 43: 193

Soter NA, Mihm MC jr (1980) Morphology of atopic eczema. Acta Derm Venereol [Suppl] (Stockh) 92: 11

Spruit D, Herweyer HE (1967) The ability of skin to change its insensible perspiration. Dermatologica 134: 364

Spruit T, Malten K (1969) Humidity of the air and water vapour loss of the skin. Dermatologica 138: 418

St Leger D, Berrebi C, Duboz C, Agache P (1979) The lipometre: an easy tool for rapid quantitation of skin surface lipids in man. Arch Dermatol Res 265: 79

Storck H (1955) Discussion to Borelli reference listed above

Storck H, Strehler E, Gysling E (1965) Abnorm geringe Aortenweite bei Patienten mit Neurodermitis disseminata. Arch Dermatol 222: 489

Storck H, Strehler E, Goor W (1972) Pathogenese der Neurodermitis disseminata: Zirkulation und neurovegetative Regulation. Arch Dermatol Forsch 244: 335

Strauss JS, Pochi PE (1961) The quantitative gravimetric determination of sebum production. J Invest Dermatol 36: 293

Stüttgen G, Atzwanger P (1961) Zur urticariogenen Wirkung des Schweißes. Hautarzt 12: 449

Stüttgen G, Krause H (1957) Zur Bewertung abnormer Hautgefäßreaktionen beim endogenen Ekzem und Asthma. Allergie Asthma 3: 206

Stüttgen G, Nassabi M, Herrmann F (1968) Einfluß trockener Wärmeexposition auf die Parotisspeichelsekretion unter besonderer Berücksichtigung der konstitutionellen Neurodermitis. Arch Klin Exp Dermatol 231: 231

Sulzberger MB, Herrmann F (1954) The clinical significance of disturbances in the delivery of sweat. Thomas, Springfield

Sulzberger MB, Herrmann F, Zak FG (1947) Studies of sweating. I. Preliminary report with particular emphasis on the sweat retention syndrome. J Invest Dermatol 9: 221

Sulzberger MB, Herrmann F, Borota A, Strauss MB (1953) Studies on sweating. VI. On the urticariogenic properties of human sweat. J Invest Dermatol 21: 293

Sulzberger MB, Herrmann F, Morill SD, Pacher F, Miller K (1959) Studies of sweat, lipids and histopathology in children with dry skin (xerosis). Int Arch Allergy Appl Immunol 14: 129

Swanbeck G (1968) A new treatment of ichthyosis and other hyperkeratotic conditions. Acta Derm Venereol (Stockh) 48: 123

Szentivanyi A (1968) The beta adrenergic theory of the atopic abnormality in bronchial asthma. J Allergy 42: 203

Tagami H, Ohi M, Iwatsuki K, Kanamaru Y, Yamida M, Ichyi B (1980) Evaluation of the skin surface hydration in vivo by electrical measurement. J Invest Dermatol 82: 188

Thiele FAJ, Senden KG van (1967) Relationship between skin temperature and the insensible perspiration of the human skin. J Invest Dermatol 47: 307

Thomsen K, Osmundsen P (1965) Guanethidine in the treatment of atopic dermatitis. Arch Dermatol 92: 418

Thomson ML, Sutarman A (1953) The identification and enumeration of active sweat glands in man from plastic impressions of the skin. Trans R Soc Trop Med Hyg 47: 412

Thune P, Kocsis M (1975) Effects of adrenergic stimulation and blocking agents on the eccrine sweat secretion in atopic dermatitis and psoriasis. Arch Dermatol Res 253: 97

Thune P, Rajka G (1974) Investigations of thurfyl nicotinate and metacholine reactions in atopic dermatitis by photoelectric reflectometry and plethysmography. Arch Dermatol Res 250: 258

Triebkorn A, Gloor M, Greiner F (1983) Comparative investigations on the water content of the stratum corneum using different methods of measurement. Dermatologica 167: 74

Uehara M, Ofuji S (1977) Abnormal vascular reactions in atopic dermatitis. Arch Dermatol 113: 627

van Staak VJBM, Kuiper JP (1971) Peripheral circulation in atopics. Dermatologica 42: 10

Warndorff JA (1970) The response of sweat glands to acetylcholine in atopic subjects. Br J Dermatol 83: 306

Warndorff J (1972 a) The response of sweat glands to beta-adrenergic stimulation. Br J Dermatol 86: 282

Warndorff J (1972 b) Continue registratie van Zweetsecretie. Thesis, Brakkenstein, University of Nijmegen

Weber RG, Roth GM, Kierland RR (1955) Further contributions to the vascular physiology of atopic dermatitis. J Invest Dermatol 24: 19

Weiss W (1956) Nicotinic acid blood levels on retention to skin responses. Am J Med Sci 231: 13

Werner Y (1986) The water content of the stratum corneum in patients with atopic dermatitis. Measurements with the corneometer CM 420. Acta Derm Venereol (Stockh) 66: 281

Werner Y, Lindberg M (1985) Transepidermal water loss in dry and clinically normal skin in patients with atopic dermatitis. Acta Derm Venereol (Stockh) 65: 102

Werner Y, Lindberg M, Forslind B (1982) The water-binding capacity of stratum corneum in dry non-eczematous skin of atopic dermatitis. Acta Derm Venereol (Stockh) 62: 334

Werner Y, Lindberg M, Forslind B (1987) Membrane-coating granules in "dry"non-eczematous skin of patients with atopic dermatitis. Acta Derm Venereol (Stockh) 67: 385

West JR, Kierland KK, Litin EM (1961) Atopic dermatitis and hypnosis. Arch Dermatol 84: 579

West JR, Johnson LA, Winkelmann RK (1962) Delayed blanch phenomenon in atopic individuals without dermatitis. Arch Dermatol 85: 227

Wheatley VR (1965) Secretion of the skin in eczema. J Pediatr 66 (part 2): 200

Whitfield A (1938) On the white reaction (white line) in dermatology. Br J Dermatol 50: 71

Wilkin KJ, Wilkin O, Kapp R, Donachie R, Chernosky ME, Buckner J (1982) Aspirin blocks nicotinic acid-induced flushing. Clin Pharmacol Ther 31: 478

Winkelmann RR, Wilhelmj CM (1963) Variations of skin reactions to vasodilators: metacholine (Mecholyl) and Trafuril. J Invest Dermatol 41: 313

Wirth H, Gloor M, Stoika D (1981) Sebaceous glands in uninvolved skin of patients suffering from atopic dermatitis. Arch Dermatol Res 270: 167

8 Pathomechanism: Attempt at Synthesis

8.1 Animal Models

One early ambition was to find a suitable animal model for AD. Although experiments on mice, guinea pigs, and rabbits may give some information on certain immunological traits also relevant for atopic allergy (e.g., Björksten and Ahlstedt 1984), the skin disease cannot be reproduced in these animals. Therefore, significant progress was made when it was discovered that dogs can suffer from atopic disease, primarily due to pollen inhalation (Patterson 1960; Anderson 1975). Of special interest for dermatologists was the fact that "the dog manifests its atopic state almost exclusively by pruritus" (Halliwell and Schwartzman 1971), mostly in facial, pedal, and axillary regions, or in a generalized form (Schwartzman 1971; Nesbitt 1978). Consequently, AD is their predominant atopic disease (Patterson 1969; Scott 1981). In 14 basenji–greyhound crossbreed dogs also demonstrating respiratory hyperreactivity, lichenified plaques and inflammatory papulonodules were registered. In these dogs it was possible to demonstrate impaired cAMP responsiveness to β-adrenergic stimuli and, after challenge with antigen aerosol, release of histamine and slow reacting substance was observed (Butler et al. 1983).

In a series of studies, Willemse and Van der Brom (1983) and Willemse (1984) investigated 208 dogs with AD, predominantly boxers, terriers, German shepherds, and poodles, and compared the localization of lesions and the diagnostic features with the human criteria of Hanifin and Rajka (1980). These included lichenification (in 84%), superficial staphylococcal pyoderma (25%), and dry seborrhea (23%); on the other hand there was no food intolerance. Intradermal testing with different inhalative allergens gave positive results, mostly to house dust, human and animal dander (including dog dandruff), and summer pollens, in 81% of the investigated dogs. Previously, a homologue of IgE had been detected in sera of atopic dogs and verified by RAST (Halliwell et al. 1972; Halliwell and Kunkle 1978). Willemse (1984) found in addition IgGd antibodies via ELISA in 84% of 62 dogs with AD, which showed properties similar to IgG S-TS antibodies in man (see Sect. 5.5.4); these were, however, classified as a secondary diagnostic feature of canine AD.

8.2 Attempt at Synthesis

As described in Chaps. 5–7, there are a number of facts and confirmed observations concerning the complex mechanisms of AD and their many aspects. A summary of the enumerated major factors is given below:

1. *Genetic constitution,* in agreement with the family history of the majority of AD patients, is a basic trait of obvious importance. This is particularly so in connection with immunological mechanisms such as impairment of the cyclic nucleotide metabolism, but there are still many unknown correlations.

2. From the broad field of immunological factors a multiple immunoregulatory defect seems plausible:

a) The *immediate-type* reaction between common environmental (atopic) allergens and in vivo/in vitro readily produced and subsequently (mast) cell-bound IgE antibodies, has a central role in atopy, even if nonimmune factors can similarly provoke atopic symptoms. Concerning AD, the role of inhalants and food allergens (except at an early age) is generally considered to be of less importance. This view, however, can be challenged on the basis of newer data: (a) the role if mite allergens may be not insignificant, (b) inhalants can act as contact allergens, (c) foods – and other allergens – can elicit IgE antibody complexes influencing, for example, T cells, mast cells, and macrophages, and (d) a late-phase reaction, previously overlooked, may develop. The author's view is that these allergens primarily act through itch provocation.

b) The impaired *delayed* reactivity demonstrable in vivo and in vitro may mostly be attributed to defective T suppressor cell function which supposedly leads to increased IgE production. Although this correlation has not been confirmed by all investigators, the concept may be a bridge between increased immediate and decreased delayed reactivity in AD. The IgE-bearing Langerhans' cells, which cooperate with eosinophils, may be considered as another possible link between type I and IV immune reactions. Impairment of NK, monocyte, and leukocyte functions leads to reduced resistance to living agents and may cause reduced T(suppressor) cell functions. The major clinical consequences are frequent staphylococcal and viral infections. Furthermore, although cytotoxic cells may be deficient in number, according to one opinion autocytotoxic cells may mediate skin damage, e.g., via fibroblast killing (see Sect. 5.7.2).

Some data also point to impairment of T helper and B cell functions in AD.

c) The *infiltrates* in AD with predominant T helper cells and antigen-presenting cells reveal the paradox that not only reduced tuberculin-type and contact allergic reactivity exists in AD but, without doubt, a type IV response, clinically expressed as an eczematous reaction.

3. The releasability of mast cells, mostly as a result of an immediate reaction, accounts for the easily liberated histamine. Histamine has an obvious relevance in the pathomechanism of AD as it elicits itch, vascular reactions, and, in addition to the inflammatory effects, also has important immunoregulatory functions via H_2-receptors, not least in increasing neutrophil and T cell functions/cell-mediated immunity. LT B_4, probably via chemoattraction of leukocytes, similar to certain complement components, may also have a not unimportant

mediator role, while some prostaglandins are considered to be itch-potentiating agents. Monokines, like interleukin-1 and interleukin-2, may participate in the activation of T cells. Interferon-γ may be involved in the anti-infectious resistance.

The role of acetylcholine, in perhaps counterbalancing adrenergic influences, is still under debate.

The fact that bone marrow transplantation from a nonatopic donor has healed the Wiskott-Aldrich syndrome indicates the significance of mononuclears and mast cells, i.e., bone marrow derived cells, in AD.

4. The cyclic nucleotide metabolism of mononuclears, mast cells, and neutrophils is faulty in AD and is the cause of a reduction in cAMP activity, which therefore cannot dampen the inflammatory reaction. This is probably represented by an increased PDE activity. Already present in cord blood, this hyperreactivity is a possible marker for AD and may perhaps explain the mast cell releasability.

5. In Chap. 7 arguments have been presented for the major pathomechanistic role of alterations of the AD skin, illustrated by several changed functions of the symptom-free skin. These alterations primarily include the increased itchiness and further morphological changes, disturbances in water exchange and sebum production, and vascular dysregulation. The alterations of the skin may be analogous to changes in other target organs involved in atopy, and one may speculate that differences between respiratory atopy and AD depend on the structure and function of the involved organ, where the immune/nonimmune alterations occur in varying degrees.

All of these pathomechanistic aspects have been mentioned earlier in this book and by several other authors; there are, however, many questions related to them, some as yet unanswered. One of these questions is, which of the factors are of primary and which of secondary character. In Table 8.1 these factors are distinguished according to whether they influence the course of AD or are

Table 8.1. Putative primary and secondary immunological and pathophysiological events in the mechanism of AD

Putative primary events (influencing the course of AD)	Putative secondary events (dependent on the course of AD)
1. Increased itch	1. Itchy skin
2. Increased PDE activity	2. High IgE production
3. Dry skin/reduced lipid secretion/stratum corneum alteration/increased TWL/reduced water content/impaired barrier function	3. Reduced cell-mediated immunity
	4. Reduced anti-infectious resistance/reduced chemotaxis
Lower resistance to irritants	5. Vascular disturbances
Increased staphylococcal colonization	6. Sweat disturbances (?)
4. Mast cell releasability(?)	
5. Disturbed metabolism of linoleic acid in serum lecithin(?)	

(?), possibly pertinent to the other group

dependent on it. Otherwise the definition "primary" is rather problematic, for there may always be an event which can be considered as preceding the assumed "primary" phenomenon. There exist excellent designs illustrating concepts concerning the mechanisms of AD, with various opinions on the importance and correlations of the different putative etiological factors (Pillsbury et al. 1961; Sulzberger 1971, 1983; Borelli and Schnyder 1965; Hanifin and Lobitz 1977; Ring 1981; Wütrich 1983; Leung and Geha 1986; and others). These are more or less adapted to the rapidly developing progress in the field, and often only cover one aspect, e.g., the immuno-(biochemical) data. The author attempts to justify his own hypothesis because his aim is to place the major symptom of the disease in the center of postulated events, and he pays great attention to the condition of skin where the different pathomechanistic phenomena take place. These are considered in an attempt to briefly define the disease: *AD is a specific dermatitis in the abnormally reacting skin of the atopic resulting in itch with sequelae, as well as in eczematous inflammation.* In creating a pathomechanistic model it is important not to overlook the last step, i.e., how the putative factors de facto elicit the clinical disease, as it is, for instance, known that demonstrable aspects of delayed hypersensitivity in AD in vitro are not entirely identical with in vivo results. Therefore the author made an attempt to place the most prominent clinical symptom, the itch, in the center of the pathomechanism. Based on the data mentioned in the previous chapters, the author's present interpretation of the pathomechanism of AD is summarized in Fig. 8.1. The aim of a design ought not to be to press all data into the Procrustean bed of the model but rather to provide input upon which others may improve. Also of relevance is the difference between the statically presented factors of the mechanism and the dynamic, changeable disease. To explain this difference, one has to imagine a vicious circle between some major stages in the mechanism, e.g., as illustrated in certain immunological events: interplay of

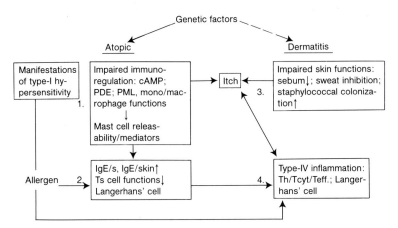

Fig. 8.1. Mechanism of AD: attempt at synthesis. *cAMP,* cyclic 3,5,-adenosine monophosphate; *PDE,* phosphodiesterase; *PML,* polymorph leukocytes; *Mono,* monocyte; *IgE/s,* IgE in serum; *Ts,* T suppressor cell; *Th,* T helper cell; *Tcyt,* cytotoxic T cell; *Teff,* T effector cell

Table 8.2. Synopsis for the clinician

Most stimuli, either on allergic or nonimmunological basis, reaching the skin outwardly or inwardly (incl. emotional influences) elicit or maintain *itch:*

In AD there is an immunological *imbalance,* and therefore:
1. Low defense against living agents
2. Many positive immediate reactions with variable clinical significance

In AD there is a *dysfunctioning* skin, and therefore:
1. The skin is less resistant to solvents and irritation
2. It is overcolonized with staphylococci
3. Sweating leads to itch

IgE and T cell functions, histamine immunoregulation, etc. (see, e.g., Ring 1981). Furthermore, some important factors influencing the course of the disease, sometimes barely discernible from etiological influences, should be considered (see Chap. 9).

For the clinician a summary is given in Table 8.2.

References

Andersson W (1975) Atopic dermatitis in the dog. Cutis 15: 955

Björksten B, Ahlstedt S (1984) Relevance of animal models for studies of immune regulation of atopic allergy. Allergy 39: 317

Borelli S, Schnyder UW (1965) Neurodermitis constitutionalis sive atopica, II. In: Miescher G, Storck H (eds) Entzündliche Dermatosen. II. Springer, Berlin Heidelberg New York, p 254 (Handbuch der Haut- und Geschlechtskrankheiten, vol II/1)

Butler JM, Peters JE, Hirshman CA, White CR, Margolin LB, Hanifin JM (1983) Pruritic dermatitis in asthmatic basenji-greyhound dogs: a model for human atopic dermatitis. J Am Acad Dermatol 8: 33

Haliwell REW, Kunkle GA (1978) The radioallergosorbent test in the diagnosis of canine atopic disease. J Allergy Clin Immunol 62: 236

Haliwell REW, Schwartzman RM, Rockey JH (1972) Antigen relationship between human. IgE and canine IgE. Clin Exp Immunol 10: 399

Haliwell REW, Schwartzman RM (1971) Atopic disease in the dog. Vet Rec 89: 209

Hanifin JM, Lobitz WC (1977) Newer concepts of atopic dermatitis. Arch Dermatol 113: 663

Hanifin JM, Rajka G (1980) Diagnostic features of atopic dermatitis. Acta Derm Venereol [Suppl 144] (Stockh) 92: 44

Leung DYM, Geha RS (1986) Immunoregulatory abnormalities in atopic dermatitis. Clin Rev Allergy 4: 67

Nesbitt CH (1978) Canine allergic inhalant dermatitis: a review of 230 cases. J Am Vet Assoc 172: 55

Patterson R (1960) Investigations of spontaneous hypersensitivity of the dog. J Allergy 31: 351

Patterson R (1969) Laboratory models of reaginic allergy. Progr Allergy 13: 322

Pillsbury DM, Shelley WB, Kligman AM (1961) A manual of cutaneous medicine. Saunders, London, p 93

Ring J (1981) Atopic dermatitis: a disease of immuno-vegetative (autonomic) dysregulation. In: Ring J, Burg G (eds) New trends in allergy. Springer, Berlin Heidelberg New York, p 237

Schwartzman RM (1971) Current veterinary therapy. IV. Saunders, Philadelphia, p 282

Scott DW (1981) Observation on canine atopy. J Am Anim Hosp Assoc 17: 91

Sulzberger M (1971) Atopic dermatitis. In: Fitzpatrick TB, Arndt KA, Clark WH jr, Eisen AZ, van Scott EJ, Vaughan JH (eds) Dermatology in general medicine, Part III. McGraw-Hill, New York, p 680

Sulzberger MB (1983) Historical notes on atopic dermatitis: its names and nature. Semin Dermatol 2: 1

Willemse A (1984) Investigations on canine atopic dermatitis. Thesis, University of Utrecht

Willemse A, van den Brom WE (1983) Investigations of the symptomatology and the significance of immediate skin test reactivity in canine atopic dermatitis. Res Vet Sci 34: 261

Wütrich B (1983) Neurodermitis atopica sive constitutionalis. Akt Dermatol 9: 1

9 Factors Influencing the Course of AD

Experience has shown that several factors may influence the course of the disease, acting as triggers or having a beneficial effect, and as most of these are known also to play some part in the obscure and complex etiology of AD, no sharp distinction can usually by drawn between etiological factors (mentioned in Sect. 5.8) and those influencing the course. However, as the latter usually have no *primary* causal importance, it seems more practical to include them in a separate chapter.

9.1 Seasonal Dependence

It is well known that there are seasonal changes in the course of the disease, many AD patients showing a tendency to improve in summer, but the data vary in different geographical areas and climates. Such seasonal changes are seen in all but a minority of patients, who usually have severe AD which runs a continuous course; in the author's experience they comprise 10% of all cases, an incidence which fits in well with the data of Schnyder (1957) but which is lower than the figure reported by other workers, including Oddoze (1959).

These seasonal variations generally consist of deterioration in winter and improvement in summmer, and they occur in such regions as Northwest Europe, the United Kingdom, Scandinavia, and the United States. It is well known that a large number of AD patients, often the majority, show this deterioration in winter even in the sunny, dry, but cold climate found in South Africa (Loewenthal 1957). It was suggested by Pirilä (1950) that, in winter, the shorter duration of daylight rather than the lower temperature plays the principal role in this common seasonal deterioration. Certainly, house dust cannot be incriminated, for the exacerbation is more common in cases in which skin tests with house dust are negative than in those with positive reactions (Schnyder 1957).

The consensus is that the improvement commonly seen in summer results chiefly from exposure to the sun and from sea bathing. Such improvement was found in 76% of the author's cases, and, on analysis of the possible causes, no association with sensitivity to allergens was found, although there was some evidence that reactivity to summer pollens was a little more common in cases that deteriorated compared with those that improved in summer; the relevant figures were 28.3% and 17.3% respectively. Clearly, various factors may be responsible for improvement or deterioration in summer, these being summarized in Table 9.1 (see also summer prurigo in Chapter 2).

Table 9.1. Factors influencing the course of AD during summer

Improvement may be due to:	Aggravation may be due to:
Better sebum and sweat secretion	Extreme sweating (strong heat)
Sun baths (infrared rays and sweating? ultraviolet rays?)	Increased exposure to sunlight
Sea bathing (keratolytic effect?)	Irritation following sea bathing of long duration
Reduced exposure to dust and mold indoors	Increased exposure to molds outdoors
Changes of environment (beneficial climatic and "allergen" conditions)	Changes of environment (unfavorable climatic and "allergen" conditions
Intake of less spiced food	Increased intake of fruits, vegetables
Holidays (elimination of irritants, allergens, beneficial psychological influences)	Increased contact with animals, pollens
Improvement of skin circulation. Nonuse of woollen clothes	
Less danger of infections in the upper respiratory tract	
Metabolic changes, such as increased activity of the adrenal cortex?	

Table 9.2. Rate of AD cases with seasonal dependence

	Schnyder (1957)	Rajka (1961)
Winter deteriorated cases	54%	48%
Summer deteriorated cases	15%	14%
Spring deteriorated cases	13%	19%
Autumn deteriorated cases	8%	9%
Cases without seasonal dependence	10%	10%

During the short spring in Scandinavia, which starts rather late, it has been found that only 5% of AD patients improve, whereas 19% deteriorate and 66% remain unchanged; the residual 10% show no seasonal variation whatsoever. The incidence of sensitivity to spring pollens, such as from trees and especially birch, is higher in cases deteriorating in spring than is the overall incidence of pollen sensitivity. The relevant figures are 36% and 20.1% respectively; thus spring pollen may well play a minor role. It should be noted that these data refer to "pure" AD patients, no atopic respiratory symptoms being evident. Most patients remain unchanged in the autumn, although 9% deteriorate. Finally, with regard to seasonal deterioration, there is remarkably good agreement between the data from Scandinavia and those from Switzerland (see Table 9.2). Young (1980) looked at the problem from another angle and registered first visits of AD patients, or their complaints, in relation to different seasons. He found an accumulation of complaints in the autumn and related this primarily to persons with house dust allergy, like asthmatics, seeking medical advice in autumn. Patients with spring and summer complaints included persons with pollen allergy. Imai et al. (1987) observed over a period of 5 years several AD patients who deteriorated during the summer and attributed this to a high relative humidity and temperature, with subsequent sweating, in this region of Japan. Types of heating may also have some relevance.

9.2 Climatic Factors

In several respects this topic is strictly correlated with the effects of season on the course of AD, as the number of cases influenced by climate corresponds to the number which vary with season. The role played by weather is very complex, the following being triggers of AD: sudden changes in temperature, high atmospheric pressure, and strong winds. A humid climate is not detrimental to all types of the disease, as cases with severe keratin plugging of sweat ducts do well in hot humid environments which hydrate the keratin; on the other hand, Sulzberger (1955) indicated that, if the sweat disturbance in AD is due to swelling of the stratum corneum and to edema of tissues surrounding the duct and its opening, a dry warm climate is more beneficial.

A sea voyage or residence at a seaside resort in a sunny climate or in the highlands has a beneficial effect on AD. Of 440 cases of the disease at a Mediterranean allergy clinic (La Roche Posay):

35% came from regions with a continental climate
23% came from regions with a highland climate
21% came from regions with an oceanic climate
17% came from regions with a Mediterranean climate.

According to these figures a sunny Mediterranean climate is twice as beneficial as a continental one (Oddoze 1966). The favorable effect of a sunny climate like that of California or Florida, or of a dry warm climate as in Arizona or Egypt, has been stressed in several reports (see also Sect. 12.2.1). An interesting observation of the incidence of AD in families living first in Singapore then moving to Germany indicates the role of the relative humidity on the course of the disease (Hindson 1976).

The author has sent questionnaires to dermatologists associated with university departments or in private practice living in Asia, Australia, New Zealand, Latin America, and Africa, i.e., to countries outside Europe and North America, where there are abundant data on AD problems in the literature. Based on answers from 34 countries there was unanimous agreement on the role of climatic factors in the disease (Rajka 1986) (see Table 9.3).

Table 9.3. Climatic factors influencing AD

Factor	Effect	Remarks
Cold dry weather	Aggravating (as a rule)	Due to dryness
Hot humid weather	Frequently aggravating	Due to perspiration and secondary infection. High relative humidity sometimes claimed as beneficial
Cold humid weather	Frequently aggravating	Example: winter in Latin America
Warm dry weather	Frequently aggravating	Example: in the Middle East. In some cases claimed as beneficial (UV effect?)

9.3 Some Environmental Factors

Further environmental factors include a change of residence or hospitalization. Nexmand (1948) noted improvement after a change of residence in 9 of 17 patients with AD, most of whom had moved from damp to dry houses or had sensitivity to house dust and molds. With regard to indoor molds, housing is of particular importance; this the author demonstrated in 30 "pure" AD cases with positive skin test responses to molds. Many of these patients lived in wooden houses, deteriorated clinically in humid summer residences, or were even worse during rainy weather. Furthermore, there are reports indicating that individual patients with AD may derive clinical improvement from moving to a house with less exposure to molds ("dry" residences).

Siemens and Jagtman (1951) emphasized the frequently confirmed observation that a period of hospitalization often may itself, in the absence of therapy, improve AD, as the new environment is free of relevant allergens and trigger factors. These authors were of the opinion that the regular occurrence in hospital of a spontaneous remission in young as well as in older cases rebuts the essential role attributed to psychic factors in this response; however, psychic factors apparently cannot be discounted entirely in some of these cases. Several authors suggest that air pollution may decrease the threshold or directly aggravate AD, although this obvious possibility has yet not been systematically studied. Among the substances nitrous gases and SO_2 are most frequently mentioned.

9.4 Socioeconomic Environment

Most AD patients are city dwellers, living usually in highly industrialized countries; these facts may be relevant to the reports by Marchionini et al. (1958) and Marchionini (1960) in which it was pointed out that cultural influences, civilization, urbanization, and "psychointellectual" stress all promote the occurrence of the disease. Whereas about 41% of all patients attending the Munich Dermatological Clinic were city inhabitants, 62% of the AD patients of this clinic were city dwellers; similar findings were reported by Pirilä (1950). Studies have been performed on groups of people who, after settling in a more developed urban environment, have shown a rise in the incidence of AD. For example, in Jamaicans who have moved to London and in emigrants from Taiwan to Honolulu or to San Francisco, AD occurs more frequently than it does in the population not only of their country of origin but also of the city in which they have settled (Davis et al. 1961; Worth 1962).

The social milieu also exerts an influence on nutritional conditions and is therefore related to the incidence of AD, which is commoner in well-nourished children. However, comparison of the weights of infantile AD cases and of controls has produced conflicting results, the atopic babies being heavier according to de Graciansky (1966) but the same weight as the controls according to Sedlis (1965). There are more arguments for, than against, a correlation between over-nutrition and AD.

Although sociological studies have been undertaken, most reports concern "exclusive" series, that is, patients attending dermatological clinics. Thus in the series from Munich quoted above, it was found that the patients or their parents tended to belong to a higher than average social class (Borelli and Schnyder 1965). There are obvious and numerous sources of error in such investigations; in consequence, this problem has not been definitely solved to date. Interestingly, the author's above-mentioned study of 34 countries could not confirm the significance of socioeconomic factors. It seems that social class has no primary influence on the development of the disease, and even the data on industrialization and urbanization are inconclusive (Rajka 1986).

9.5 Occupation

The occupation and the socioeconomic status of the individual are closely interrelated. According to statistical surveys (Fuchs 1956; Borelli 1970), AD occurs more frequently in occupations in which exposure to dust, wool, textiles, hairs, or lipid solvents is relatively common; yet, in working conditions under which contact dermatitis often occurs, there is no parallel incidence of AD. The greatest sufferers from the disease are tradesmen, followed by industrial and agricultural workers. Fuchs (1956) listed: textile workers, furriers, and hairdressers as the occupational groups most "threatened" by AD. According to the author's experience the following occupational factors are mostly negative for AD patients: work in a hot environment, wet work, work with strong defatting substances, strong chemical/mechanical irritants (including wool), strong inhalant allergens, and working places with a high risk of infection (see also Table 11.1). The results of the quoted questionnaires sent to dermatologists from 34 countries pointed to the following occupations as potentially aggravating the course of AD:

Farming/working outdoors (including building)
Business/studying/intellectual work

i.e. a list which was, in part, contrary to expectations. A possible explanation might be as follows: farmers were highly represented in the clientele of the doctors participating in the study, and in intellectual workers psychological stress may be an important trait. Involvement of the hand in housewives with AD, primarily due to irritants (e.g., detergents, wet work), is a very frequent and well-known occurrence (Rystedt 1985 and others). In summary, although various occupations have been implicated as representing a risk for AD patients, there is no doubt that some are particularly hazardous, such as hairdressing (Wilkinson and Hambly 1978; Cronin and Kullavanijaya 1979), baking (Järvinen et al. 1980), and wet work in hospitals.

Atopics have a 13.5 times greater risk of developing an occupational skin problem according to Keil and Shmunes (1983). These skin problems predominantly affect the hands, and a correlation between (mostly irritative) occupational hand eczema and AD has been reported by several authors (Glickman and Silvers 1967; Agrup 1969; Adams 1981). Lammintausta and Kalimo (1981) and Lammintausta et al. (1982) reported that among hospital workers, hand dermatitis occurred in 65% of persons with atopic symptoms and in 75% of those with dry itchy hands (and atopic relatives), and that this hand dermatitis most frequently developed during the first year of their service. In a thorough study of 2452 newly employed hospital workers the chance of developing hand eczema either in wet or in dry work was three times greater for AD subjects, and they also suffered the disease more severely (Nilsson et al. 1985). The predicted probability of developing hand eczema was 91% in subjects with a combination of atopy, earlier hand involvement, and metal dermatitis (Nilsson 1986).

A retrospective study comprising 549 previously hospitalized AD patients showed a large number with hand eczema, and in most of these cases it had been present since childhood. The role of moisture and of contact with chemicals was hard to evaluate on objective grounds, but was an important complaint of the patients and had led to change of work – mostly spontaneous – in 55 cases. The majority of these patients had felt better therefore, but healing occurred in only one-quarter. These data thus provide evidence for the deleterious effect of wet work and chemicals on AD, and especially on hand lesions (Rystedt 1981, 1985).

Of contact allergens nickel was primarily mentioned, but junior hairdressers already had a high prevalence of nickel allergy at the start of their apprenticeship, probably due to ear-piercing (van der Burg et al. 1986). Interestingly, positive patch tests showed the same frequency for AD patients with or without hand involvement and could not explain the development of hand afflication (Forsbeck et al. 1983).

The consequences of hand involvement due to occupational factors in AD patients are quite serious with regard to the possibility of them continuing their work. Table 9.4 shows the data of Marchionini et al. (1958), of the author (Rajka 1961), and of Borelli (1970). Forsbeck et al. (1983) also emphasized that AD patients with hand lesions changed job more often than those with unaffected hands. Shmunes and Keil (1984) stated that atopy was represented in 93% of those who lost their jobs due to a work-related cause. Among 31 patients with

Table 9.4. The influence of AD on the occupational activity of the patients

	Marchionini et al. (1958)	Rajka (1961)	Borelli (1970)
Patients hindered in occupational activity	33%	20%	57%
Patients hindered in occupational career	29%		46%
Patients who changed occupation (once)	20%	3%	19%

AD only 35% had no reported difficulty, while 16% experienced limited career opportunities, 42% functional difficulty, and 19% interpersonal difficulty (Jowett S and Ryan T personal communication).

9.6 Psychological Factors

The very complex question of the influence of psychological factors will be dealt with only briefly here. No specific psychic disturbance characteristic of the disease has been found, and no predisposition to a particular personality could be established (Kuypers 1968), although there is a preponderance of the emotionally labile type (Kepecs et al. 1951). However, as in many other psychosomatic disturbances, it is generally possible to find evidence that the patient tends to repress his emotions, in that he has difficulty in expressing aggression towards the outside world, and that he not infrequently directs it towards himself instead; in this respect, scratching could be interpreted as an attempt at self-punishment (Kierland and Walsh 1950). According to another study, however, outward expression of aggression was a common as in controls, although latent hostility was greater in AD patients (Jordan and Whitlock 1972). The influence of maternal rejection has often been discussed (Miller and Baruch 1948; Williams 1951; Privat and Ferran 1972) and is of importance during the critical first months after birth (Musaph 1964); on the other hand, maternal overprotection is also often to be found.

Ring et al. (1986) and Ring and Palos (1986) investigated psychosomatic aspects in 55 children with AD via psychological tests. One of these, the Freiburger Personality Inventory, revealed that the mothers of children with AD were less spontaneous and less emotional than were the mothers of controls. The style of education was in general more strict and the mothers favored adult behavior in their children. In children's drawings the mothers were drawn larger than the fathers, a friendly atmosphere was lacking, and unpleasant, dangerous animals were drawn. This expresses that although there is no typical atopic child personality, these children more often display aggressive thoughts towards their parents than do controls. Furthermore, when the patient and his environment are at loggerheads, a state of tension may result and exacerbate his skin disease. These psychological disturbances, in the view of the author and others, including Jagtman (1951), elicit or act on the key symptom of AD, namely the pruritus; then the typical skin lesions ensue.

Jordan and Whitlock (1972) assume that AD patients develop scratch responses more readily and that these subside more slowly. As Whitlock (1976) concludes: "Once again let it be said that the fundamental problem in this disorder from the psychophysiological point of view is the inherent tendency of the skin to itch with small provocation."

The sequence of the psychosomatic events may be triggered by other psychological symptoms as well, e.g., fear and tension, which can influence blood vessels; such vascular responses have, in fact, been reproduced by suggestion (Schnyder and Borelli 1965). The influence of emotion on sweat glands also deserves mention in this context. According to Borelli and Schnyder (1965), psychic influences together with education, stress, and socioenvironmental factors may lead to autonomic dysregulation (Korting 1954), and here the asthenic overreactivity or fear reaction, as a consequence of relative sympathetic hypertonia of the skin, plays a role in the pathological vascular responses. Follow-up interviews 20 years after initial diagnosis showed that stress was the primary trigger of symptoms (Hanifin et al. 1986). Based on animal experiments and observations on gastric hemorrhagia, Reimann et al. (1981) concluded that histamine may be a stress mediator. It is essential, however, not to overlook the converse situation, clearly pointed out by Sulzberger (1955), in which violent pruritus, insomnia, and serious disfigurement of the skin, which is known to play an important role in communication with environment, combine to produce secondary psychological disturbances; if the skin disease improves, the psychopathological features described above are frequently seen to disappear. Whitlock (1976) also comments that abnormal personality traits are variable and dependent upon age and the clinical state of the patient's skin at the time of examination. He further suggests that these abnormal patient features cannot be considered as the primary cause of AD. These arguments support the concept that somatic factors play a primary role, yet no clinician with many years' experience of this disease can dispute the influence psychological factors have on AD despite the unsatisfactory results of psychotherapy in such patients reported by Borelli and Schnyder (1965), or the only exceptionally beneficial responses recorded by Brown and Bettley (1971). It is in fact impossible to have a definite opinion as to whether psychological or somatic factors play the main role in this complex disease, but from a practical point of view the interrelation between these two factors, psychological and somatic, often creates a vicious circle in the patient during certain phases of his disease. From the practical point of view, over 70% of the dermatologists from the 34 countries suggested that psychic stress is a frequent aggravating factor for AD patients (Rajka 1986).

9.7 Other Factors

9.7.1 Military Service and Sports

The effect of military service on the course of AD also merits mention, as difficulties frequently arise for male patients in the armed forces due, for example, to changes in living and working conditions and to the presence of different allergens. Approximately 20% of male cases deteriorate; the results of an analysis of 19 such patients are shown in Table 9.5.

Unfortunately sports and different kinds of physical efforts so important for young people (though not only for them) very frequently elicit sweating with subsequent itch and temporary deterioration of the condition.

Table 9.5. Analysis of 19 of 100 male AD patients who showed deterioration during military service

	Results of immediate skin tests							Owing to the skin disease the patient was	
Reg. no.	Animal hair	Dust, mold	Food	Pollen	Others	The patient suspects as deteriorating factors:	Other manifestations	Placed in a lower class	Exempted from military service
53/111	+	+	+	+	II/9–10	Dust, wool, straw, fumes			
119					IV/5	Petroleum			
132		+					Rhinitis		
136[a]		Negative							
183[a]	+	+	+						
56/ 93		Negative						+	
103		+			II/10				
108	+	+	+	+					
135	+	+		+			Rhinitis	+	
140		Negative							
151	+					Grooming			
57/ 79	+	+		+	II/9–10	Dust, straw		+	
100				+			Rhinitis		+
104	+	+		+		Straw, tidying			
111					II/9–10	Navy blue uniform		b	
130				+		Sweating			
58/ 86	+	+	+	+			Rhinitis		+
87	+		+	+			Rhinitis		
89		Negative				Heat, moisture, uniform			

[a] Had a recurrence of AD in military service
[b] Placed in a lower class for scoliosis
II/9–10: staphylococcal extracts
IV/5: lycopodium extract

9.7.2 Hormonal Influences

The influence of the endocrine system on the course of AD is frequently discussed, but there is usually difficulty in separating this from related influences such as autonomic nervous system function or psychological factors. There is, however, convincing evidence that the level of certain hormones has a direct effect on the disease (Table 9.6), the course of which may sometimes appear to alter after major endocrinological changes. Thus, AD may improve around the time of onset of puberty (Lomholt 1944), especially in male patients. According to the author's statistics, symptom-free periods are significantly less frequent around the time of menarche; a percentage of girls in fact show pronounced deterioration of their dermatitis at that time. During puberty, there are numer-

Table 9.6. Effect of menstruation on the course of AD in 40 women

Better during menstruation	10 cases
Worse during menstruation	14 cases
Worse during the premenstrual period	13 cases
Worse during the postmenstrual period	3 cases

ous associated psychological difficulties and altercations with authority which may have a detrimental effect on AD in teenagers, especially in those who later have problems in selecting an occupation or a marital partner. This shows in the peak ages on admission to hospital for AD; these were found to be 15–16 years for females, and 17–18 years for males (Pirilä 1950).

There is controversy about the course of AD during pregnancy (Brunsting 1936; Nexmand 1948; Hellerström and Lidman 1956; Eichenberger 1963), but it seems that improvement and deterioration occur with about the same frequency; the effect was beneficial in 14, and detrimental in 11 of the author's 25 cases. In addition, the course of the disease in a single pregnancy may fluctuate, and in different pregnancies in the same patient, the disease may follow different courses. Premenstrual changes and pregnancy have not been shown to produce parallel effects on AD in the same patient. Finally, the course of the disease may change during lactation (Pirilä 1950; Rajka 1961; Eichenberger 1963).

9.7.3 Infections

Bacterial infections and vaccines may frequently elicit or exacerbate AD (for viral infections, see Chap. 2). Deterioration subsequent to upper respiratory tract infections has been reported in different studies, which recorded the following incidences: 39% (Norrlind 1946), 23% (Storck 1959), 27%–30% (Rajka 1961), and 47% (Hellerström and Lidman 1956). Such deterioration clearly cannot be caused by a single factor, and the roles of different bacteria, of viruses, and possibly of alterations in host resistance have to be taken into account; of relevance here is the statement by Urbach that infection is a predisposing factor in allergy (Urbach and Gottlieb 1946). Of all these possible factors, pyococci have provided the most fruitful source of information; a preponderance of staphylococci was found in the nose and the throat of AD patients by Herlitz (1956), but the results of such studies cannot entirely answer the questions which ask what effects upper respiratory tract infections have on AD and how they achieve them.

Investigating the development of atopic respiratory allergy, Backman et al. (1984) stated that infections in infancy do not facilitate it. The role of staphylococcal infection on the skin has been discussed earlier (see Chap. 2), and its relevance in the deterioration of the clinical state is well known.

9.7.4 Problems with Schooling in Young AD Patients

The fairly common problem of schooling in children with AD has been somewhat neglected by most authors. In detailed studies by the author it was found that about 30 of 40 schoolchildren with AD showed a tendency for schooling and the disease to have an adverse effect on each other. Thus, for most of these children, school presents a source of difficulty (Rajka 1961; Sonneck et al. 1967). The most frequently encountered problems were:

1. Difficulty in concentration due to pruritus
2. Deterioration of the skin disease due to sweating induced by physical training
3. The necessity of eating unsuitable foods
4. Absence from school due to the disease

According to Borelli (1970), the disease prevented or interfered with tuition at school in no less than 35% of a large series of AD children; such frequent absences from school may lead to future difficulties in occupational training. Counseling in cases of itch following physical efforts is difficult; often the unpopular advice of choosing between "health" and sports has to be given and the latter is, understandably, preferred by the child.

Some practical measures in connection with factors causing deterioration in the course of AD will be discussed in Chaps. 11 and 12.

References

Adams R (1981) High risk dermatoses. J Occup Med 23: 829

Agrup G (1969) Hand eczema and other hand dermatoses in South Sweden. Acta Derm Venereol [Suppl] (Stockh) 49: 61

Backman A, Björksten F, Ilmonen S, Juntinen K, Suoniemi I (1984) Do infections in infancy affect sensitization to airborne allergens and development of allergic diseases? Allergy 39: 309

Borelli S (1970) Dermatologische Klimatherapie und ihre Erfolgsbeurteilung. In: Braun Falco O, Bandmann HJ (eds) Fortschritte der Dermatologie, vol 6. Springer, Berlin Heidelberg New York, p 141

Borelli S, Schnyder UW (1965) Neurodermitis constitutionalis sive atopica. II. In: Miescher G, Storck H (eds) Entzündliche Dermatosen. II. Springer, Berlin Heidelberg New York, p 254 (Handbuch der Haut- und Geschlechtskrankheiten, vol II/1)

Brown DG, Bettley FR (1971) Psychiatric treatment of eczema: a controlled trial. Br Med J II: 729

Brunsting LA (1936) Atopic dermatitis (disseminated neurodermitis) of young adults. Arch Dermatol Syph 34: 935

Cronin E, Kullavanijaya P (1979) Hand dermatitis in hairdressers. Acta Derm Venereol [Suppl] (Stockh) 85: 47

Davis LR, Marten RH, Sarkany I (1961) Atopic eczema in European and Negro West Indian infants in London. Br J Dermatol 73: 41

de Graciansky P (1966) Eczéma constitutionnel. Soc Med Hop Paris 117: 765

Eichenberger ME (1963) Über Vorkommen, Verlauf, Testresultate und Therapie der Neurodermitis. Inauguraldissertation. Juris, Zürich

Forsbeck M, Skog E, Åsbrink E (1983) Atopic hand dermatitis. A comparison with atopic

214   Factors Influencing the Course of AD

dermatitis without hand involvement, especially with respect to influence of work and development of contact sensitization. Acta Derm Venereol (Stockh) 63: 9

Fuchs O (1956) Der Einfluß des Berufs auf das endogene Ekzem. Berufs Dermatosen 4: 225

Glickman FS, Silvers SH (1967) Hand eczema and atopy in housewives. Arch Dermatol 95: 487

Hanifin JM, Cooper KD, Roth HL (1986) Atopy and atopic dermatitis. Periodic synapsis. J Am Acad Dermatol 15: 703

Hellerström S, Lidman H (1956) Studies of Besnier's prurigo (atopic dermatitis). Acta Derm Venereol (Stockh) 36: 11

Herlitz G (1956) Bacterial infection and infantile eczema. Int Arch Allergy Appl Immunol 8: 160

Hindson TC (1976) Discussion to Vickers CHF et al. Br J Dermatol (Suppl 12): 130

Imai S, Takeuchi S, Mashiko T (1987) Jahreszeitliche Änderungen im Verlauf des atopischen Ekzems. Hautarzt 38: 599

Jagtman GG (1951) Symptomatische en Experimenteel-therapeutische Onderzoekingen over het Eczema pruriginosum faciei-flexurarum (Lichen Vidal disseminatus, Prurigo Besnier, Neurodermitis disseminata, Spätexsudatives ekzematoid, atopic dermatitis). Haasbek, Alphen a d Rijn

Järvinen KAI, Pirilä V, Björksten F, Keskinen H, Lehtinen M, Stubb S (1980) Unsuitability of bakery work for a person with atopy: a study of 234 bakery workers. Ann Allergy 42: 192

Jordan JM, Whitlock FA (1972) Emotions and the skin: the conditioning of scratch responses in cases of atopic dermatitis. Br J Dermatol 86: 574

Keil J, Shmunes E (1983) The epidemiology of work-related skin disease in South Carolina. Arch Dermatol 119: 650

Kepecs JG, Rabin A, Robin M (1951) Atopic dermatitis. A clinical psychiatric study. Psychosom Med 13: 1

Kierland RR, Walsh MN (1950) Correlation of the dermatologic and psychiatric approaches to the treatment of neurodermitis. Med Clin North Am 34: 1009

Korting GW (1954) Zur Pathogenese des endogenen Ekzems. Thieme, Stuttgart

Kuypers BRM (1968) Atopic dermatitis: some observations from a psychological viewpoint. Dermatologica 136: 387

Lammintausta K, Kalimo K (1981) Atopy and hand dermatitis in hospital wet work. Contact Dermatitis 7: 301

Lammintausta K, Kalimo K, Aantaa S (1982) Course of hand dermatitis in hospital workers. Contact Dermatitis 8: 327

Loewenthal LJA (1957) Atopic dermatitis. Geographical, climatic and racial factors. Acta Derm Venereol (Stockh) III: 14

Lomholt S (1944) Hudsygdommene og deres behandling. Gads, Copenhagen

Marchionini A (1960) Neuere Untersuchungen über die Neurodermitis constitutionalis. In: Marchionini A (ed) Fortschritte der praktischen Dermatologie, vol 3. Springer, Berlin Heidelberg New York

Marchionini A, Borelli S, Eichhoff D (1958) Konstitutions-, Umwelt- und Klimafaktoren bei der konstitutionellen Neurodermitis. In: 3ème Cong d'Allergol. Flammarion, Paris, p 609

Miller H, Baruch D (1948) Psychosomatic studies of children with allergic manifestations. Psychosom Med 10: 275

Musaph H (1964) Itching and scratching. Psychodynamics in dermatology. Karger, Basel

Nexmand PH (1948) Clinical studies of Prurigo Besnier. Rosenkilde and Bagger, Copenhagen

Nexmand PH (1958) Occupational problems for patients with Besnier's prurigo. In: Occupational allergy. Stenfert Kroese, Leiden

Nilsson E (1986) Individual and environmental risk factors for hand eczema in hospital workers. Thesis no 168, University of Umeå, Sweden

Nilsson E, Mikaelsson B, Anderson S (1985) Atopy, occupation and domestic work as risk factors for hand eczema in hospital workers. Contact Dermatitis 13: 216

Norrlind R (1946) Prurigo Besnier (atopic dermatitis). Acta Derm Venereol [Suppl] (Stockh) 13

Oddoze L (1959) Notre statistique sur l'étiologie du prurigo de Besnier en France. Acta Allergol 13: 410

Oddoze L (1966) L'éczema atopique. In: Huriez C (ed) Actualites sur les eczémas. Revue Medicine Suppl, p 11

Pirilä V (1950) Prurigo Besnier. Acta Derm Venereol (Stockh) 30: 114

Privat Y, Ferran J (1972) Psychosomatic reflexions on atopic dermatitis. In: Charpin J, Coutin C, Aubert J, Frankland AW (eds) Allergology. Proceedings, 8th European Congress on Allergy. Excerpta Medica, Amsterdam, p 161

Rajka G (1961) Prurigo Besnier (atopic dermatitis) with special reference to the role of allergic factors. III. The role of some factors in the course of prurigo Besnier. Acta Derm Venereol (Stockh) 41: 363

Rajka G (1986) Atopic dermatitis. Correlation of environmental factors with frequency. Int J Dermatol 25: 301

Reimann HJ, Meyer HJ, Wendt P (1981) Stress and histamine. In: Ring J, Burg G (eds) New trends in allergy. Springer, Berlin Heidelberg New York, p 50

Ring J, Palos E (1986) Psychosomatische Aspekte der Eltern-Kinder-Beziehung bei atopischem Ekzem im Kindesalter. II. Hautarzt 37: 609

Ring J, Palos E, Zimmermann F (1986) Psychosomatische Aspekte der Eltern-Kinder-Beziehung bei atopischem Ekzem im Kindesalter. I. Hautarzt 37: 560

Rystedt I (1981) Dermatological problems in the work environment following childhood skin disease. Acta Derm Venereol [Suppl] (Stockh) 95: 43

Rystedt I (1985) Hand eczema and long-term prognosis in atopic dermatitis. Acta Derm Venereol [Suppl] (Stockh) 117: 34

Schnyder UW (1957) The importance of intracutaneous tests in various types of constitutional neurodermitis. Int Arch Allergy Appl Immunol 11: 64

Schnyder UW, Borelli S (1965) Neurodermitis constitutionalis sive atopica. In: Miescher G, Storck H (eds) Entzündliche Dermatosen. II. Springer, Berlin Heidelberg New York, p 228 (Handbuch der Haut- und Geschlechtskrankheiten, vol II/1)

Sedlis E (1965) Natural history of infantile eczema: its incidence and course. J Pediatr 66 (2): 158

Shmunes E, Keil J (1984) The role of atopy in occupational dermatoses. Contact Dermatitis 11: 174

Siemens HW, Jagtman GG (1951) Spontane Heilung von Ekzemen bei Aufnahme ins Krankenhaus. Hautarzt 2: 99

Sonneck HJ, Goetzki H, Adam J (1967) Das konstitutionelle Ekzem und der Einfluß der Schule. Dtsch Gesundheitswes 22: 73

Storck H (1959) Über bakterielle Allergie. In: Schuppli R (ed) Aktuelle Probleme der Dermatologie, vol I. Karger, Basel, p 252

Sulzberger MB (1955) Atopic dermatitis: its clinical and histopathological picture. In: Baer RL (ed) Atopic dermatitis. Lippincott, Philadelphia, p 11

Urbach E, Gottlieb PM (1946) Allergy, 2nd edn. Grune and Stratton, New York

Van den Burg CKH, Bruynzeel DP, Vreeburg KJJ, von Blomberg BME, Scheper RJ (1986) Hand eczema in hairdressers and nurses: a prospective study. Contact Dermatitis 14: 275

Whitlock FA (1976) Psychophysiological aspects of skin disease. Saunders, London, p 133

Wilkinson DS, Hambly EM (1978) Prognosis of hand eczema in hairdressing apprentices. Contact Dermatitis 4: 63

Williams DH (1951) Management of atopic dermatitis in children. Control of the maternal rejection factor. Arch Dermatol Syph 63: 545

Worth RM (1962) Atopic dermatitis among Chinese infants in Honolulu and San Francisco. Haw Med J 22: 31, quoted by Sedlis E

Young E (1980) Seasonal factors in atopic dermatitis and their relationship. Acta Derm Venereol [Suppl] (Stockh) 92: 111

10 Diagnosis and Grading (Severity)

10.1 Diagnostic Criteria

Although the diagnosis of AD appears to be quite straightforward, and AD is considered as being self-evident, the situation is more complex than it may seen (Archer 1986). There exist atypical "borderline" cases resulting in differential diagnostic problems. Considering that about 15% of the population may have atopy, and over 10% of children may have AD, it is not surprising that any disease may include AD subjects among its sufferers, leading some clinicians to try to link various diseases to atopy or AD. Sometimes only certain positive immediate reactions, or high IgE, are used as major arguments for "atopy/AD," which obviously leads to false deductions (see also below). The necessity for strict and uniform diagnostic criteria is very clearly shown in the work by Malten (1971) on nickel sensitivity and AD. Using a history of atopy as the sole diagnostic criterion, 48% of his patients could be classified as atopic; if positive skin tests to inhalants were considered, the figure became 33%; and if both were taken into account, 57% could be called atopic. Therefore it is necessary to adopt accurate criteria to avoid such false or loosely stated correlations originating not infrequently from nondermatologists. In order to provide uniform criteria in the diagnosis of AD, a list was worked out that reflected and summarized American and European points of view (Hanifin and Rajka 1980) (see Table 10.1). Although this is not a perfect list and some details may be debatable, including the rank of order of the enumerated minor criteria, looking at the most recent AD literature, it seems to have been generally accepted. Therefore, although some suggestions have been noted, e. g., the inclusion of eosinophilia and Hertoghe's sign or the omission of keratoconus, the list has not yet been revised.

Most traits are mentioned in Chap. 2 and few comments are necessary. The major criteria for infants should not be interpreted rigidly, since the chronicity is not yet obvious, they usually lack respiratory allergies, and the family history may be negative in a proportion of cases (E. Bonifazi, personal communication). Another remark is that RAST may be added to the criteria of immediate-type reactivity.

The validity of the adapted criteria on AD materials is an important point. The highest scores in the proband group were registered for white dermographism, dry skin/xerosis, irritation by textiles, and facial pallor/erythema (Svensson et al. 1985). Xerosis and facial pallor, in addition to a positive history

Table 10.1. Guidelines for the diagnosis of AD

Must have 3 or more basic features:

Pruritus
Typical morphology and distribution:
a) Flexural lichenification or linearity in adults
b) Facial and extensor involvement in infants and children
Chronic or chronically relapsing dermatitis
Personal or family history of atopy (asthma, allergic rhinitis, AD)

Plus 3 or more minor features:

Xerosis
Ichthyosis/palmar hyperlinearity/keratosis pilaris
Immediate (type I) skin test reactivity
Elevated serum IgE
Early age of onset
Tendency toward cutaneous infections (esp. *Staph. aureus* and herpes simplex)/impaired
cell-mediated immunity
Tendency toward nonspecific hand or foot dermatitis
Nipple eczema
Cheilitis
Recurrent conjunctivitis
Dennie-Morgan infraorbital fold
Keratoconus
Anterior subcapsular cataracts
Orbital darkening
Facial pallor/facial erythema
Pityriasis alba
Anterior neck folds
Itch when sweating
Intolerance to wool and lipid solvents
Perifollicular accentuation
Food intolerance
Course influenced by environmental/emotional factors
White dermographism/delayed blanch

and early onset, were also found in an investigation of 372 Chinese patients, which is an important contribution to the global picture of AD (Kang and Tian 1987). These authors suggest a modification in dividing minor criteria into genetic, immunological, and physiopharmacological groups. Diepgen et al. (1989) compared diagnostic criteria on 110 AD patients with 527 persons of the normal populations. Based on statistical evaluation, they give a score system showing the highest values for the following features: itch when sweating, intolerance to wool, xerosis, white dermographism and Hertoghe's sign.

The existence or lack of major symptoms and the heterogeneity of AD suggest that, for one or another major trait, there might exist diverging subgroups in AD. They may be based on clinical differences (presence or absence of respiratory symptoms, prurigo response, ichthyosis, etc.). Other subgroups may be based on immunological differences (e.g.), high/low IgE production, grade of cell-mediated immunity, low/high threshold histamine releasers) or on pathophysiological characteristics (e.g., presence or absence of paradoxical vascular reactivity). There are analogies to other heterogeneous atopic diseases such as bronchial asthma (Aas 1981).

In the author's opinion, distinguishing subgroups within AD may increase the interest of certain findings for some patients and may, possibly, sometimes be useful in the selection of a given therapy. On the other hand, it should not be forgotten that AD is a dynamic disease and this casts some doubt on the value of a strictly applied classification depending on *one* clinical/immunological symptom *at a given period of time.*

The diagnostic situation would be easier if a basic and specific marker of AD could be clearly established. The suggested markers are mentioned in Table 8.1, first column.

10.2 Differential Diagnosis

Although providing no firm basis from the point of view of establishing the diagnosis of AD, the *lack* of some traits may have some differential diagnostic value, such as:

1. *Intense pruritus* (present, of course, in other eczematous processes too).
2. *Positive immediate skin tests/RAST.* If these tests are properly conducted (see Sect. 5.2.2), the absence of positive results is an indication, but not a weighty argument, against atopy/AD. In this connection egg reactivity in in-

Table 10.2. Differential diagnosis between infantile atopic and seborrheic dermatitis

	AD	Seb. D.
Localization: Face	Sides	Central
Retroauricular area	+	+ +
Scalp	+ − + +	+ +
Folds/napkin area	+	+ +
First manifestation after birth/1 month	+ − + +	+ +
Frequent familial history	Atopy	Seborrhea
Inquietude/sleeplessness (1–2 months)	+ +	+
Scratching/rubbing (> 2 months)	+ +	−
Frequent high IgE/s	+ +	−
RAST/prick test positivity (milk, egg etc.)	+ +	−
Symptoms of food intolerance	+ +	−
Colonization with staphylococci	+ +	+
Colonization with *Candida*	(+)	+ − + +
Exacerbation by heat/humidity	+ +	+ +
Abnormal Th/Ts ratio (> ca. 4 months)	+ +	−
Association with immunopathies	Wiskott-Aldrich syndrome Ataxia telangiectasia, etc.	Hyper-IgE
Histology: Epidermodermal inflammation	+ +	+ +
Signs of scratching (> 2 months)	+ +	−
Response to treatment	Poor	Good

Abbreviations: IgE/s, IgE in serum; Th, T helper cell; Ts, T suppressor cell

fant and pollen in adult atopics are most frequently quoted; recently the significance of mite reactivity has been mentioned.

3. *Paradoxical vascular responses* (see Sect.7.4). Although nonspecific for differential diagnostic distinction, these are present in quite a high percentage of AD patients (e.g., white dermographism in 100%, Svensson et al. 1985; the combination of white dermographism, nicotinate reactions, and delayed blanch in 90%, Rajka 1960).

4. *Nickel patch positivity*. Although not infrequent in AD, such positivity is also present in a high percentage of healthy women and, of course, in contact dermatitis patients.

The most important differential diagnostic problems, involving the infantile phase of AD versus seborrheic dermatitis, are summarized in Table 10.2 (see also Sect.2.2.2). Chronic acral dermatitis (Winkelmann and Gleich 1973) should also be considered. In this therapy-resistant condition the IgE is strongly elevated but no atopic history is present and the usual immunological traits of AD are lacking.

10.3 Grading (Severity)

No uniform criteria exist to characterize the status, i.e., the clinical condition in AD. In most reports the extent and/or severity are separately estimated. Several approaches are used for characterization of the clinical state at the time of the clinical or research investigation:

1. A simple judgment of the intensity of the clinical state
2. Scoring systems based on certain important, mostly morphological parameters, including the extent of skin involvement (Rogge and Hanifin 1977; Zachary and MacDonald 1983)
3. Scoring systems based on clinical facts and history, as well as on some investigations, such as IgE or vascular tests (Queille-Roussel et al. 1985; Svensson and Möller 1986)

At the Third International Symposium on Atopic Dermatitis (1988, Oslo), the present author and J.M.Hanifin took the initiative in organizing a workshop with invited participants to elaborate simple systems for the grading of AD. The aim was to recommend uniform designs for basic and clinical investigations. The baseline grading, which may be carried out on the basis of a single consultation, permits distinction between mild moderate, and severe AD by means of a score summation using the "rule of nine" to characterize the involved skin areas (Rajka and Langeland 1989) (Table 10.3, Fig.10.1). This grading system can be considered as an improved version of earlier suggestions (Rajka 1983; Langeland 1983).

At the same workshop, Hanifin (1989) suggested a standardized grading of subjects for cliniclal research studies in AD. The objectives were to establish parameters for grading response to therapy and to optimize clinical trial designs (Table 10.4) and has been based on earlier studies of his group (Seymour et al. 1987).

Table 10.3. Grading (severity) of AD

I. *Extent*
A) *Childhood and adult phase*
   Less than approx. 9% of body area   =1
   Involvement evaluated as more than score 1, less than score 3   =2
   More than approx. 36% of body area   =3
B) *Infantile phase*
   Less than approx. 18% of skin involved   =1
   Involvement evaluated as more than score 1, less than score 3   =2
   More than 54% of skin involved   =3

II. *Course*
   More than 3 months remission during a year[a]   =1
   Less than 3 months remission during a year[a]   =2
   Continuous course   =3

III. *Intensity*
   Mild itch, only exceptionally disturbing night sleep   =1
   Itch, evaluated as more than score 1, less than score 3   =2
   Severe itching, usually disturbing night sleep   =3

Score summation
   3–4:   mild
   4.5–7.5: moderate
   8–9:   severe

When in doubt, score 1.5 or 2.5 may also be used
[a] May be adjusted in infants or if onset was less than 1 year before grading

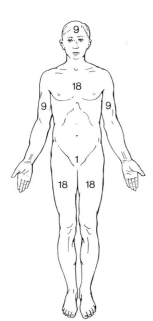

Fig. 1. "Rule of 9": calculation of body area involved. Head 9%, upper extremity 9%, anterior trunk 18%, posterior trunk 9%, lower extremity 18%, genital area 1%

Table 10.4a. Parameters used in grading severity of dermatitis (Hanifin 1989)

1. Erythema[a]
2. Induration/papulation[a]
3. Pruritus/excoriation[a]
4. Lichenification[b]
5. Scaling/dryness[b]
6. Erosion/oozing/weeping[c]

[a] Requisite basic parameters
[b] May be helpful for systemic trials or for more extensive or long-term evaluations.
[c] Requisite for younger pediatric populations; otherwise generally not relevant to adult populations.

Table 10.4b. Scoring of atopic dermatitis signs and symptoms in a target area (Hanifin 1989)

Erythema	Induration	Pruritus
0.0 = none	0.0 = none	0.0 = none
0.5	0.5	0.5
1.0 = mild	1.0 = mild	1.0 = mild
1.5	1.5	1.5
2.0 = moderate	2.0 = moderate	2.0 = moderate
2.5	2.5	2.5
3.0 = severe	3.0 = severe	3.0 = severe

References

Aas K (1981) Heterogeneity of bronchial asthma. Allergy 36: 3

Archer CB (1986) Atopic dermatitis – an obvious diagnosis? Clin Exp Dermatol 11: 560

Diepgen TL, Fartasch M, Hornstein OP (1989) Evaluation and relevance of atopic basic and minor features in patients with atopic dermatitis and in the general population. Acta Derm Venereol (Suppl 144) (Stockh) (in press)

Hanifin JM (1989) Standardized grading of subjects for clinical research studies in atopic dermatitis. Acta Derm Venereol (Stockh) [Suppl 144] (in press)

Hanifin JM, Rajka G (1980) Diagnostic features of atopic dermatitis. Acta Derm Venereol [Suppl] (Stockh) 92: 44

Kang K, Tian R (1987) Atopic dermatitis. An evaluation of clinical and laboratory findings. Int J Dermatol 26: 27

Langeland T (1983) A clinical and immunological study of allergy to hen's egg white. I. A clinical study of egg allergy. Clin Allergy 13: 371

Malten KE (1971) Nickel allergic contact dermatitis and atopy. Dermatologica 142: 113

Queille-Roussel C, Raynaud F, Saurat JH (1985) A prospective computerized study of 500 cases of atopic dermatitis in childhood. I. Initial analysis of 250 parameters. Acta Derm Venereol [Suppl] (Stockh) 114: 87

Rajka G (1960) Prurigo Besnier (atopic dermatitis) with special reference to the role of allergic factors. I. The influence of atopic heredity factors. Acta Derm Venereol (Stockh) 40: 285

Rajka G (1983) Atopic dermatitis. In: Rook A, Maibach HI (eds) Recent advances in dermatology. Churchill-Livingstone, Edinburgh, p 108

Rajka G, Langeland T (1989) Grading of the severity of atopic dermatitis: Acta Derm Venereol (Stockh) [Suppl 144] (in press)

Rogge JL, Hanifin JM (1977) Immunodeficiencies in severe atopic dermatitis. Arch Dermatol 112: 1391

Seymour JL, Keswick BH, Hanifin JM, Jordan WP, Milligan MC (1987) Clinical effects of diaper types on the skin of normal infants and infants with atopic dermatitis. J Am Acad Dermatol 17: 988

Svensson A, Möller H (1986) Eyelid dermatitis: the role of atopy and contact allergy. Contact Dermatitis 15: 178

Svensson A, Edman B, Möller H (1985) A diagnostic tool for atopic dermatitis based on clinical criteria. Acta Derm Venereol [Suppl] (Stockh) 114: 33

Winkelmann RK, Gleich JG (1973) Chronic acral dermatitis: association with extreme elevations of IgE: JAMA 225: 378

Zachary CB, MacDonald DM (1983) Quantitative analysis of T-lymphocyte subsets in atopic eczema, using monoclonal antibodies and flow cytometry. Br J Dermatol 108: 411

11 Prophylaxis

The problems of preventing AD are related to its multiple etiology and to factors modifying the course of the disease. Its prophylaxis can be viewed from different angles, e.g., following the development of the disease. Below it is grouped according to major etiological factors. Of these, allergens play a significant role.

Consideration of prophylactic measures against allergens raises the question of whether "pure" AD patients should be tested for type I reactivity; it is difficult to give practitioners generally valid advice on this problem, which has provoked so much discussion among allergologists, dermatologists, and pediatricians. In the author's opinion, such testing should be regarded as only one of several investigations which can give some information on an AD patient, and it should not be performed if there is reluctance on the part of the patient (or of his parents, if he is a child) to allow it to be done. The crucial point is that no conclusions should be drawn from test results which are not verifiable as relevant; thus a positive reaction may be only an "immunological marker" of minimal significance in a given case and ought to be treated as important only if there is a history of the allergen having provoked symptoms, if it does so in exposure tests, or if its elimination produces clinical improvement. *Verification clinically and by the history is essential,* otherwise many disagreable and unnecessary dermatological, psychic, economic, and related consequences of faulty deductions can befall the AD patient. It is relevant to note here that the RAST, which is an expensive procedure, may lessen some problems, such as the inconvenience of test methods requiring injections, but that, because of the lack of reliable food allergens, for example, does not essentially alter the principles of evaluation mentioned here.

11.1 Food Avoidance

Few topics arouse such divided opinions as the relation between food avoidance and the development of AD. Based on some well-performed studies selected from a vast amount of literature, the following short summary can be given.

11.1.1 Sensitization in Utero

Prenatal sensitization to food allergens has in general been considered a possibility (Matsumara et al. 1975; Kuroume et al. 1976). Langeland (1982) found that egg allergy in AD infants mostly developed before the introduction of egg into the diet. There are several reports that neonates have shown positive skin tests to egg or milk (Balyeat 1928; Kaufman 1971), or that the RAST has been positive from the cord blood (Michel et al. 1980; Businco et al. 1983; Sianfarikas and Glaubitt 1983). On the other hand, Hamburger et el. (1983) and Björksten (1983) found no specific reactions to food allergens in cord blood. When maternal abstention from milk, dairy products, egg, fish, beef, and peanuts was advised, and was also continued during lactation, a reduction of the incidence of AD was reported (Chandra et al. 1986). Fälth-Magnusson and Kjellman (1987) excluded egg and milk from the maternal diet in late pregnancy (from the 28th week) and some mothers continued with this restriction after birth. The authors were unable to establish any differences in the occurrence of atopy, or in IgE levels, between those with a restrictive diet and those without. Furthermore, the decrease of specific IgG antibodies involved atopics and controls to the same extent. It may be commented that the diet excluded only two major allergens and was not adopted before late pregnancy, whereas fetal cells produce IgE from the 11th week onward (Miller et al. 1973).

Although some data therefore seem to confirm, although they cannot clearly prove, the possibility of intrauterine sensitization of the fetus to foods, present opinion tends more towards the suggestion that atopic mothers show high levels of specific antibodies to foods (Dannæus et al. 1978; Dannæus and Inganäs 1981), which, after being passively transferred across the placenta, protect the offspring from developing the relevant food allergy. This is another argument against the necessity of diet restriction during pregnancy. Fälth-Magnusson et al. (1988) remark that "high levels of maternal IgG, IgA or IgM antibodies to food at delivery did not appear to protect the baby against development of atopic disease". These things considered, there is an obvious need for thorough studies in this field in order to confirm or exclude the possibility of intrauterine sensitization of the fetus to foods. On the other hand, the spontaneous desire of an atopic mother to abstain from certain food allergens is difficult to contradict for psychological reasons.

11.1.2 Breast Feeding

The effect of breast feeding, recommended by Grulee and Sandford as long ago as 1936, on the development of AD is a highly controversial issue due to differences in the duration of the feeding, the period of observation, selection of patient material, etc., as well as the frequent lack of appropriate controls (Burr 1983; Kovar et al. 1984). Quite often, whether or not breast-feeding mothers adhere to any diet is not considered; this is a major error since, in contrast to conditions during pregnancy, it has been clearly proven that maternal dietary proteins easily pass into the breast milk and cause skin symptoms in the infants

(Talbot 1918; Shannon 1921; Donnally 1930; Hemmings and Kulangara 1978; Gerrard 1979; Bahna and Heiner 1980; Kilshaw and Cant 1984; Cant et al. 1985). In other words, the suckling infant, without maternal allergen avoidance, is not on an allergen-free diet. This is further indicated by studies showing that small quantitites of, for example, cow's milk, demonstrable in human milk, elicit high levels of specific IgE antibodies in infants (Björksten and Saarinen 1978). The same authors also reported that breast-fed neonates might be given cow's milk formulas during the night in certain hospitals.

Analyzing some careful studies with more extensive patient material, with a longer registration period of breast feeding compared with bottle feeding, and with maternal allergen avoidance, a protective effect on the development of AD and/or atopy was noted (Matthew et al. 1977; Saarinen et al. 1979; Chandra 1979; Juto et al. 1982; Businco et al. 1983). A lack of effect from breast feeding has almost always been observed when relevant allergen avoidance was not clearly advised to the mother (Halpern et al. 1973; Hide and Guyer 1981; Fergusson et al. 1981; Kramer and Moroz 1981; Golding et al. 1982; Gruskay 1982; Mahoud et al. 1982; Van Asperen et al. 1984) or was only partial (Fälth-Magnusson and Kjellman 1987; Fälth-Magnusson et al. 1987).

A common argument against the protective effect of breast feeding in AD is the not insignificant occurrence of the disease in this infants. Such infants may also develop cow's milk allergy, although it is uncertain in several reports whether or not the mother and the child were on a totally milk-free diet. One report states that AD has become more frequent in breast-fed children in recent years (Taylor et al. 1984); this study has, however, been criticized (Peters et al. 1985). The delayed introduction of solids has mostly been combined with breast feeding (Saarinen et al. 1979) and is therefore difficult to evaluate, but a clear protective effect of this measure was shown in the studies of Kajosaari and Saarinen (1983).

Thus, a critical evaluation shows that the balance of reports tends to favor the concept of the protective effect of breast feeding on the incidence of AD, although the issue must be considered unresolved. The uncertainty over this topic is also reflected in the data which the author collected from dermatologists in 32 countries, mostly from the Third World; of these, only 25% presumed a correlation between breast feeding and the development of AD (Rajka 1986, and additional data).

The mechanism of the effects of breast feeding in atopy is unclear, but the findings of a specific IgG response (Dannæus et al. 1978; Firer et al. 1981) as well as a reduction of specific IgA antibodies (Machtinger and Moss 1986) are of considerable interest. Furthermore, human milk factors may promote maturation of neonatal immune functions (Björksten 1984).

The anti-infectious capacity of human milk is well-documented and includes, in addition to secretory IgA, migrating lymphocytes from the enteromammary circle, macrophages and neutrophils, as well as nonspecific resistance factors such as lactoferrin, lysozyme, and interferon (Goldman and Smith 1973). This indicates a considerable protection from gastrointestinal or respiratory infections for the infant.

11.1.3 Avoidance Diets

It is difficult to make a sharp distinction between prophylaxis and therapy by means of diet. If diet is applied in the case of an infant with already manifested AD, this is an obvious treatment method to improve the skin condition. It seems, however, more practical to include such cases here, and under therapy (Chap. 12), only the effect of drugs on food allergy or intolerance will be mentioned.

Elimination of some suspected or obviously noxious foods in connection with AD has long been practiced by different physicians, primarily by dermatologists and pediatricians. In addition to numerous anecdotal cases, evaluation of the effect of avoidance of certain food items has been registered in several studies (Rowe and Rowe 1951; Kesten 1954; Sedlis 1965; Hagerman 1966; Hammar 1977; Hathaway and Warner 1983). There are, however, few controlled, basic studies in this area, and therefore the value of food allergen-free diets for infants with potential AD, i.e., those with one or two atopic parents and/or one or more atopic siblings, is debatable. The sources of error in dietary trials are even more frequent than those mentioned in relation to breast feeding, which makes comparison and evaluation difficult. As already described in Sect. 5.3, the more important problems here include: the inadequacy of skin tests and of unrepeated challenge tests without adequate placebo, imperfect compliance, and the fact that itch and late reactions are sometimes omitted from the evaluations. Due to the multiple etiology of AD, challenge may cause deterioration, while elimination does not lead to improvement of the condition. Because of regional and national eating habits, a universally valid basic formula cannot be given.

Regarding carefully performed studies on the effect of exclusion diet on AD, the recommendation of Atherton (1981) and Atherton et al. (1978), should be mentioned. They gave a basic diet for 8 weeks and then separately introduced beef, milk, egg, and chicken (the latter two may share allergenic components, Langeland 1983), allocating a week for each; they also provided explanation and diet sheets for the parents and, due to negative nutritional aspects, included cooperation with a dietician. In addition, food items mentioned in the patient's history were excluded. If milk proved to be an allergen (and boiling does not solve the problem), soya milk preparations (such as Prosobee, Wysoy, New Velactin, or S formula) were tried as substitutes. Soya preparations had been tried earlier by Glaser and Johnstone (1952) and Glaser (1965), but they often have an unpleasant odor and not infrequently sensitize. Goat's milk may also be chosen as a substitute but it may be infected or cross-react with human milk. With cases still not improving, oligoallergenic diets were tried in accordance with similar principles, and in his 1981 report, Atherton gave examples of such diets. With this regimen he observed a beneficial effect in 14 of 20 participating infants.

Juto et al. (1978) proposed similar elimination diets: egg and fish were avoided for the first year, even if symptoms were absent, and the infants received casein hydrolysate (Nutramigen) or soya milk formulas and vitamins. Of

21 infants, 7 healed and 12 improved, and at the age of 2 years the disease cleared in 17 patients. Hill and Lynch (1982) reported a favorable effect of an elemental diet (Vivonex) in eight infants with severe AD. Neild et al. (1986), on the other hand, could not register any difference in clearing, through egg and milk exclusion diets, in the 40 infants involved in their study.

Strict elimination of fish and citrus fruits – based on positive challenge – did not change the incidence of these food allergies when evaluation was performed at the age of 3 years, indicating that food allergy can only be postponed and not prevented by elimination (Saarinen and Kajosaari 1980).

David et al. (1984) also reminded us of the need for complete calcium intake during exclusion diets. In 25 *adult* patients with severe AD, despite data indicating food intolerance in their histories, no differences were noted in a double-blind study carried out during 3 weeks of hospitalization, using an antigen-free preparation (Vivisorb) and a placebo (Munkvad et al. 1984). On the other hand, an uncontrolled follow-up study 1–3 years after an initial restrictive diet, lasting 1 month and resulting in improvement in 262 of 675 eczematous patients, frequently showed long-term improvement in atopic patients (Veien et al. 1987).

An interesting point is the effect of the early introduction of allergenic foods into the diet of AD infants. In breast-fed infants, small quantities of cow's milk or other food proteins may lead to higher levels of specific IgE antibodies than in infants fed on cow's milk (Björksten and Saarinen 1978), indicating that minute amounts of food allergens result in IgE formation (Juto and Björksten 1980; Firer et al. 1981). As compared with breast feeding, early and transient feeding with cow milk formula resulted in a reduced incidence of allergic symptoms in infants followed-up to 18 months of age (Lindfors and Enocksson 1988).

These observations, confirming the animal experiments of Jarrett (1977, see Sect. 5.3.1), may challenge the predominant concept of the value of food elimination (from an early age) for children with atopy/AD.

Comments: In families which display atopic heredity and/or which already have a child with atopy, food avoidance may be indicated (particularly if the infant is already suffering from AD) but should not be forced since the role of foods in the individual AD case may be inconclusive. Dietary measures are not routinely indicated for the majority of AD patients and should not be continued indefinitely; rather gradual reintroduction of the offending food(s) is often appropriate (The Task Force on Pediatric Dermatology 1986). The value of avoidance of certain food items during pregnancy cannot be clearly proven and such avoidance should not, therefore, be required of the mother. On the other hand, the breast-feeding mother who wishes to have dietary measures for her child has to avoid the same allergenic food proteins as her child. If the parents prefer to perform challenge trials on her child, tests should be carried out with only one food at a time and after a long avoidance of the suspected item. A challenge, if positive, should be repeated twice before more definite conclusions are drawn. Possible reactions should be observed from 15 min after exposure (itch) until 2 days (itch, aggravation of dermatitis, or new skin lesions). If urticarial (angioedema, contact urticaria) or gastrointestinal symptoms appear, they indicate a causal relationship and that food needs to be avoided by the atopic child, but these symptoms are no proof of the etiology of AD.

The individual susceptibility to foods cannot be predicted and may only partially be delineated by the previously mentioned methods. When there is evidence of an established individual intolerance, it is necessary to pay attention to idiosyncratic reactivities in addition to general recommendations. Based on the clinical evidence that common foods frequently aggravated AD in childhood, the following general avoidance list may be of value for parents who wish to take such an approach for their infant:

1. Avoidance primarily recommended (possibly until 1 year of age): eggs, cow's milk, fish (in regions where it is a common food)

2. Avoidance possibly recommended (particularly when there is a considerable family history of atopy or when the infant already has skin inflammation): shellfish, nuts, peanuts, cocoa/chocolate, pork, dairy products, citrus fruits, strawberry, sour fruits (such as sour apples), tomatoes, peas, soyabeans, carrots

3. Careful observation or avoidance may also be advisable for: cereals (wheat, oat), pears, plums, peaches, celery, rutabaga, cheese (such as Roquefort-type)

In principle, the same items apply for children as for infants, but possible allergens in sweets and beverages should also be noted. In addition, some further idiosyncrasy-eliciting foods, particularly if the AD is active, are spices (pepper, mustard, paprika, curry), vinegar-containing foods, and smoked meats.

Adults must avoid any food known to cause clinical sensitivity (realizing the results of skin tests or RAST have little significance). In active disease it is advisable to avoid foods able to elicit idiosyncrasy (Rajka 1983).

11.2 Inhalant Allergens

Even if the causal relationship between inhalant allergens and AD is not convincing for the majority of AD patients (see Sect. 5.2), for individual cases and for the respiratory symptoms prophylactic measures against airborne allergens merit attention. Thus a child with AD should be warned against keeping pet dogs, cats, or guinea pigs and against contact with other animals such as horses, cows, or pigs. The reason for this is that there is a significantly greater possibility that skin, pulmonary, or nasal symptoms, in any combination, may develop in these cases than in non-atopic children. A correlation between cats and dogs in the home and a positive skin or challenge test has been shown (Björksten 1986).

The discovery of the role of house dust mites in AD, by inhalation and particularly by contact (see Sect. 5.2.6), requires prophylactic measures. These include, in addition to thorough cleaning, some special measures such as removal of bedroom carpets and dust-attracting curtains, the covering of matresses with impermeable fabric, use of polyester-filled pillows, washing the bed clothes with hot water, avoidance of upholstered furniture, and possible use of acaricide chemicals (Platts-Mills and Chapman 1987; Zimmermann 1987). Concerning the latter, although several such preparations have been tested, there is still no ideal substance available. Most substances used have several disadvantages.

One should pay attention to avoiding intense exposure to molds (old houses, moist localities or storerooms, stables, etc.). On the other hand, pollen allergy is a minor problem for pure AD subjects. It is important to give clear advice in writing, and to instruct the mother of an atopic child how to observe and to analyze the role potential inhalant and food allergens are playing in her child's AD. The effectiveness of these measures, designed to avoid allergens, is augmented if exclusion of stimuli which promote pruritus is used as the foundation of prophylaxis; the beneficial effects of such an approach, as observed by many clinicians, bear witness to the importance of pruritus in AD.

11.3 Occupational Prophylaxis

In young persons the choice of a suitable occupation requires consideration, but the well-known tendency of the disease to heal spontaneously around the age of 30 naturally must not influence this choice at an earlier age. It is a mistake to regard AD patients as a uniform group, for this has led to differences of opinion regarding occupations suitable for these patients. The author consequently divided his patients into three groups: one with and one without sensitization, and the third with both AD and respiratory allergy (see Table 11.1)

Table 11.1. Contraindicated occupations for persons with AD[a]

Persons with	Relatively contraindicated to work with/at	Absolutely contraindicated to work with
1. AD	(a) Strong inhalation allergens (dust, hair, animal hair, flour, certain chemicals, etc.) (b) Wool (c) Heavy physical work. Warm damp place of work. Exposure to cold for long periods (d) Wet work (e) Strong defatting substances (organic solvents, detergents) (f) Strong chemical and mechanical irritants and contact allergens (e.g., nickel) Workplace with high infection risk.	
2. AD with relevant inhalational/epicutaneous sensitization	(a) (b) (c) (d) (e) (f)	Corresponding/ cross allergens
3. AD with respiratory allergy	(a) (b) (c) (d) (e) (f). Substances irritating respiratory passages. Moderate to heavy physical work in asthma	Corresponding/ cross allergens

[a] Some unsuitable occupations for AD patients, particularly if hands are involved: hairdressing, nursing, domestic work/cleaning, cooking/restaurant trade, food handling

(Rajka 1967). In this table the contraindications are based on prophylaxis against allergy (a) and on known pathological disturbances (b–e); these often occur in combination. In the author's experience, contact allergy and contact irritation are not infrequent in AD but do not always lead to very significant occupational problems, although the principles of assessment used for other chronic inflammatory skin conditions (f) must also be applied to some extent in these cases. Several authors have emphasized that the AD patient can, by scratching, introduce allergens and irritants into an already inflamed skin, with all the usual consequences. These principles should be followed when advising young patients with AD who have difficulties in choosing an occupation.

Hobbies present a related problem as they can have very detrimental effects on the course of the disease; grooming or contact with animals and working with photographic developers are examples.

11.4 Other Measures

Genetic factors have a major impact on the development of atopic disease and, therefore, genetic counseling for parents with an atopic background is of importance. Young severely affected atopics/AD subjects have already experienced the disadvantages of their disease but also need genetic information in connection with family planning.

Although the time of birth has some relevance for the development of allergy to mites or pollens, it is difficult for a physician to take a nonpermissive standpoint here. Adverse climatic or meteorological conditions are very difficult to combat, but, if possible, this should be attempted (see also Sect. 12.2.1); in particular, steps should be taken to guard against cold and against rapid changes in temperature. Patients with AD should be careful about, and in some cases avoid, circumstances such as gymnastics and sports, exercises, overheating, and hot or spiced foods and drinks, which can lead to intense sweating and possibly provoke pruritus.

Of environmental factors the negative effect of tobacco smoke has been emphasized in the development of respiratory atopy. Air pollution was mentioned briefly under Sect. 9.3.

Respiratory or gastrointestinal viral infections may have a negative effect on the skin of infants with AD, but the only possibility of avoiding such infections is breast feeding, which has a certain protective role in this connection (see Sect. 11.1.2). Close relatives with active herpes (labialis) should be seriously warned against kissing or having close contact with infants with AD. Viral vaccines may increase the allergic "breakthrough" and thus represent a certain risk for atopic children, also owing to their content of traces of egg, horse serum, or antibiotics. These disadvantages should, however, be balanced against the need for immunization.

Overheating should be avoided. The prophylactic use of creams, for example on the hands of AD patients who have a dry skin, should in general be encouraged, but a suitable preparation should be prescribed by the doctor; applications should not be selected simply on the recommendations of a layman or advertisements. Other measures helpful for a dry skin include humidification of the room and the use of baths.

Woollen garments and rough textiles should be avoided, and a mild soap, with thorough rinsing, should be used for washing clothing, linen, and nappies; detergents, bleaches, enzymes, and water softeners should preferably not be used. The detrimental effects of emotional stress on AD patients should not be ignored but offer little scope for effective management. To quote Sulzberger (1971): "Tensions, stresses and emotional upsets should be avoided, but this is usually much easier said than done. Psychoanalysis and psychotherapy also do not seem to be feasible approaches in most patients."

Practicable preventive measures include not only registration of patients and in the case of pregnant women with AD, subsequent observation of the children they produce, but also rehabilitation centers for AD sufferers (Richter 1961; Harnack 1961).

References

Atherton DJ (1981) Allergy and atopic eczema. II. Clin Exp Dermatol 6: 317

Atheron DJ, Sewell M, Soothill JF, Wells RS, Chilvers CED (1978) A double blind controlled crossover trial of an antigen avoidance diet in atopic eczema. Lancet I: 401

Bahna SL, Heiner DC (1980) Allergies to milk. Grune and Stratton, New York

Balyeat RM (1928) Hereditary factor in allergic diseases, with special reference to general health and mental activity of allergic patients. Am J Med Sci 176: 332

Björksten B (1983) Does breast-feeding prevent the development of allergy? Immunol Today 4: 215

Björksten B (1984) Atopic allergy in relation to cell-mediated immunity. Clin Rev Allergy 2: 95

Björksten F (1986) Early allergen contacts. J Allergy Clin Immunol 78: 1010

Björksten F, Saarinen UM (1978) IgE antibodies to cow's milk in infants fed breast milk and milk formula. Lancet II: 624

Burr ML (1983) Does infant feeding affect the risk to allergy? Arch Dis Child 58: 561

Businco L, Marchetti F, Pellegrini G, Perlini R (1983) Predictive value of cord blood IgE levels "at risk" newborns and influence of type of feeding. Clin Allergy 13: 505

Cant AM, Marsden RA, Kilshaw PJ (1985) Egg and cow's milk hypersensitivity in exclusively breast fed infants with eczema and detection of egg proteins in breast milk. Br Med J 291: 932

Chandra RK (1979) Prospective studies of the effect of breast feeding on incidence of infection and allergy. Acta Pædiatr Scand 68: 691

Chandra RK, Puri S, Suraiya C, Cheema PS (1986) Influence of maternal food antigen avoidance during pregnancy and lactation on incidence of atopic eczema in infants. Clin Allergy 16: 539

Dannæus A, Inganäs M (1981) A follow-up study of children with food allergy. Clinical course in relation to serum IgE and IgG antibody levels to milk, egg and fish. Clin Allergy 11: 533

Dannæus A, Johansson SGO, Foucard T (1978) Clinical and immunological aspects of food allergy in childhood. II. Development of allergic symptoms and humoral immune response to foods in infants of atopic mothers during the first 24 months of life. Acta Pædiatr Scand 67: 497

David TJ, Waddington E, Stanton RHJ (1984) Nutritional hazards of elimination diets in children with atopic eczema. Arch Dis Child 59: 323

Donnally HH (1930) The question of the elimination of foreign protein (egg white) in woman's milk. J Immunol 19: 14

Fälth-Magnusson K, Kjellman NIM (1987) Development of atopic disease in babies whose mothers were receiving exclusion diet during pregnancy - a randomized study. J Allergy Clin Immunol 80: 869

Fälth-Magnusson K, Kjellman NIM, Magnusson KE (1988) Antibodies IgG, IgA and IgM to food antigens during the first 18 months of life in relation to feeding and development of atopic disease. J Allergy Clin Immunol 81: 743

Fälth-Magnusson K, Öman H, Kjellman NIM (1987) Maternal abstention from cow milk and egg in allergy risk pregnancies. Allergy 42: 64

Fergusson DM, Horwood LJ, Beautrais AL, Shannon FT, Taylor B (1981) Eczema and infant diet. Clin Allergy 11: 325

Firer MA, Hosking CS, Hill DJ (1981) Effect of antigen load on development of milk antibodies in infants allergic to milk. Br Med J 283: 693

Gerrard JW (1979) Allergy in breast fed babies to ingredients in breast milk. Ann Allergy 42: 69

Glaser J (1965) The prevention of eczema. J Pediatr 66 (2): 262

Glaser J, Johnstone DE (1952) Soybean milk as a substitute for mammalian milk in early infancy with special reference to prevention of allergy to cow's milk. Ann Allergy 10: 433

Golding J, Butler NR, Taylor B (1982) Breast-feeding and eczema/asthma. Lancet I: 910

Goldman AS, Smith CW (1973) Host resistance factors in human milk. J Pediatr 82: 1082

Grulee CG, Sanford HN (1936) The influence of breast and artificial feeding on infantile eczema. J Pediatr 9: 223

Gruskay FL (1982) Comparison of breast, cow and soy feedings in the prevention of onset of allergic disease. A 15-year prospective study. Clin Pediatr (Phila) 21: 486

Hagerman G (1966) The importance of food factors in atopic dermatitis. In: Collvin K, Nilzén Å, Skog E (eds) Sven Hellerström 65 years. Berlingska boktryckeriet, Lund, p 81

Halpern SR, Sellars WA, Johnson RB, Anderson DW, Saperstein S, Reisch JS (1973) Development of childhood allergy in infants fed breast, soy or cow's milk. J Allergy Clin Immunol 51: 139

Hamburger RN, Heller S, Mellon MH, O'Connor RD, Zeiger RS (1983) Current status of the clinical and immunological consequences of a prototype allergic disease prevention program. Ann Allergy 51: 281

Hammar H (1977) Provocation with cow's milk and cereals in atopic dermatitis. Acta Derm Venereol (Stockh) 57: 159

Harnack K (1961) Wege zur Eindämmung und Behandlung des endogenen Ekzems sowie zur Rehabilitation der Erkrankten. Dtsch Gesundheitswes 16: 128

Hathaway MJ, Warner JO (1983) Compliance problems in the dietary management of eczema. Arch Dis Child 58: 463

Hemmings WA, Kulangara AC (1978) Dietary antigens in breast milk. Lancet II: 275

Hide DW, Guyer BM (1981) Clinical manifestations of allergy related to breast and cow's milk feeding. Arch Dis Child 65: 172

Hill DJ, Lynch BC (1982) Elemental diet in the management of severe eczema in childhood. Clin Allergy 12: 313

Jarrett EEE (1977) Activation of IgE regulatory mechanisms by transmuscosal absorption of antigen. Lancet I: 223

Juto P, Björksten B (1980) Serum IgE in infants and influence of type of feeding. Clin Allergy 10: 593

Juto P, Engberg S, Winberg J (1978) Treatment of infantile atopic dermatitis with a strict elimination diet. Clin Allergy 8: 493

Juto P, Möller C, Engberg S, Björksten B (1982) Influence of type of feeding on lymphocyte function and development of infantile allergy. Clin Allergy 12: 409

Kajosaari M, Saarinen UM (1983) Prophylaxis of atopic disease by six months' total solid food elimination. Acta Pediatr Scand 72: 411

Kaufman HS (1971) Allergy in the newborn: skin test reactions confirmed by the Prausnitz-Küstner test at birth. Clin Allergy 1: 363

Kesten B (1954) Allergic eczema. N Y State J Med 54: 2441

Kilshaw PJ, Cant AJ (1984) The passage of maternal dietary proteins into human breast milk. Int Arch Allergy Appl Immunol 75: 8

Kovar MG, Serdula MK, Marks JS, Fraser DW (1984) Review of the epidemiologic evidence for an association between infant feeding and infant health. Pediatrics 74 (Suppl): 65

Kramer MS, Moroz B (1981) Do breast feeding and delayed introduction of solid foods protect against subsequent atopic eczema? J Pediatr 98: 546

Kuroume T, Oguri M, Matsumara T, Iwasaki I, Kanbe Y, Yamada T, Kawabe S, Negishi K (1976) Milk sensitivity and soybean sensitivity in the production of eczematous manifestations in breast-fed infants with particular reference to intra-uterine sensitization. Ann Allergy 37: 41

Langeland T (1982) A clinical and immunological study of allergy to hen's egg white. Allergy 37: 323

Langeland T (1983) A clinical and immunological study of allergy to hen's egg white. VI. Occurrence of proteins crossreacting with allergens in hen's egg white as studied in egg white from turkey, duck, goose, seagull and hen's egg yolk, and hen's and chicken's sera and flesh. Allergy 38: 399

Lindfors A, Enocksson E (1988) Development of atopic disease after early administration of cow milk formula. Allergy 43: 11

Machtinger S, Moss R (1986) Cow's milk allergy in breast-fed infants: the role of allergen and maternal secretory IgA antibody. J Allergy Clin Immunol 77: 341

Mahoud JM, Church RE, Bleehen SS, Harrington CI (1982) The effect of breast feeding on the subsequent development of atopic eczema: a case control study. Br J Dermatol (Suppl 22): 15

Mathew DJ, Norman AP, Taylor B, Turner MW, Soothill JF (1977) Prevention of eczema. Lancet I: 321

Matsumara T, Takayashi K, Oguri M, Iwasaki I (1975) Egg sensitivity and eczematous manifestations in breast-fed newborns with particular reference to intrauterine sensitization. Ann Allergy 35: 221

Michel FB, Bousquet J, Greillier P, Robinet-Levy M, Coulomb Y (1980) Comparison of cord blood IgE concentrations and maternal allergy for prediction of atopic disease in infancy. J Allergy Clin Immunol 65: 422

Michel FB, Bousquet J, Dannæus A, Hamburger RN, Bellanti JA, Businco ML, Soothill J (1986) Preventive measures in early childhood allergy. J Allergy Clin Immunol 78: 1022

Miller DL, Hirvonen T, Gitlin D (1973) Synthesis of IgE by the human conceptus. J Allergy Clin Immunol 52: 182

Munkvad M, Danielsen L, Hoy L, Povlsen CO, Secher L, Svejgaard E, Bundgaard A, Larsen PO (1984) Antigen-free diet in adult patients with atopic dermatitis. Acta Derm Venereol (Stockh) 64: 524

Neild VS, Marsden RA, Bailes JA, Bland JM (1986) Egg and milk exclusion diets in atopic eczema. Br J Dermatol 114: 117

Peters T, Golding J, Butler NR (1985) Breast-feeding and childhood eczema. Lancet I: 49

Platts-Mills TAE, Chapman MD (1987) Dust mites: immunology, allergic disease and environmental control. J Allergy Clin Immunol 80: 755

Rajka G (1967) Occupational choice for persons with chronic common dermatoses and pathological skin functions. Acta Derm Venereol (Stockh) 47: 15

Rajka G (1983) Dietary associations in atopic dermatitis. In: Hanifin JM (ed) Atopic dermatitis and other endogenous eczemas, Sem Dermatol vol 2. Thieme-Stratton, New York, p 30

Rajka G (1986) Atopic dermatitis. Correlation of environmental factors with frequency. Int J Dermatol 25: 301

Richter U (1961) Erfahrungen in der Dispensaire-Behandlung des endogenen Ekzems (lecture). Hautarzt 12: 286

Rowe AH, Rowe AH (1951) Atopic dermatitis in infants and children. J Pediatr 39: 80

Saarinen UM, Kajosaari M (1980) Does dietary elimination in infancy prevent or only postpone a food allergy? Lancet I: 166

Saarinen UM, Backman A, Kajosaari M, Siimes MA (1979) Prolonged breast-feeding as prophylaxis for atopic disease. Lancet II: 163

Sedlis E (1965) Some challenge studies with food. J Pediatr 66 (2): 235

Shannon WR (1921) Eczema in breast fed infants as a result of sensitization to foods in the mother's diet. Am J Dis Child 23: 392

Sianfarikas K, Glaubitt D (1973) RAST mit Nahrungsmittelallergenen bei Neugeborenen. RAST 3 Berichtsband. Grosse, Berlin, p 172

Sulzberger MB (1971) Atopic dermatitis. In: Fitzpatrick TB, Arndt KA, Clark WH jr, Eisen AZ, van Scott EJ, Vaughan JH (eds) Dermatology in general medicine. Part III. McGraw-Hill, New York, p 680

Talbot FB (1918) Eczema in childhood. Med Clin North 1: 985

Taylor B, Wadsworth M, Wadsworth J, Peckham C (1984) Changes in the reported prevalence of childhood eczema since the 1939-45 war. Lancet II: 1255

The Task Force on Pediatric Dermatology: Caputo RV, Frieden I, Krafchik BR et al. (1986) Diet and atopic dermatitis. J Am Acad Dermatol 15: 543

Van Asperen PP, Kemp AS, Melis CM (1984) A prospective study of the clinical manifestations of atopic disease in infancy. Acta Pediatr Scand 73: 80

Veien NK, Hattel T, Justesen O, Nörholm A (1987) Dietary restrictions in the treatment of adult patients with eczema. Contact Dermatitis 17: 223

Zimmermann T (1987) Reduzierung des Hautstaubmilbenallergens nach Zimmer- und Bettsanierung. Untersuchung mit einem Teststreifensystem (Acarex). Allergologie 10: 31

12 Management of AD

Rapport between the physician and AD patients (or their parents if they are children) is sometimes difficult as psychological factors, superimposed on the skin disease, can make them very demanding patients who expect the physician to cure their severe pruritus and the inflammatory changes. In addition, past therapeutic failures may have led them to adopt an indifferent or even a sceptical attitude towards their physician, in whom they may even totally have lost all confidence. Thus, physicians caring for AD patients do well to have a sound practical training in psychology to help them to manage these patients effectively.

Many details of the management of AD, and particularly dietary measures, have already been discussed in the predicting chapter on prophylaxis. An evaluation of the more important therapeutic results achieved up to recent years follows.

12.1 Specific and Immunological Therapy

To influence the course of AD by specific therapy has been a long-standing ambition of clinicians. Just how hyposensitization (desensitization) works in respiratory atopies is not fully understood; however, provided that the relevant allergen is used in adequate concentration, it is found that after the initial phase in a course of hyposensitization, when injections of the antigen are frequent, the serum IgE level is initially elevated but later decreases during the period of long-term hyposensitization (Berg and Johansson 1971; Johansson et al. 1972). This is an agreement with earlier studies based on biological titration using passive transfer techniques, which demonstrated an initial increase and a subsequent decrease in circulating reagins (Cooke et al. 1935; Sherman et al. 1939).

These findings led to the concept of blocking antibodies which act against reagins (IgE). There is some evidence that such blocking antibodies exist; however, despite a suspicion that they correspond to a certain subclass of IgG antibodies, their nature remains unknown. Equally obscure is the exact correlation between these blocking antibodies and IgE. Some authors believed that, as there is insufficient correlation between the clinical effects of hyposensitization and the serum levels of blocking antibody, the latter plays no great role in the former (Lichtenstein et al. 1968). More recent studies on the mechanism of specific therapy implicate not only IgG antibodies (Prahl et al. 1981) but also the generation of antigen-specific T suppressor cells (Canonica et al. 1979; Rocklin et al. 1980; Tamir et al. 1987). Furthermore, induction of anti-idiotypic antibodies and a decrease in mediator releaseability is under debate. Several clinicians have studied the effects of hyposensitization in these cases, using more or less reliable criteria, and it is characteristic that Becker (1932), who was one of the first to report on this method, was already critical of this effectiveness. A large number of dermatologists and allergologists who subsequently have evaluated this method in AD patients, have produced reports which have ranged from enthusiastic to sceptical; relatively favorable results have been achieved by the use of inhalants, whereas success has been rare when employing the subcutaneous or peroral routes for food hyposensitization. Studies in which results were subjected to critical analysis showed that a temporary or quantitative effect of hyposensitization could be achieved in only a minority of treated cases (Nexmand 1948); for example no difference was found in mold-sensitive AD patients whether they were "hyposensitized" with the relevant allergen or with a placebo (Rajka, unpublished observations). Thus the generally disappointing response to hyposensitization in AD is keeping with the inadequate theoretical basis mentioned already, but this does not mean that in certain AD cases, with a proven reaginic background, hyposensitization can a priori be expected to be valueless. Thus favorable results were seen in 15 carefully selected cases (Di Prisco de Fuenmayor and Champion 1979), in 8 of 50 cases (Korossy 1980), in nine mite-positive patients (Zachariæ et al. 1980), and furthermore in two monozygotic twins treated over 2 years (Ring 1982). It is, however, inadvisable to extrapolate these few beneficial results to be the majority of "pure" AD patients, but with purified allergens (semidepot, tyrosine-adsorbed vaccines or modified allergens: allergoids) and better methods of evaluating the results, the possibility of specific therapy should not be totally overlooked. On the other hand, patients who have AD combined with asthma and/or atopic rhinitis often derive considerable benefit from specific hyposensitization as far as their respiratory symptoms are concerned and this sometimes includes the skin condition (Bergquist and Nilzén 1972; Jarisch et al. 1979; Seidenari et al. 1986).

Of other immunological methods, the result of attempted immune stimulation by levamisole was disappointing (Alomar et al. 1978). In another study, the clinical condition, as well as the immunological parameters, improved (Jarisch et al. 1979). Transfer factor was applied in some severe cases. In general only slight benefit was registered, while the immunological values sometimes showed improvement (Strannegård et al. 1975; Hovmark and Ekre 1978; Zachariæ et al. 1980). A suppressor cell increase was observed after giving dialyzable leukocyte extract, which contains, among other things, transfer factor (Herlin et al. 1981). In two severe AD cases leukophoresis was carried out in our clinic without lasting benefit but with some improvement of the impaired immune parameters (Amundsen, unpublished observations). Similarly, a short effect was seen using plasma separation (Nielsen et al. 1984). On the other hand, thymopoietin pentapeptide had a beneficial effect on clinical and immunological parameters in a double-blind trial in 18 AD patients (Kang et al.

1983), Thymosine was proposed for AD patients to improve deficient T cell response (Byrom 1980) but clinical results have not yet been reported.

By thymostimulin (TP-1) administration clinical but no immunological improvement was seen compared with placebo (Harper 1989).

Although immunostimulant therapy has not yet led to any great benefit in AD, this trend, including measures counteracting IgE, seems a logical approach for the future.

12.2 General Measures

12.2.1 Climatotherapy

The favorable effects on AD of certain climatic and weather conditions, such as temporary residence in the mountains, at the seaside, or in a dry warm climate, have been discussed in Chap. 9, and form the rationale for the frequent use of climatotherapy in the management of this disease. Authors such as Marchionini et al. (1958) reported that German and Turkish AD patients benefitted from residence in the mountains, and Nexmand (1948) noted a dramatic improvement in Danish patients during their stay in the Norwegian mountains. An interesting variation on seaside holidays is a sea cruise (Linser 1967). Especially valuable in this context are reports in which objective parameters are used to evaluate improvement of the AD. Such studies were undertaken on the island of Norderney in the North Sea, and the excellent improvement reported was exemplified by the fact that almost all the AD patients on systemic corticosteroid therapy were able to abandon it during their stay (Pürschel 1962, 1987, Grabowski 1956). Residence at Davos also was reported to give fairly good results, including the ability to stop systemic corticosteroid therapy, and the return to normal of previously abnormal responses to mediators and to cholinergic substances (Borelli 1970, Kneist and Rakoski 1987). The time taken to produce this beneficial effect is about 6 weeks, which therefore is taken as the optimal duration of such a stay. Another important result was an improvement in these patients' ability to work; before their stay, this had been impaired in 50%, whereas 1 year later some disability remained in only 8.3% (Borelli 1970). Unfortunately, improvement usually lasts only until the patient returns to his original environment; some clinicians therefore recommend that patients with severe and intractable AD, who have previously improved during a short stay, should consider untertaking long-term climatotherapy in the form of a change in residence.

AD patients moving to so-called mini-risk houses with a better indoor climate (concerning air exchange rate, relative humidity, temperature etc) showed clinical improvement compared to non-moving control AD cases (Beck et al. 1989).

12.2.2 Hospitalization

Hospitalization may be helpful especially in the treatment of severe cases, but also as a change of environment for the AD patient under psychological stress and for children whose mothers are worn out by managing their treatment or are overprotective; however, such separation of mother from child is not always a success and may, in fact, create new psychological problems. After discharge, the benefits of hospitalization are generally short-lived; nevertheless, it is usually worth-while if the nurses and physicians in hospital give mothers instruction on adequate care and on the local therapy which will subsequently have to be used at home. Minihospitalization at home, with bed rest during weekends, close supervision, and daily lukewarm baths followed by emollient and sedation, etc. has also been recommended (Roth 1978).

12.3 Systemic Therapy

Almost every conceivable internal remedy which has been used anywhere in the world for resistant skin disease has been tried in AD, but only a few drugs and methods have withstood the test of time.

12.3.1 Antipruritics

The best way to test the efficacy of an antipruritic drug or method is to study its effect on experimental itch (Shelley and Arthur 1957; Rajka et al. 1956; Rajka 1968; Ekblom et al. 1984) or on scratching (Savin et al. 1973, 1975; Felix and Shuster 1975) (see also Chap. 3). These methods are, however, complicated and therefore simpler methods are mostly used, based on clinical assessment; the latter frequently employ a double-blind technique, but apply grading of the intensity of itch. The result of the use of these simpler methods is that there are few properly conducted studies in this field (Savin 1980).

12.3.1.1 Antihistamines

The anti-inflammatory effect of antihistamine preparations is unconvincing but their antipruritic action is undoubted; their frequent and successful use for the relief of itch not only is of crucial importance in the treatment of AD; it is also further proof of the central role played by pruritus in this disease. The choice of a particular antihistamine is dictated by the experience of the individual physician, by the range of preparations available (which in turn depends on the pharmaceutical companies serving the region), and especially by published reports of beneficial results from the drugs compared with a placebo. Clinical evaluation of antipruritic drugs should be based on randomized, double-blind studies on selected patients and suitable controls (Cormia and Dougherty 1959). It is important to consider carefully the very significant antipruritic effect of a placebo (Epstein and Pinski 1964; Fischer 1968; and others).

Antihistamines are available as tablets, capsules, elixirs, and preparations for injection; they are grouped according to their chemical structure, to their duration of action, (short, intermediate, or long), and to whether they are for day or night use.

The latest day antihistamines such as terfenadine and astemizole are very potent histamine blockers, and thus efficacy against itch can be expected from their use. In fact, the author has seen considerable benefit in AD patients from their use (Rajka, unpublished observations), similar to observations of Bazex et al. (1982), although Krause and Shuster (1983) believe that only sedative antihistamines have any effect in AD. Antihistamines for day use have few side-effects. The number of antihistamines suitable for night use is vast and as preparations with a sedative effect are often indicated for the AD patient, the choice of drug should be based on the desired ratio of clinical efficacy to unwanted side-effects, primarily sedation (Hägermark et al. 1985). A combination of day and night antihistamines may be of the benefit, and based on clinical experience, is the standard method used by the author. On the other hand, the H_2-antagonist cimetidine blocked histamine-induced itch and vascular phenomena only moderately (Hägermark et al. 1980) and was clinically inferior to a control H_1-antagonist preparation in personal pilot studies (Rajka 1980), although it is dubious whether H_1-receptors can transmit itch. This was in agreement with most reports of a negative or slight effect of H_2-antagonists on itch (Foulds and MacKie 1981; Frosch et al. 1984); thus cimetidine does not seem to have an important role in the antipruritic therapy of AD.

Ketotifen, a new drug with antihistaminic potency, has not given better results in our hands than the usual antihistamines (Rajka, unpublished observations). Not all clinicians use antihistamines in AD, but, despite their purely suppressive action, there is, in the author's opinion, good reason to prescribe them to prevent or to help control pruritus and thus to interrupt the vicious circle of itch and inflammation. This indication applies equally to children with insomnia or nocturnal restlessness due to pruritus. These drugs are also useful temporarily in the management of AD patients in whom systemic corticosteroids have just been discontinued.

Even psychotropic drugs, especially tranquilizers, may be used for short periods in AD, and, in choosing one, chloral hydrate, that long established and very useful sedative and hypnotic, should not be forgotten. In addition, antidepressive drugs can be tried against nocturnal itch (Gupta et al. 1987). The norepinephrine-releasing chemical guanethidine has been reported to have an antipruritic action (Vigliolia 1962), but no further evidence on this has been forthcoming (Thomsen and Osmundsen 1965).

In order to counteract scratching (registered by a golf-counter), Melin et al. (1986) employed a behavioral treatment, in accordance with Rosenbaum and Ayillon (1981), in AD patients, together with hydrocortisone cream. A significant improvement was registered when this treatment was evaluated against the cream alone. By using a combined group and behavioral self-control approach (including relaxation training), improvement in scratching and in some clinical parameters was reported in ten AD patients by Cole et al. (1988). Autogenic training is considered a useful complementary psychosomatic therapy for AD patients (Kämmerer 1987).

12.3.2 Anti-Inflammatory Agents

Corticosteroids and cytostatics should be mentioned first. These drugs not only counteract inflammation but also influence the impaired immune mechanism in AD.

The indications and contraindications of systemic corticosteroid therapy are well known. Their use as standard treatment during the long periods of AD cannot in general be recommended, but it must be accepted that their use, short-term and in low dosage, can be invaluable in helping some patients with severe intractable AD (including erythroderma) in their social and occupational activities. Every practicing physician uses this type of therapy and has to try to avoid serious side-effects by restricting the indications for its use, by limiting the duration and total dose of a course, and by weaning the patient off the drug concerned with care. The accepted view is that the use of systemic corticosteroids should be limited and that colleagues who tend to overprescribe them should be informed of this opinion. As corticosteroids inhibit growth, their administration is generally contraindicated in children (Lancet, Editorial 1969, and others). For this clientele, however, combined oral and nasal beclomethasone diproprionate, which caused only a slight decrease in urinary cortisol values during treatment, was recommended (Atherton et al. 1984).

Depot preparations of synthetic ACTH seem to benefit AD, but they produce undesirable side-effects similar to those of corticosteroids. Cyclophosphamide and azathioprine were tried in nine severe AD cases unresponsive to steroid therapy. After several months' application, an improvement with long-term remission was recorded (Morrison and Schulz 1978); however, only two of seven AD cases treated with azathioprine cleared in the study of August (1982). Colchicine treatment had no effect in ten AD patients (Zachariæ et al. 1985), whereas cyclosporin in low dose improved two patients (van Joost et al. 1987). Beneficial clinical results and histological alterations were seen after 6 weeks administration of 6 mg/kg/day cyclosporin A (Cooper et al. 1989). As regards other anti-inflammatory drugs, a favorable effect was reported with chloroquine (Döring and Müllejans-Kreppel 1987) and with some anticholinergics (J. M. Hanifin, personal communication).

Ionizing radiation is also used by some dermatologists in AD. Conventional superficial X-ray therapy was more effective than grenz rays in 25 AD patients with hand involvement (Fairris et al. 1985).

12.3.3 Light Therapy

As first reported by Morison et al. (1978) and evaluated by the author in a first series of eight patients (Rajka 1980), PUVA therapy gave favorable effects especially on eczematous areas and if maintenance therapy was given. Similar results have been reported by Sannwald et al. (1979) and by several other authorities at various meetings. The problem is, however, that due to the need for cumulative dosage in this chronic disease and taking into consideration the average age of the AD clientele, this therapy is not justified on account of the known long-term risks. In other words, even if improvement is frequently seen, the benefit/rsik ratio is not acceptable for the average AD case, at least for long-term treatment. On the other hand, its use can be justified in children with severe AD and growth hindrance due to steroids (Carabott et al. 1987), whereas others use these two methods in adult cases in combination (Morison 1985). It may also be used in adolescents with severe AD (Atherton et al. 1988).

UV-B or combined UV-B + UV-A phototherapy, an earlier used method recommended by Nexmand (1948), among others, has had a renaissance in recent years in Scandinavian countries, where the level of exposure to sun is relatively small (Hannuksela et al. 1985; Middelfart et al. 1985, Jekler and Larko 1988, Falk 1989). Earlier complete remission and less frequent or later relapses were achieved in 77 AD patients treated with UV-A plus UV-B than in 85 AD patients treated only with UV-B (Falk 1989). German authors have also had favorable experience with phototherapy in AD (Pullmann et al. 1985). Several possible explanations are put forward for the effect of phototherapy in AD, including (a) thickening of the stratum corneum, (b) reduced mast cell activation (Georgii et al. 1987), (c) depletion of Langerhans cells, (d) killing of bacteria, and (e) antipruritic and sedative clinical effect (Nexmand 1948). Mostly frequent (2-3× weekly) and long-term (several months) treatment is necessary in order to achieve benefit. In the opinion of the author, based on his own favorable experiences, this treatment is of considerable benefit for AD patients living in a climate with little sunshine.

Phototherapy given to certain skin area corresponds to local treatment.

12.3.4 Chromones

Chromones, i.e., cromoglycate used orally (Nalcrom) for its stabilizing effect on mast cells of the gut, gave some protection against food sensitivity in AD in two cases reported by Brostoff et al. (1979). This was, however, not confirmed in the study of Daugbjerg et al. (1984). Favorable results of chromone on the course of AD were reported by Molkhou and Waguet (1981), and in an open study Lever and MacKie (1984) observed improvement in 9 of 19 young adult AD patients. Previously MacKie (1981) had reported a drop in IgE values in two children with AD after this treatment.

On the other hand, several authors have been unable to report significant improvement in AD after using sodium chromoglycate (Atherton et al. 1982; Lindskov and Knudsen 1983; Graham et al. 1984) or a further chromone product, FPL 57787 (Larsen and Schultz Larsen 1979; Schultz Larsen and Jacobsen 1980; Kavli and Larsen 1981).

12.3.5 Essential Fatty Acids

Two families of essential fatty acids in plasma phospholipids have therapeutic relevance for AD:

1. The n-3 series (e.g., α-linolenic acid and eicosapentaenoic acid).
2. The n-6 series (e.g., linoleic acid, γ-linolenic acid, and arachidonic acid).

Hansen (1933) found a decrease of essential fatty acids in the serum of AD patients. In a thorough study, Manku et al. (1984) stated that the major dietary n-6 fatty acid, i.e., linoleic acid, was elevated and the n-3 fatty acid α-linolenic acid somewhat raised in the serum of AD patients, whereas the metabolites were decreased. This was interpreted not as an essential fatty acid defect but rather as due to the existence of an abnormal metabolism, presumably in both cases, owing to impairment of the enzyme δ-6-desaturase.

Most researchers have studied the efficacy of n-6 series products, mostly contained in the diet of Western countries. Hansen (1933) demonstrated early on that AD improved when corn oil, rich in linoleic acid, was added to the diet, although this was not confirmed by Taub and Zakon (1935). In recent years, evening primrose oil (Efamol), rich in linoleic acid and γ-linolenic acid, has been tried in the management of AD. Favorable results have been reported in AD patients by various authors (Lovell et al. 1982; Wright and Burton 1982; Manku et al. 1984; Wright 1985; Schalin-Karilla et al. 1987; Meigel et al. 1987), including in respect of hyperreactivity associated with AD in children (Guenther and Wexler 1987). Other authors, however, could not confirm these favorable therapeutic results in AD (Bamford et al. 1985; Skogh 1986). Concerning the n-3 series, eicosapentaenoic acid, contained in oils of marine fish, produces less inflammatory eicosanoids than do essential fatty acids of the n-6 series (see also Sect. 6.4). By adding eicosapentaenoic acid to the diet, competitive inhibition of n-6 eicosanoids might occur; therefore it is worthwhile trying this product (Max-Epa) in the treatment of AD and other conditions. Working with nutrition researchers we gave Max-Epa to 31 AD patients in a 12-week double-blind study (the compliance being monitored by analysis of the fatty acid pattern) and observed an improvement in itch, scaling, and overall subjective severity; however, a significant clincial improvement could not be reported (Björneboe et al. 1987). Since itch was decreased in these studies, similar to trials in psoriasis, where erythema and scaling also improved (Bittiner et al. 1988), it is not impossible that larger doses might improve the clinical condition.

12.3.6 Anti-Infectious Agents

A cornerstone of the management of AD is the counteraction of the effect on the AD skin of the ever-present *Staphylococcus aureus,* which easily, e.g., after minor common traumas, increases to levels eliciting clinical symptoms. In the experience of the author, however, this aspect is not infrequently omitted by the therapist. Systemic antibiotics, primarily penicillin, are usually required for treatment. Due to the frequent resistance, penicillinase-resistant penicillins are needed; however, it must be remembered that penicillin may, in atopics, elicit type I sensitivity, including anaphylactic shock. Moderate efficacy and development of resistance make erythromycin an unpopular choice, particularly for pediatricians and bacteriologists; thus in some cases other antistaphylococcal antibiotics to which the infecting microorganism has been shown to be sensitive may be considered. Furthermore, trimethoprim has also been claimed as effective (Harrison 1987). In the case of toxicity and fever, hospitalization may be necessary. When there are frequently recurring secondary infections, long-term use of systemic antibiotics has to be considered. This may involve several months' treatment, although this prophylactic measure is varyingly practiced by dermatologists (see also Sect. 12.4).

The treatment of *eczema herpeticum Kaposi* is now dominated by the intravenous (and later possibly oral) application of acyclovir. Its efficacy in reducing possible mortality and significantly shortening the course of the disease is beyond dispute and in accordance with personal experience. There is a vast amount of literature concerning favorable casuistics (Swart et al. 1983; Woolfson 1984; Jawitz et al. 1985; Taieb et al. 1985; Muellemann and Doyle 1986; and others).

The presence of *Pityrosporon orbiculare* on the head and neck in AD motivated the introduction of systemic ketokonazole with favorable results (Clemmensen and Hjorth 1983).

12.4 Topical Therapy

Obviously it is impossible to enumerate all the varieties of topical therapy used by dermatologists, pediatricians, and general practitioners in different parts of the world. The choice of methods and remedies is influenced by such factors as the traditions in various schools of dermatology, personal experience, information published in locally or widely distributed medical periodicals, and advertisements issued by pharmaceutical companies serving the region; fashion, of course, plays a great part. Evaluation of different methods of treatment is usually made by comparing a pair of preparations used simultaneously, each on a different site; however, the possibility of seasonal fluctuations and spontaneous remissions in the course of the disease has to be taken into account. The following discussion is, therefore, only a very general review of the most widely used methods.

12.4.1 Antipruritics and Tars

The most important facet of topical therapy in AD is to apply remedies with an antipruritic effect, a fact which underlines the importance of itch in the mechanism of the disease. There is an unlimited choice of baths, dressings, lotions, shake-lotions, creams, and ointments, and the only restrictions to their use are their sensitizing potential, as with menthol, resorcinol, antihistamines, and several local anesthetics, and their locally irritant properties, as with phenol and resorcinol. Antipruritics act either by producing anesthesia or by replacing pruritus by other stimuli; the latter include the sensation of mild burning, as is induced by crotamiton, and, more commonly, the sensation of cold as is elicited by the direct or indirect application of cold water, by the evaporation of water from cold creams, lotions, and other preparations, or by the application of such substances as menthol.

Some patients with pruritus of their own volition apply heat, which induces pain and subsequently compensatory cooling, or they use mechanical stimulation, which may exhaust the local depots of histamine or traumatize the itch receptors. Of the excellent antipruritics recognized empirically by earlier dermatologists, tars are a good example. However, in making a selection from the jungle of recommended topical preparations, it is advisable to use objective itch parameters to evaluate their antipruritic effect, which is then compared with an assessment, by blind studies, of their clinical efficacy; their appraisal should not be made exclusively on the basis of apparent clinical effectiveness. Melton and Shelley (1950) tested 54 preparations, and Shelley and Arthur (1957) applied other compounds as well; none was found to produce any effect on experimentally elicited histamine pruritus. However, a decrease of sensitivity was found experimentally by Haas (1947) using histamine, and by Rajka et al. (1956) using morphine. Furthermore, the author employed the trypsin duration method (see Fig. 12.1 and Chap. 3) and found that the topical use of corticosteroids, anesthetics, antihistamines, or anti-inflammatory preparations had an effect in about 50% of the cases, that some members of these groups of substances were less effective, and that other preparations, recommended in pharmacopeias, had no effect at all (Table 12.1). Unfortunately, side-effects constitute a considerable disadvantage in the long-term topical use of antihistamines or of potent corticosteroids. Of the local anesthetics with a low sensitizing potential, lidocaine preparations, which contain the base and not the effective salts (Dalili and Adriani 1972), have a documented antipruritic effect and can be used for temporary relief; however, topical corticosteroids with an anti-inflammatory effect are preferable for short-term use.

Used in baths, paints, liniments, ointments, and pastes, *tars* are indispensable in the management of the subacute and chronic, and possibly even acute phases of AD, in which they act as antipruritic, disinfectant, and desquamating agents and also help to counter lichenification. As tars may be cosmetically objectionable in therapy on account of their color and odor, several purified preparations have been made available.

Some physicians prefer wood tars such as pine, birch, beech, and cade (pix pini, betulae, fagi, and juniperi respectively), but most use coal and bituminous tars. Coal tars are different distillates of coal and consequently are of complex and variable composition; a mixture of 11 hydrocarbons (Kinmont 1958) or certain polycyclic hydrocarbons such as naphthalene, anthracene, and phenanthrene (Sedlis 1965) may represent the most effective ingredients of coal tar. However, the use of crude coal tar is therapeutically more effective than dis-

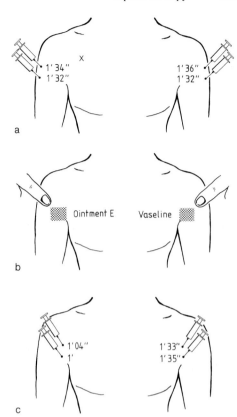

Fig. 12.1a–c. Method of evaluating antipruritic effect of topically applied agents, e. g., by testing ointment E on a patient. *x:* itch duration after intracutaneously applied trypsin

Table 12.1. The influence of ten ointments on experimental itch

Ointment code	Relevant therapeutic indication in relation to itch or inflammation	Antipruritic effect on experimental itch in investigated subjects
A	Pruritus vulvae et ant	2/10
B	Pruritus anogenitalis	3/10
C	Superficial inflammatory infiltrations	3/10
D	Pruritus ani	4/10
E	Various types of pruritus	4/10
F	(Experimental anti-inflammatory preparation)	4/10
G	Pruritus senilis, ani et vulvae	9/20
H	Pruritic dermatoses	10/20
I	Pruritus anogenitalis	10/20
J	Pruritus	11/20

tilled tar, possibly on account of its content of heavy oils. Coal tar (pix carbonis or liquida) is applied undiluted or in a concentration of 1%–10%. Several coal tar products in different vehicles, such as liquor carbonis detergents, pix carbonis preparata, and liquor picis carbonis, as well as many proprietary preparations, are widely used.

Coal tars are photosensitizers, but their carcinogenic effect in man seems to be very low. Bituminous tars from shale also are frequently applied in the treatment of AD, the most commonly used preparation being ichthammol (ichthyol); this distillate of certain bituminous schists, which have been sulfonated and neutralized with ammonia, is applied in a concentration of 2%–3% in various ointments or pastes.

12.4.2 Topical Corticosteroids

Topical corticosteroids, primarily the more potent ones, such as the difluorinated or the fluorochlorinated preparations, are the most effective form of topical therapy in AD but, as discussed in connection with their systemic use, they should be prescribed only if there are strong indications and should be stopped before the frequently met local side-effects, such as skin atrophy, appear. Adrenocortical suppression, which has been observed during their use (Scoggins 1962; Taylor et al. 1965; Keczkes et al. 1967), is intermittent or incomplete; however, if topical corticosteroids are used under polythene occlusion or on large or denuded areas over long periods, they cannot be considered as harmless, a fact which applies also to the less potent preparations recommended for children. The physician should not prescribe them exclusively but should alternate their use with other topical therapy, and should apply them only during periods of considerable inflammation and pruritus; on no account should these preparations be recommended for dry skin with minimal inflammation. When they are stopped, the major part of therapy ought to consist of other topical applications which contain no corticosteroids. In other words, a graded use may be recommended. The author, for example, uses a four-step approach:

1. Start with a very strong or strong topical steroid for 1–2 weeks
2. Follow with a moderately potent steroid alternating with an antibacterial preparation (or a combination) for 3–4 weeks
3. Apply a mild topical steroid, such as hydrocortisone, alternating with a lubricant for several weeks
4. Finally, stop steroid treatment and use only lubricants (possibly alternating with antibacterials)

The length of the scheduled periods, particularly of 2 and 3 may vary according to the severity of AD, and also depend on the extent of the skin disease and the area involved as absorption differs considerably in various skin areas (Feldmann and Maibach 1967).

Other approaches include the choice of the weakest effective topical steroid in the individual case, or the application of the initial potent steroid until total clearance occurs, followed by a switch to weaker ones (Vickers 1982). Once daily application is sufficient and, according to most experiments, equal in effectiveness to several daily applications (Sudilovski et al. 1981; Kligman 1986;

Roth 1987). It should preferably be applied in the evening, as recommended by Marghescu (1987), because of the circadian biorhythm of cortisol production. On the other hand, intermittent use of topical steroids may also be tried (cf. Marghescu 1983). This is often motivated by avoidance of steroid tachyphylaxis (Du Vivier and Stoughton 1975), which the author, however, in accordance with the opinion of Kligman (1986) and the experiences of Jegasothy et al. (1985), has never observed clinically. The importance of the vehicle in topical steroid preparations is often overlooked, although it may significantly enhance the penetration and thus the efficacy and also the absorption or local irritation (e.g., of hydrocortisone) and, not least, may have a therapeutic effect in its own right (Kligman 1986).

12.4.2.1 Hazards

To avoid local atrophy, telangiectasia, persistent erythema, and/or significant absorption, very strong or strong topical steroids should principally be avoided:

1. On some body regions. The author never applies such preparations to the face (although it is often lichenified/thickened), genitals, axillae, inguinal areas, or antecubital/popliteal flexures.
2. In late pregnancy and in infants.

Even lower-strength steroids should be applied cautiously to the buttocks of infants (due to the risk of granuloma gluteale infantum) and particularly under napkins and impermeable pants. Furthermore, regardless of age caution is necessary when steroids are applied long-term on the eyelids or around the eyes, due to some small risk of the development of glaucoma or cataract (Cubey 1976; Sevel et al. 1977). Occlusion should be avoided or applied for only a short time on certain skin regions (folds should be avoided), otherwise the absorption will be considerable (see p.240). Adequate information on steroids and good contact with the patients/parents are, in the author's opinion, absolute prerequisites to avoid insufficient use based on fear and, particularly, misuse. Failure in these respects may cause patients not to improve or to develop addiction based on rebound redness after stopping the steriod, driving him/her back to the steroid (Sneddon 1979; Kligman 1986). In the author's experience the best way to try to break this addiction is a longer hospitalization with intense, nonsteroid local therapy and strict follow-up of the patient. The physician should keep a record of quantities prescribed and convince the patient not to turn to other doctors to iterate the prescription of strong steroids or to use steroids prescribed for other family members or friends. On the combination of topical steroids with other active ingredients, see below. Some recalcitrant lichenified plaques may be helped by intralesional injections of corticosteroids.

12.4.3 Treatment of Acute Eczematous Reaction

For patients with AD in a exudative phase, the preferred treatment, as in other eczemas, comprises wet dressing, changed frequently (at least every 4 h) with Burow's solution or with saline, and the use of tepid or colloid baths.

Corticosteroid lotions are often used and, if there is evidence of infection, a topical antibiotic, antibacterial, or antimycotic preparation is also employed, though a potassium permanganate is to be preferred due to the efficacy and lack of side-effects, apart from coloring.

12.4.4 Measures Against Dryness

Local applications, which improve the ichthyotic and keratotic condition of the AD skin, should be preferred as basic therapy, these include salicylic acid, lactic acid, lactate (Dahl and Dahl 1983), and creams with a suitable content of fat, water, and effective emulsifiers. Urea 10%–20% in a cream base is an effective substitution therapy for dry skin (Swanbeck 1968) and has a fairly significant antipruritic effect (Swanbeck and Rajka 1970). It may be formulated with hydrocortisone cream and this preparation has exerted as good, or almost as good, effects as fluorinated steriod creams (Laurberg 1975). Otherwise, combination with nonpotent steroids can be indicated in dry skin, where signs of mild inflammation can usually be shown (see Sect. 2.6.1). Tars have been mentioned above.

One of the cornerstones of topical therapy in AD is an adequate cream base but this is difficult to find. Those which have been successful in certain cases include hydrophilic, vanishing, or emollient creams. A range of bland emollients are used by the AD patients who tend to vary in their tolerance of individual creams and ointments. Generally, O/W emulsions (type milk; day cream) are better tolerated by the inflamed and basically dry skin of the AD patients but lead to increased dryness due to the evaporative effect of water.

On the other hand, a W/O emulsion (type butter; night cream, ointments), by producing an impermeable film, inhibits water loss and, despite its greasiness, is a better therapeutic choice for dry skin. It can, however, be added that in patients in whom sweating is a strong flare factor, occlusive ointments are contraindicated.

A compromise may be to start, during the subacute phase of AD, with creams from which ingredients, including steroids, are more readily released, but later, when inflammation subsides and dryness of the skin becomes the primary problem, to switch over to bland ointments (possibly to zinc paste) or to other emollients which, like petrolatum (Kligman 1986), staying in place, provide an extracutaneous reservoir.

It is important to be aware that ingredients such as perfumes and preservatives, and possibly lanolin, are potential sensitizers. The use of hydrating bath oils was mentioned under prophylaxis; emollients after a bath may be beneficial as they increase and are aimed to preserve hydration. However, opinions concerning the usefulness of bathing and soaps, particularly for children with

AD, are strongly divided, as (excessive) exposure to water and skin lipid solvents may aggravate the particularly dry skin of AD patients (White et al. 1987; and others). The best known recommendation in this connection is the regimen of Scholtz (1964), who advocated that only short showers, without soap, should be used on the skin of AD children (except in axillae and the groin, and on unaffected hands), and that a grease-free emollient should be used for cleansing. He also recommended propylene glycol as a suitable base for topical corticosteroids. Although he reported beneficial results, the regimen was occasionally too drying. This method and its modifications are obviously indicated for warm climates (such as Western and Southern parts of the United States), where sweating is a frequent flare factor; however, its efficacy has been debated (Buckley 1983; Rhodes 1986). Furthermore, it is important not to use too hot water as longer baths in hot water can lead to itch. Soaps are useful in reducing the staphylococcal colonization of the AD skin, but are, in general, considered to be irritating to the dry atopic skin (Hellerström and Rajka 1967; Sulzberger 1975); this could also be proven by patch and chamber testing (Rostenberg and Sulzberger 1937; Frosch and Kligman 1979), which is, however, different from the way soaps are used. In a recent study, 130 AD patients were allowed to use common toilet soap and, immediately after bathing, topical medication (steroid creams and for patients with dry skin, petrolatum) was applied. The study was conducted over two consecutive years but after just a week 91% of the patients showed a considerable improvement in the skin lesions; no deterioration was observed, and thus the topical medications were found to be more effective than they were before the use of soap (Uehara and Takada 1985). It is possible that, in this interesting study, the potentially irritative effect of soaps was counteracted by topical steroids. In any case, its shows that short use of soaps can, in general, not be considered as contraindicated in the management of AD patients. Several clinicians recommend soap substitutes (soapless cleansers) or neutral, acid and soft/mild soaps, or water with colloidal additives, such as soda, corn starch, or oatmeal. It seems uncertain whether or not detergents are more appropriate for AD skin than soaps; they are nonalcalic but remove skin lipids more efficiently than soaps. Arachis oil or paraffin oil may be used to clean off, for example, pastes from the skin.

12.4.5 Antibacterial and Antimycotic Agents

If the skin is frequently superinfected, the temporary use of antiseptics and disinfectants, including, for example, chlorhexidine, is recommended. However, infection by dermatophytes and especially *Candida* often occurs, e.g., after long-term systemic of topical corticosteroid therapy, and, as this may be overlooked, agents with both an antibacterial and an antimycotic action are to be preferred. Dyes of the methylrosaniline group and baths or dressings with potassium permanganate or hydroquinolines are examples, but the latter have the disadvantage of being quite common sensitizers. Similar problems of sensitization arise with the neomycin group of antibiotics; thus they and potentially cross-reacting drugs should be used with caution and only for short periods.

Opinions are divided as to whether corticosteroids and antimicrobial agents should be used in combination or separately. The former opinion is mostly practiced based on the possibility of a mutual potentiation of the two ingredients (Polano et al. 1960; Wachs and Maibach 1976; Leyden and Kligman 1977). There is a problem with sensitization, e.g., regarding neomycin, which is, however, considered to be exaggerated (Leyden and Kligman 1977). In opposition to this combination it is argued that resistant organisms may be produced after topical antibiotics have been used over a prolonged period (Rasmussen 1984). Through a newer effective topical antibiotic (mupirocin), significant clinical improvement and a reduction in the number of *Staphylococcus aureus* on the skin was reported; recolonization occurred after 2 weeks in only half of the studied 42 patients (Lever et al. 1986; Morton et al. 1988).

12.4.6 Special Points for Infantile Eczema

As mentioned above, compresses with Burow's solution or saline are recommended for lesions which weep frequently, and they can be applied over a film of a corticosteroid preparation as suggested by some workers, including Waisman (1972). Other authors warn against the use of topical steroids in the napkin region (Bonifazi 1987, see also Sect. 12.4.2.1). The necessity of applying antibacterial, antimycotic preparations or both to intertriginous areas should not be forgotten. Tubular gauze (see below) and the application of a bland lubricant have their uses. Restraining bandages are a cruel procedure but may have to be used for short periods in hospital departments to protect the infant with intensely pruritic lesions from the consequences of scratching. AD is the napkin area [also labeled diaper rash, although this is based, in the strictest sense, on maceration induced by plastic panties (Bonifazi 1987)] is a difficult therapeutic problem. New type disposable diapers containing absorbent gelling materials have reduced TWL, are closer to normal skin pH, and have caused less cases of napkin dermatitis, particularly when compared with normal infants on a double-blind basis (Campbell et al. 1987; Seymour et al. 1987).

Tubular gauze or elasticated tubular net is the method of choice for covering ointments or dyes applied to the skin of an AD patient of any age; it is comfortable, is readily adjustable to the body contours, allow evaporation, produces no friction, and, up to a point, prevents staining of clothes or linen. For hand eczema, the use of lightweight cotton cloves at night is often recommended.

Furthermore, it is necessary to convince the mothers of the sick children with good information and judgement to follow the therapeutic guidelines (Yamamoto 1989).

12.4.7 Newer Topical Therapy

Topical application of chromones (sodium cromoglycate cream or ointment 4%–10%) was initially claimed to have a beneficial effect in AD (Haider 1977), but later authors could find some improvement in mild but not in severe AD (Ariyanayagam et al. 1985) or no improvement at all (Zachariæ et al. 1980; Kjellman and Gustafsson 1986), including in respect of a newer chromone preparation (FPL 57787, Söndergaard et al. 1980).

PDE inhibition has been a very interesting development since it involves a central biochemical defect in AD (see Sect.6.3). Initially Kaplan et al. (1978)

Table 12.2. Practical advice for the clinician in the management of AD patients

Infants
1. Consider anti-inflammatory measures: wet dressings (e.g., with Burow's solution), graded application of steroids (potent ones, if at all, for only a very short time, particularly if large skin areas are involved; or moderately potent ones). *Cave:* face, flexures, genitalia, napkin area. Inform parents about steroids, keep a record of prescribed quantities.
2. Consider counteracting itch with antihistamine mixtures or solutions.
3. Consider frequent use of emollients after the acute phase. Advise infrequent and short bathing with bath oils and brief use of soaps, with application of emollients immediately afterwards. Consider the use of tars in subacute/long-lasting cases.
4. Consider antibacterial treatment [penicillinase-resistant penicillins or other systemic antibiotics according to microbe sensitivity, possibly topical desinfectants and steroid-antibacterial combinations (caution with neomycin, due to sensitization possibility)].
5. Consider avoidance of major food allergens (also for the mother if lactating) and food intolerance eliciting items (spices, etc.).
6. Advise avoidance of overheated rooms, woollen clothes, occlusive textiles, pets, greater house dust (mite) exposure; humidification of bedroom can be tried.
7. Advise avoidance of cold, and rapid changes of temperature.
8. Consider the possibility of herpetic infection (then hospitalize the patient). Advise avoidance of family members with active (labial) herpes.
9. Advise lactation until about 6 months (for anti-infectious prophylaxis and possibly to postpone development of food allergies).

Children/youngsters
See 1–8 above. Special remarks:
Ad 1. Somewhat more liberalism on topical steroid application.
Ad 2. Consider day antihistaminics and in the evening H_1-antagonists.
Ad 3. Consider the application of ointments in chronic phase.
10. Advise caution in gymnastics and exercises that will lead to sweating and subsequent itch.
11. Advise avoidance of playing with snow or water.

Adults
Also consider occupation and/or housework.

For severe cases
A) Consider phototherapy (for adults possibly short photochemotherapy).
B) Dietary measures (like point 5, or basic diets).
C) Antihistaminic all day, in the evening with stronger sedative effect.
D) Long-term topical steroids (at the beginning even potent ones).
E) Hospitalization ("minihospitalization" can be tried).
F) Short cure with systemic steroids.
G) Climatotherapy

found an alleged effect of topically applied caffeine on the cAMP level of cells in AD, which later could not verified. The PDE inhibitor Ro 20-1724 reduced hyper-IgE synthesis by AD cells in vitro (Cooper et al. 1985) and a preliminary study indicated some therapeutic effect (Hanifin 1987). Systemic administration of the effective PDE blocker theophylline had no effect in AD, which argues against such a view (Ruzicka 1980), but Hanifin, who confirms this result, interprets as a tachyphylactic effect of long-term theophylline. In Baer's (1985) opinion the earlier established effect of papaverine in AD is based on counteracting of PDE. All this means that, even if at the moment there is no certain proof of the therapeutic effect of PDE inhibitors, it is worthwhile following this trend in the future.

According to the report of Archer and MacDonald (1987) the β_2-adrenoceptor salbutamol, in 1% ointment, reduced the erythema but no other clinical parameters when applied in 20 AD patients in a double-blind trial; some degree of systemic absorption even occurred.

12.5 Concluding Remarks

Although a breakthrough in the treatment of AD has not yet occurred, a number of therapeutic trends seem to promise more effective future management of AD patients. The more promising of these trends may include:

1. New "antiallergic substances"
2. New immunostimulants
3. New anti-inflammatory drugs
4. New PDE inhibitors
5. New antistaphylococcal drugs

Finally, for the clinician some practical advice is given for the management of AD patients (see Table 12.2).

References

Alomar A, Gimenez-Camarasa JM, de Moragas JM (1978) The use of levamizole in atopic dermatitis. Arch Dermatol 114: 1316

Archer CB, MacDonald DM (1987) Treatment of atopic dermatitis with salbutamol. Clin Exp Dermatol 12: 323

Ariyanayagam M, Barlow TJG, Graham P, Hall-Smith SP, Harris JM (1985) Topical sodium cromoglycolate in the management of atopic eczema - a controlled trial. Br J Dermatol 112: 343

Atherton DJ, Soothill JF, Elvidge J (1982) A controlled trial of oral sodium cromoglycate in atopic eczema. Br J Dermatol 106: 681

Atherton DJ, Carabott F, Glover MT, Hawk JLM (1988) The role of psoralene photochemotherapy (PUVA) in the treatment of severe atopic eczema in adolescents. Br J Dermatol 118: 791

Atherton DJ, Heddle RJ, Soothill JF (1984) Beclomethasone diproprionate for atopic eczema (abstract). Br J Dermatol (Suppl 26): 9

August PJ (1982) Azathioprine in the treatment of eczema and actinic reticuloid. Br J Dermatol 107 (Suppl 22): 23

Baer RL (1985) Papaverine therapy in atopic dermatitis. J Am Acad Dermatol 13: 806

Bamford JTM, Gibson RW, Renier CM (1985 Atopic eczema unresponsive to evening prim-rose oil. J Am Acad Dermatol 13: 395

Bazex J, Sans B, Rostin M (1982) Comparative study of terfenadin in allergic skin of patients in France. Arzneimittelforschung 32: 1196

Beck HI, Bjerring P, Harving H (1989) Atopic dermatitis and the indoor climate. Acta Derm Venereol (Suppl 144) (Stockh) (in press)

Becker SW (1932) Dermatoses associated with neurocirculatory instability. Arch Dermatol Syph 25: 655

Berg T, Johansson SGO (1971) In vitro diagnosis of atopic allergy. II. IgE and reaginic anti-bodies during and after rush desensitization. Int Arch Allergy Appl Immunol 41: 434

Bergquist G, Nilzén Å (1972) The release of histamine from blood corpuscles by antigen-anti-body reactions. IV. The histamine release from whole blood before and after treatment of patients allergic to animal dander with staphylococcal vaccine. Acta Allergol 27: 381

Bittiner SB, Tucker WFG, Cartwright I, Bleehen SS (1988) A double-blind, randomized place-bo-controlled trial of fish oil in psoriasis. Lancet I: 378

Björneboe A, Söyland E, Björneboe GEA, Rajka G, Drevon CA (1987) Effect of dietary sup-plementation with eicosapentaenoic acid in the treatment of atopic dermatitis. Br J Der-matol 117: 463

Bonifazi E (1987) Skin problems in the napkin area. In: Happle R, Grosshans E (eds) Pediat-ric dermatology. Advances in diagnosis and treatment. Springer, Berlin Heidelberg New York, p 103

Borelli S (1970) Dermatologische Klimatherapie und ihre Erfolgsbeurteilung. In: Braun-Falco O, Bandmann HJ (eds) Fortschritte der Dermatologie, vol 6. Springer, Berlin Heidelberg New York, p 141

Brostoff J, Carini C, Wraith DG (1979) Production of IgE complexes by allergen challenge in atopic patients and the effect of sodium cromoglycate. Lancet I: 1268

Buckley RH (1983) Atopic dermatitis: a new therapeutic regimen. JAMA 250: 2926

Byrom NA (1980) Thymosine inducible "null cells" in atopic children. Acta Derm Venereol [Suppl] (Stockh) 92: 63

Campbell RL, Seymour JL, Stone LC, Milligan MC (1987) Clinical studies with disposable diapers containing absorbent gelling materials: evaluation of effects on infant skin condi-tion. J Am Acad Dermatol 17: 978

Canonica GW, Mingari MC, Melioli G, Colombatti M, Moretta L (1979) Imbalances of T cell subpopulations in patients with atopic disease and effect of specific immunotherapy. J Im-munol 123: 2669

Carrabott F, Atherton DJ, Glover M, Hawk JLM (1987) The role of photochemotherapy (PU-VA) in the treatment of children with severe atopic dermatitis and short stature. Br J Dermatol 117 (Suppl): p 14

Clemmensen OJ, Hjorth N (1983) Treatment of dermatitis of the head and neck with ketokon-azole in patients with type I sensitivity to *Pityrosporon orbiculare.* Semin Dermatol 2: 26

Cole WC, Roth HL, Sachs LB (1988) Group psychotherapy as an aid in the medical treatment of eczema. J Am Acad Dermatol 18: 286

Cooke RA, Barnard JJ, Hebald S, Stull A (1935) Serological evidence of immunity with co-existing sensitization in a type human allergy. J Exp Med 62: 733

Cooper KD, Kang K, Chan SC, Hanifin JM (1985) Phosphodiesterase inhibition by Ro 20-1724 reduces hyper-IgE synthesis by atopic dermatitis cells in vivo. J Invest Derma-tol 84: 477

Cooper KD, Taylor RS, Baadsgaard O, Headington JT, Voorhees JJ (1989) Atopic dermatitis: treatment with cyclosporine A and demonstration of T cells reactive to autologous epider-mal cells. Acta Derm Venereol (Suppl 144) (Stockh) (in press)

Cormia FE, Dougherty JW (1959) Clinical evaluation of antipruritic drugs. Arch Dermatol 79: 172

Cubey RB (1976) Glaucoma following application of corticosteroid to skin. Br J Dermatol 95: 207

Dahl MV, Dahl AC (1983) 12% lactate lotion for the treatment of xerosis. Arch Dermatol 119: 27

Dalili M, Adriani J (1972) The efficacy of local anaesthetics in blocking sensations of itch, burning and pain in normal and "sunburned" skin. Clin Pharmacol Ther 12: 913

Daubjerg PS, Bach-Mortensen N, Österballe O (1984) Oral sodium cromoglycate treatment of atopic dermatitis related to food allergy. Allergy 39: 535

Di Prisco Fuenmayor MC, Champion RH (1979) Specific hyposensitization in atopic dermatitis. Br J Dermatol 101: 697

Döring HF, Müllejans-Kreppel U (1987) Chloroquin-Therapie der atopischen Dermatitis. Z Hautkr 62: 1205

Du Vivier A, Stoughton RB (1975) Tachyphylaxis to the action of topically applied corticosteroids. Arch Dermatol 111: 581

Ekblom A, Fjellner B, Hansson P (1984) The influence of mechanical vibratory stimulation and transcutaneous electric nerve stimulation on experimental pruritus induced by histamine. Acta Physiol Scand 122: 361

Epstein E, Pinski JB (1964) A blind study. Arch Dermatol 89: 548

Fairris GM, Jones DH, Mack DP, Rowell NR (1985) Conventional superficial X-ray versus Grenz ray therapy in the treatment of constitutional eczema of the hands. Br J Dermatol 112: 339

Falk E (1989) Phototherapy in atopic dermatitis. Acta Derm Venereol (Stockh) (Suppl 144) (in press)

Feldmann R, Maibach H (1967) Regional variation in percutaneous penetration of ^{14}C-cortisol in man. J Invest Dermatol 48: 181

Felix R, Shuster S (1975) A new method for the measurement of itch and the response to treatment. Br J Dermatol 93: 303

Fischer RW (1968) Comparison of antipruritic agents administered orally. JAMA 203: 418

Foulds IS, MacKie RM (1981) A double-blind trial of the H_2-receptor antagonist cimetidine and the H_1-receptor antagonist promethazine hydrochloride in the treatment of atopic dermatitis. Clin Allergy 11: 319

Frosch PJ, Kligman AM (1979) The soap chamber test: a new method for assessing the irritancy of soaps. J Am Acad Dermatol 1: 35

Frosch PJ, Schwanitz HJ, Macher E (1984) A double blind trial of H_1 and H_2 receptor antagonist in the treatment of atopic dermatitis. Arch Dermatol Res 276: 36

Georgii A, Przybilla B, Ring J, Hörwick E (1987) Hautreaktionen durch Mastcellenaktivierung: Beziehung zur Atopie und Effekt von UV-Bestrahlung (abstract). Allergologie 10: 412

Grabowsky HG (1956) Die Beeinflussung der kindlichen Neurodermitis durch das Nordsee-Klima. Kinderärztl Prax 24

Graham P, Hall-Smith SP, Harris JM, Price ML (1984) A study of hypoallergenic diets and oral sodium cromoglycate in the management of atopic eczema. Br J Dermatol 110: 457

Guenther L, Wexler D (1987) Efamol in the treatment of atopic dermatitis. J Am Acad Dermatol 17: 860

Gupta MA, Gupta AK, Ellis CN (1987) Antidepressives in dermatology. Arch Dermatol 123: 647

Haas TH (1947) Über den Juckreiz. Klin Wochenschr 24/25: 353

Hägermark O, Strandberg K, Grönneberg R (1980) Effects of histamine receptor antagonists on histamine-induced responses in human skin. Acta Derm Venereol [Suppl] (Stockh) 92: 116

Hägermark O, Levander S, Ståhle M (1985) A comparison of antihistaminic and sedative effects of some H_1-receptor antagonists. Acta Derm Venereol [Suppl] (Stockh) 114: 155

Haider S (1977) Treatment of atopic eczema in children; clinical trial of 10% sodium cromoglycate ointment. Br Med J 1: 1570

Hanifin JM (1987) Veränderte Phosphodiesterase-Aktivität der Leukozyten bei atopischem Ekzem. Hautarzt 38: 258

Hannuksela M, Karvonen J, Husa M, Jokela R, Katajamæki L, Leppisaari M (1985) Ultraviolet light therapy in atopic dermatitis. Acta Derm Venereol [Suppl] (Stockh) 114: 137

Hansen AE (1933) Serum lipid changes and therapeutic effects of various oils in infantile eczema. Proc Soc Exp Biol Med 31: 160

Harper JI (1989) Newer clinical examples of immunological changes in atopic dermatitis (HIV infection, Thymostimulin & Cyclosporin). Acta Derm Venereol (Suppl 144) (Stockh) (in press)

Harrison PV (1987) Trimethoprim and acute exacerbations of eczema. Clin Exp Dermatol 12: 238

Hellerström S, Rajka G (1967) Clinical aspects of atopic dermatitis. Acta Derm Venereol (Stockh) 47: 75

Herlin T, Jensen JR, Thestrup-Pedersen K (1981) Dialyzable leucocyte extract stimulates cAMP in T lymphocytes. Allergy 36: 337

Hovmark A, Ekre HP (1978) Failure of transfer factor therapy in atopic dermatitis. Acta Derm Venereol (Stockh) 58: 497

Jarisch R, Sandor I, Götz M, Kümmer F (1979) Immunotherapie allergischer Erkrankungen. Hautarzt 30: 365

Jawitz JC, Hines HC, Moshell AN (1985) Treatment of eczema herpeticum with systemic acyclovir. Arch Dermatol 121: 274

Jegasothy B, Jacobson C, Levine N et al. (1985) Clobetasol propionate versus fluocinonide cream in psoriasis and eczema. Int J Dermatol 24: 461

Jekler J, Larkö O (1988) UVB phototherapy of atopic dermatitis. Br J Dermatol 119: 697

Johansson SGO, Berg T, Foucard T (1972) IgE and specific reagins after hyposensitization. In: Charpin J, Boutin C, Aubert J, Frankland AW (eds) Allergology. Proceedings, 8th Europ Cong d'Allergie. Excerpta Medica, Amsterdam, p 359

Kämmerer W (1987) Die psychosomatische Ergänzungstherapie der Neurodermitis atopica - Autogenes Training und weitere Maßnahmen. Allergologie 12: 536

Kang K, Cooper KD, Hanifin JM (1983) Thymopoietin pentapeptide (TP-5) improves clinical parameters and lymphocyte subpopulation in atopic dermatitis. J Am Acad Dermatol 8: 372

Kaplan RJ, Daman L, Rosenberg W, Feigenbaum S (1978) Topical use of caffeine with hydrocortisone in the treatment of atopic dermatitis. Arch Dermatol 114: 60

Kavli G, Larsen PÖ (1981) Double-blind crossover trial comparing systemic chromone-carboxylic acid with placebo in patients with atopic dermatitis. Allergy 36: 597

Keczkes K, Frain-Bell W, Honeyman AL, Sprunt G (1967) The effect of adrenal function of treatment of eczema and psoriasis with triamcinolone acetonide. Br J Dermatol 79: 475

Kinmont PDC (1958) Clinical trial. Arch Dermatol 77: 635

Kjellman NIM, Gustafsson IM (1986) Topical sodium cromoglycate in atopic dermatitis. Allergy 41: 423

Kligman AM (1986) Topical steroids: perspectives and retrospectives. In: Ring J, Burg G (eds) New trends in allergy. II. Springer, Berlin Heidelberg New York, p 342

Kneist W, Rakoski J (1987) Neurodermitis atopica - Klimatherapie im Hochgebirge. Allergologie 10: 531

Korossy S (1980) Allergic reactivity in persistent atopic dermatitis. Acta Derm Venereol [Suppl] (Stockh) 92: 135

Krause LB, Shuster S (1983) Mechanisms of action of antipruritic drugs. Br Med J 287: 1199

Lancet (editorial) (1969) Corticosteroid therapy and growth. Lancet I: 393

Larsen PÖ, Schultz Larsen F (1979) Clinical trial of a new choromone compound for systemic treatment of atopic dermatitis: Acta Derm Venereol (Stockh) 59: 270

Laurberg G (1975) Topical treatment with urea-hydrocortisone in atopic dermatitis. Dermatologica 151: 30

Lever RS, MacKie R (1984) The use of sodium cromoglycate in young adults with severe chronic atopic dermatitis. Clin Exp Dermatol 9: 143

Lever R, Downey D, Hadley K, Baber L, Hannigan C, MacKie R (1986) A double-blind study of the effect of topical mupirocin in chronic atopic dermatitis (abstract). Br J Dermatol (Suppl 30): 27

Leyden JL, Kligman AM (1977) The case for steroid-antibiotic combination. Br J Dermatol 96: 179

Lichtenstein LM, Norman PS, Winkenwerder WL (1968) Clinical and in vitro studies on the role of immunotherapy in ragweed hay fever. Am Med J 44: 514

Lindskov R, Knudsen L (1983) Oral disodium cromoglycate treatment of atopic dermatitis. Allergy 38: 161

Linser K (1967) Bericht über die erste mit 450 Ekzem- und Asthma-Kranke auf einem schwimmenden Sanatorium durchgeführte Hochseeklimakur. Hautarzt 18: 423

Lovell CR, Burton JL, Horrobin DF (1982) Treatment of atopic eczema with evening primrose oil. Lancet I: 278

MacKie RM (1981) Intestinal permeability and atopic disease. Lancet II: 155

Manku MS, Horrobin DF, Morse NL, Wright S, Burton JL (1984) Essential fatty acids in the plasma phospholipids of patient with atopic eczema. Br J Dermatol 110: 643

Marchionini A, Borelli S, Eichhoff D (1958) Konstitutions-Umwelt- und Klimafaktoren bei der konstitutionellen Neurodermitis. In: Halpern BN, Holtzer A (eds) 3ème Congrès International d'Allergologie. Flammarion, Paris, p 609

Marghescu S (1983) Externe Kortikoidtherapie: Kontinuierliche versus diskontinuierliche Anwendung. Hautarzt 34: 1114

Marghescu S (1985) Treatment of atopic dermatitis with steroids. Acta Derm Venereol [Suppl] (Stockh) 114: 157

Marghescu S (1987) Die örtliche Behandlung der Neurodermitis atopica. Allergologie 10: 519

Meigel W, Dettke T, Meigel EM, Lenze U (1987) Additive orale Therapie der atopischen Dermatitis mit ungesättigten Fettsäuren. Z Hautkr (Suppl 1): 100

Melin L, Frederiksson T, Norén P, Swebilius BG (1986) Behavioral treatment of scratching in patients with atopic dermatitis. Br J Dermatol 115: 467

Melton FM, Shelley WB (1950) The effect of topical antipruritic therapy on experimentally induced pruritis in man. J Invest Dermatol 15: 325

Middelfart K, Stenvold SE, Volden G (1985) Combined UVB and UVA phototherapy of atopic eczema. Dermatologia 171: 95

Molkhou P, Waguet JC (1981) Food allergy and atopic dermatitis in children: treatment with oral sodium cromoglycate. Ann Allergy 47: 173

Morison WL (1985) PUVA combination therapy. Photodermatology 2: 229

Morison WL, Parrish JA, Fitzpatrick TB (1978) Oral photochemotherapy of atopic eczema. Br J Dermatol 98: 25

Morrison GL, Schulz EJ (1978) Treatment of eczema with cyclophosphamide and azathioprine. Br J Dermatol 98: 203

Morton F, Lever RS, Hadley KM, MacKie RM (1988) The importance of staphylococcal colonization in atopic dermatitis (abstract). Br J Dermatol 118: 280

Muelleman PJ, Doyle JA (1986) Eczema herpeticum treated with oral acyclovir. J Am Acad Dermatol 15: 716

Nexmand PH (1948) Clinical studies of Prurigo Besnier. Rosenkilde and Bagger, Copenhagen

Nielsen H, Thomsen B, Djurup R, Söndergaard E et al. (1984) Plasma separation in patients with bronchial asthma, atopic dermatitis and hyperimmunoglobulinaemia E. Allergy 39: 329

Polano MK, Vries de HR, Delver A (1960) Analysis of the results obtained in the treatment of atopic dermatitis with corticosteroid and neomycin containing ointments. Dermatologica 120: 191

Prahl P, Skov P, Minuva U, Weeke B, Nexö B (1981) Estimation of affinity and quantity of human antigen-specific serum IgG (blocking antibodies). Allergy 36: 555

Pullman H, Möres E, Reinbach S (1985) Wirkungen von Infrarot- und UVA-Strahlen auf die menschliche Haut und ihre Wirksamkeit bei der Behandlung des endogenen Ekzems. Z Hautkr 60: 171

Pürschel W (1962) Zum konstitutionellen Ekzem mit/ohne Asthma bronchiale. Z Haut Geschlechtskr 32: 321

Pürschel W (1987) Neurodermitis atopica – Klimabehandlung am Meer. Allergologie 10: 526

Rajka E, Korossy S, Gozony M (1956) Zur Pathogenese des urtikariell-entzündlichen Juckens. III. Quantitative Untersuchung der das lokale Morphium-Jucken beeinflussenden Arzneimittel. Dermatologia 112: 81

Rajka G (1963) Studies in hypersensitivity to molds and staphylococci in prurigo Besnier (atopic dermatitis). Acta Derm Venereol (Suppl 54)

Rajka G (1968) Evaluation of drug influence on the itch duration in the skin of patients with atopic dermatitis, various eczemas and psoriasis. II: Experiments in unaffected skin. Comparisons with itch threshold technique and clinical evaluation. Acta Derm Venereol (Stockh) 48: 98

Rajka G (1980) Recent therapeutic events: Cimetidine and PUVA. Acta Derm Venereol (Stockh) [Suppl 92] p 117

Rasmussen JE (1984) Recent developments in the management of patients with atopic dermatitis. J Allergy Clin Immunol 74: 771

Rhodes AR (1986) Treatment of atopic dermatitis: old and new modalities. Clin Rev Allergy 4: 87

Ring J (1982) Successful hyposensitization treatment in atopic eczema: results of a trial in monozygotic twins. Br J Dermatol 107: 597

Rocklin RE, Scheffer AL, Greneider DK, Melmon KL (1980) Generation of antigen-specific suppressor cells during allergy desensitization. N Engl J Med 302: 1213

Rosenbaum MS, Ayillon T (1981) The behavioural treatment of neurodermitis through habit-reversal. Behav Res Ther 19: 313

Rostenberg A, Sulzberger MB (1937) Some results of patch tests. A compilation and discussion of cutaneous reactions to about five hundred different substances as elicited by over ten thousand tests in approximately one thousand patients. Arch Derm Syph 35: 433

Roth HL (1987) Atopic dermatitis revisited. Int J Dermatol 26: 139

Ruzicka T (1980) Effect of theophylline in atopic dermatitis: a double-blind cross-over study. Arch Dermatol Res 269: 109

Sannwald C, Ortonne JP, Thivolet J (1979) La photochimiothérapie orale de l'eczéma atopique. Dermatologia 159: 71

Savin JA (1980) Do systemic antipruritic agents work? J Dermatol 102: 113

Savin JA, Peterson WD, Oswald I (1973) Scratching during sleep. Br J Dermatol 93: 296

Savin JA, Peterson WD, Oswald I, Adam K (1975) Further studies of scratching during sleep. Br J Dermatol 93: 297

Schalin-Karilla M, Mattila L, Jansen CT, Uotila P (1987) Evening primrose oil in the treatment of atopic eczema: effect on clinical status, plasma phospholipid fatty acids and circulating blood prostaglandins. Br J Dermatol 117: 11

Scholtz J (1964) Management of atopic dermatitis. Calif Med 100: 103

Schultz Larsen F, Jacobsen KU (1980) Atopic dermatitis and systemic treatment with a new chromone compound (FPL 57787), a double blind clinical trial. Acta Derm Venereol [Suppl] (Stockh) 92: 128

Scoggins RB (1962) Decrease of urinary corticosteroid following application of a fluocinolone acetonide under an occlusive dressing. J Invest Dermatol 39: 473

Sedlis E (1965) Some controlled observations with topical therapy. J Pediatr 66 (2): 255

Seidenari S, Mosca M, Taglietti M, Manco S (1986) Specific hyposensitization in atopic dermatitis. Dermatologica 172: 229

Sevel D, Weinberg EG, Van Niekerk CH (1977) Lenticular complications of long-term steroid therapy in children with asthma and eczema. J Allergy Clin Immunol 60: 215

Seymour JL, Keswick BH, Hanifin JM, Jordan WP, Milligan MS (1987) Clinical effects of diaper types of the skin of normal infants with atopic dermatitis. J Am Acad Dermatol 17: 988

Shelley WB, Arthur RP (1957) The neurohistology and neurophysiology of the itch sensation in man. Arch Dermatol 76: 296

Sherman WB, Stull A, Cooke R (1939/1940) Serologic changes in hay fever cases treated over a period of years. J Allergy 11: 225

Skogh M (1986) Atopic eczema unresponsive to evening primrose oil (linoleic and gamma-linolenic acid). J Acad Dermatol 15: 114

Sneddon IB (1979) Adverse effects of topical fluorinated corticosteroids in rosacea. Br Med J I: 671

Söndergaard J, Kassis V, Knudsen L, Wadskov S, Wünscher B, Weismann K (1980) Cromones in atopic dermatitis. Arch Dermatol Res 267: 223

Strannegård IL, Hansson L, Lindholm L et al. (1975) Transfer factor in severe atopic diseases. Lancet II: 702

Sudilovski A, Muir JG, Bocobo FC (1981) A comparison of single and multiple applications of halcinonide cream. Int J Dermatol 20: 609

Sulzberger MB (1975) Atopic dermatitis. In: Maddin S (ed) Current dermatologic management. Mosby, St. Louis, p 106

Swanbeck G (1968) New treatment of ichthyosis and other hyperkeratotic conditions. Acta Derm Venereol (Stockh) 48: 123

Swanbeck G, Rajka G (1970) Antipruritic effect of urea solutions. Acta Derm Venereol (Stockh) 50: 225

Swart RNJ, Vermeer BJ, van der Meer JWM, Enschede FAJ, Versteeg J (1983) Treatment of eczema herpeticum with acyclovir. Arch Dermatol 119: 13

Taieb A, Fontan I, Maleville J (1985) Acyclovir therapy for eczema herpeticum in infants. Arch Dermatol 121: 1380

Tamir R, Castracane JM, Rocklin RE (1987) Generation of suppressor cells in atopic patients during immunotherapy that modulate IgE synthesis. J Allergy Clin Immunol 79: 591

Taub SJ, Zakon SJ (1935) Use of unsaturated fatty acids in the treatment of eczema. JAMA 105: 1675

Taylor LS, Malkinson FD, Sak C (1965) Pituitary-adrenal function following topical triamcinolone acetonide and occlusion. Arch Dermatol 92: 174

Thomsen K, Osmundsen PE (1965) Guanethidine in the treatment of atopic dermatitis. Arch Dermatol 92: 418

Uehara M, Takada K (1985) Use of soap in the management of atopic dermatitis. Clin Exp Dermatol 10: 419

van Joost T, Stol E, Heule F (1987) Efficacy of low-dose cyclosporine in severe atopic skin disease. Arch Dermatol 123: 166

Vickers CFH (1982) Treatment of severe atopic eczema with potent steroids (abstract). Br J Dermatol 107 (Suppl 22): 39

Viglioglia PA (1962) Guanethidine as an antipruritic. Arch Dermatol 85: 472

Wachs GN, Maibach HI (1976) Co-operative double-blind trial of an antibiotic/corticoid combination in impetiginized atopic dermatitis. Br J Dermatol 95: 323

Waisman M (1972) Atopic dermatitis. In: Conn HF (ed) Current therapy. Saunders, Philadelphia

White MI, Jenkinson DM, Lloyd DH (1987) The effect of washing on the thickness of the stratum corneum in normal and atopic individuals. Br J Dermatol 116: 525

Woolfson H (1984) Oral acyclovir in eczema herpeticum. Br Med J 288: 531

Wright S (1985) Atopic dermatitis and essential fatty acids: a biochemical basis for atopy? Acta Derm Venereol [Suppl] (Stockh) 114: 143

Wright S, Burton JL (1982) Oral evening primrose-seed oil improves eczema. Lancet II: 1120

Yamamoto K (1989) How doctor's advice is followed by mothers of atopic children. Acta Derm Venereol (Suppl 144) (Stockh) (in press)

Zachariæ H, Thestrup-Pedersen K, Thulin H et al. (1980) Experimental treatment in atopic dermatitis: immunological background and preliminary results. Acta Derm Venereol [Suppl] (Stockh) 92: 121

Zachariæ H, Cramer M, Herlin T, Jensen J, Kragballe K, Ternowitz T, Thestrup-Pedersen K (1985) Non-specific immunotherapy and specific hyposensitization in severe atopic dermatitis. Acta Derm Venereol [Suppl] (Stockh) 114: 48

Subject Index

Acetylcholine   164, 175-76
Acral vasoconstriction   188
Allergens (atopic)   78-110
Alopecia areata   34
Alteration of skin structure   172
Anhidrotic ectodermal dysplasia (see
   Genetic disorders)
Animal hair   86-87
Animal models   197
Antibiotics   242
Antihistamines   238-239
Antimycotic agents   249
Antipruritics   238-239, 243-245
Associated conditions   35-39
Asthma, bronchial   35-37
Ataxia teleangiectasia   42
Atopic cataract   35
Atopic correlations   35-38
Atopic erythroderma   34
Atopic rhinoconjunctivitis   37
Atopic winter feet   25
Atopy, definition of   1-2

β-blockade theory   160
β-receptors   159-162
Body localization   23
Breast feeding   224-225

Candida   33
Candida allergens   110
Cardiovascular changes   188-189
Celiac disease (adult)   44
Chromones   241, 250
Clearing of AD   14-15
Climatic factors   205
Climatotherapy   237
Coexistence of AD with common skin
   diseases   46
Complement   163
Conjunctivitis (see Rhinoconjunctivitis)
Contact dermatitis
- allergic   46, 120-123
- irritative   46, 123-124
Corticosteroids, internal   239-240

- hazards of   240
Corticosteroids, local   246-247
- hazards of   247
Course of AD   7-12
Cow's milk allergen   100
- avoidance of   226
Cyclic nucleotides   159-162, 199

Dandruff (see Human dandruff)
Definition of AD   1, 200
- of atopy   1-2
Delayed blanch   184-187, 190
Delayed reactivity   124-132, 198
- in respiratory atopics   131-132
- in vitro   125-130
- in vivo   124-125
- to bacterial agents, decreased   124
- to viruses, decreased   130
Dennis-Morgan fold   22
Dermatitis herpetiformis   44
Dermatophyte allergens   110
Dermatophytosis   33
Diagnosis   216-219
- differential   218-219
Diapers, disposable   250
Diets (see Avoidance diets)
Distribution and etiological factors   29
- of first lesions   7
Drug reactions of immediate type   41
Dry skin   26-27, 180-181, 199
- prophylaxis   230-231
- therapy   248-249
Dyshidrosis   24, 44-45

Eczematous lesions   10, 19-20
Egg allergens   100-102
Eicosanoids   162-163
Electron microscopic findings   71
Endocrine alterations   190
Environmental factors   206
Eosinophils   70, 96, 158-159, 162
Essential fatty acids   72, 242

Fish allergens   79, 95, 101